Band of Brothers

Creators of Modern Vascular Surgery

W. ANDREW DALE, M.D.

Band of Brothers

Creators of Modern Vascular Surgery

Edited and with a Foreword by

GEORGE JOHNSON, JR., M.D. &
JAMES A. DEWEESE, M.D.

Photo Credits: pages 41 and 49, Jack A. Cannon, M.D.; page 115,
Photography Unit, University of Rochester Medical Center; page 123,
Cress; pages 153 and 165, Bachrach; page 195, Bassano & Vandyk Studios,
London; pages 205 and 471, Elson-Alexandre, Los Angeles; page 259,
Pryde Brown Photographers; and page 305, Pach Bros., N.Y.

ISBN 0-9649826-1-7

Contents

Foreword

Dr. W. Andrew Dale died of leukemia on September 22, 1990. For several years before his death, he interviewed individuals whom he considered to have made significant contributions to the field we know today as vascular surgery. He was interested in learning about the early training and experiences that led to their lives in vascular surgery, rather than their contributions that are common knowledge. When Andy learned of his terminal illness, he asked one of us, George Johnson, to finish his endeavor. I agreed, with two conditions: that he allow me to interview him, and that Jim DeWeese and I be coeditors.

Andy acknowledged that many people had not been included in this volume. We interviewed only those on his list. The process of editing was tedious at times, and portions of interviews had to be deleted by necessity; however, we strove to ensure that the original flavor of the interviews was not lost. Copyright was obtained for each interview published, with the understanding that editing would need to be done.

Shirley Simpson, Andy's secretary for years, typed the original interviews that Andy conducted, and Ivis Bohlen typed and edited the remainder. We express our gratitude to both of them. Corinne Dale has been very helpful in filling in the gaps and in helping us understand Andy's wishes.

We hope that Andy's intent has been carried out.

George Johnson, Jr.
James A. DeWeese

vii

Introduction

It is sad that the great surgeons have not recounted their own stories. They had so many things to tell us. We who are their inheritors know nothing about them except what is obvious externally.

—René Leriche, 1945

The history of surgery dates to antiquity. We know of Egyptians trephining skulls, East Indians transferring nasal flaps, and war injuries worldwide that required manipulation and repair. Centuries later, between 1846 and 1848, fortunately in time for the Civil War, the surgeon's great ally, anesthesia, appeared. The late nineteenth century brought the recognition of microorganisms as the cause of infections. Combated initially with antiseptic chemicals, they were later excluded from wounds as aseptic methods began to be applied. Skilled operators soon developed techniques for ablation of lesions and repairs of dysfunction, even within the cavities of the body. A golden age began for the art and science of surgery.

Just before the turn of the century, the hit-or-miss apprenticeship for young surgeons was forever changed, at first single-handedly, by William S. Halsted of the Johns Hopkins University. His introduction of the residency system, a progressive system of learning consisting of stages of increasing responsibility, is all the more remarkable when we recall his lifelong addiction to cocaine and morphine. The father of the residency program unsuccessfully fought his dependency, brought about by anesthesia experiments he carried out on himself, for his entire life. But he won his other war and led surgery into a new age of skill, responsibility, and achievement.

During the first decade of the twentieth century, Alexis Carrel and Charles Guthrie built a firm background for vascular surgery in their experimental laboratories in New York and Pittsburgh, where they reconstructed a variety of arteries and veins and even transplanted the head of a dog, preceding a later Russian claim by fifty years. Carrel received a Nobel Prize in 1912; Guthrie and his friends were disappointed and critical of the political selection of a laureate whose defects of character surfaced later when he became a Nazi collaborator in World War II. Whatever the merits of their complaint, the medical world soon settled into a dark age as the field awaited ancillary advances.

One of the few worthwhile results of modern warfare has been progress in surgery and its allied fields. Until recently, bloody conflicts were the only training ground for surgeons, and their expertise was thus largely limited to ablations and wound management. Repairs and reconstructions remained unknown. World War I brought a miserable stagnation of progress everywhere: No political lessons were learned and no scientific advances occurred, yet the youth of Europe were decimated in the cold, muddy fields of Flanders. Surgeons made no advances. World War II, on the other hand, was the most important occurrence of our century. In the aftermath of that war, the seeds planted so long ago by a few surgery pioneers—Carrel and Guthrie in America, J. H. Pringle in Glasgow, José Goyanes in Madrid, and Erich Lexer in Königsberg—finally burst into bloom. As a generation of young surgeons emerged from the animal laboratories and training programs in hospitals across North America, clinical advances here and in Europe created the new field of vascular surgery.

The importance of university training programs, well known today, went largely unrecognized for a score or more years after World War II. But the young men knew, and they contested vigorously for university positions. It was somewhere between unusual and impossible to become a first-rate surgeon outside that training system—not because of exclusion, but due to the system's inherent superiority.

The evolution of modern surgery, and in particular the subspecialty of vascular surgery, cannot entirely be deduced from books and articles published in scientific journals, since so much of it lies in the lives of the men who developed the field. It was my good fortune to be associated in one way or another with many of these men, to participate in their endeavors, and to know them as friends as well as professional colleagues. Although their personalities are diverse, they can be generally characterized as entrepreneurs among surgeons—curious, independent, proud, quietly or overtly aggressive men seeking a grail with considerably more longing for achievement than for material rewards. In their careers lies the history of modern vascular surgery.

Several years ago it struck me that their passage would obliterate most of the background and certainly all of the personal events that lay behind their great achievements. If personal histories were to be preserved, I felt then, it must be begun now. Hence the impetus to obtain taped interviews. Years later, these thirty-odd stories have resulted.

Several criteria for selection produced a shortlist from the large number of possibilities available. The memberships of the two national North American vascular groups, the Society for Vascular Surgery and the North American Chapter of the International Society for Cardiovascular Surgery, were reviewed. I made no attempt to include surgeons from outside North America, except for the few who were members of the above. Selection was based upon national and international recognition as a contributor to the development of peripheral vascular (as separate from cardiac) surgery. Local recognition, large numbers of cases, or newspaper fame were not counted. Finally, three surgeons already selected for the group reviewed the list, resulting in the addition of two others.

Each interview was conducted informally, and the resultant tape was edited. There was considerable correction and change of words, with the intent of presenting smooth prose without distracting pauses while preserving the individuals' own characteristics with colloquialisms natural to them. Neurologist Oliver Sacks wrote that "speech—does not consist of words alone. . . . It consists of utterance—an uttering-forth of one's whole meaning with one's whole being—the understanding of which involves infinitely more than mere word-recognition."

The title *Band of Brothers* originated in Shakespeare's *Henry V*. In that play, the English king, speaking before the Battle of Agincourt, proclaims, "We few, we happy few, we band of brothers; For he today that sheds his blood with me Shall be my brother." Later, English Admiral Horatio Nelson used the term "band of brothers" to refer to the captains who fought with him in the Battle of the Nile. Even later, Ernest K. Gann used it as the title of his book about a group of air pilots. "Band of brothers" thus denotes a group of individuals who may be diverse in origin but who are joined in life by shared interests and common goals. It is a fitting title for the pioneers of vascular surgery.

W. Andrew Dale
January 15, 1989

Band of Brothers
Creators of Modern Vascular Surgery

Wiley Barker

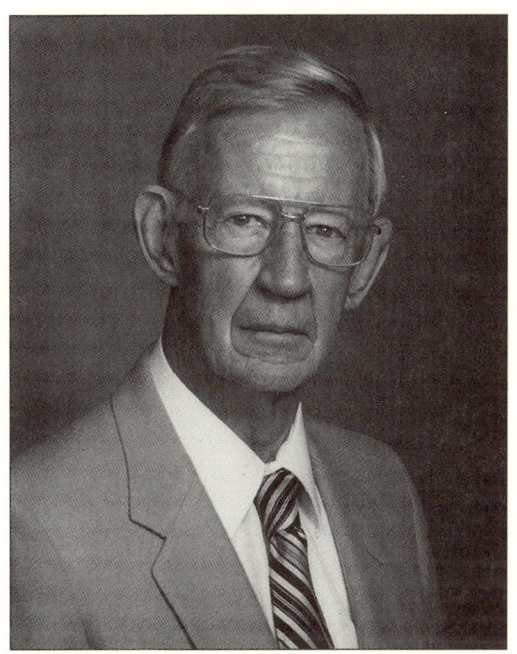

W ILEY BARKER combines the laid-back, friendly informality of his western origin with the polished urbanity
of his Boston education. His career has been a succession of intellectual achievements: Phi Beta Kappa, magna cum laude
both in college and medical school, awards, and membership in
many learned societies. Nevertheless, he has maintained an unas-
suming personality, as well as a sense of humor about it all.

His career began at the University of California at Los Angeles, and he soon became chief of General Surgery at the Wadsworth VA Hospital. He later became professor of surgery and chief of the General Surgical Section at UCLA from 1954 to 1972, as well as chief of the Peripheral Vascular Service from 1964 to 1972.

Barker's wide knowledge and perceptive understanding of issues led to his appointment as chief of staff at the Sepulveda VA Medical Center in 1979 and thereafter as assistant dean of the UCLA Medical School. During those years he also served as a consultant to four nearby hospitals. He has been elected by his peers to all the local, national, and international associations, and his leadership qualities have led to many elected offices, including governor and vice president of the American College of Surgeons and president of the Society for Vascular Surgery, the International Society for Cardiovascular Surgery, the Society of Clinical Surgeons, the Pacific Coast Surgical Association, and the Pan-Pacific Surgical Association.

Publication of 160 scientific articles and books, service as visiting professor at numerous places, many invited discussions, and radio and television appearances have made Barker widely known and respected among surgeons. He was interviewed December 13, 1987.

Dale: Wiley, what was your early background?

Barker: I was born in 1919 in Santa Fe, New Mexico, where my father was an attorney. He was originally a geologist and had not attended law school. He became involved in the civil land laws of New Mexico as it was becoming a state, so he was allowed to practice law in that restricted area. He read law further, in Judge Holloman's office, and after that he was finally admitted to court practice before the bar. After that, he practiced for fifty years before he died at ninety-one.

Dale: Did your father urge you to be a doctor?

Barker: I don't believe so. I think he expected me to be an engineer or an artist. I wound up going to Harvard instead of the University of New Mexico because a fellowship there made it less expensive for me to go to Harvard for undergraduate school.

Dale: You must have had a good high school record.

Barker: It was a small western high school; there were only one hundred students in my class. Nonetheless, it had good academic standing, and practically all of the boys in the school participated in the three athletic events we had—football, basketball, and track.

Dale: Was it a culture shock when you went to Boston?

Barker: It was a distinct culture shock to leave the small Santa Fe high school for Boston. I haven't recovered yet! Actually, although it was a distinct change, I enjoyed the thirteen years I spent in Boston. I thought I was going to become an engineer. Soon that changed to a career as a biochemist. By the time I was deeply into biochemistry, I also became interested in biology in general. One of my advisors suggested that if I went to medical school, I'd be a better biochemist. But once I began to deal with patients, it was good-bye biochemistry!

Then I went into the navy, during which time you may recall that I met you at Maxwell Field, Alabama. After my service time, I returned to Boston as an Arthur Tracy Cabot Fellow, to which I had been appointed by Elliott Cutler. He planned for me to go on through his residency program, but unfortunately, he died. His replacement, Francis Moore, told me, "Sure, we'll keep the agreement. You'll be chief resident someday, but first I want you to spend time in the laboratory; then come back for your clinical training about 1956." It was then 1948! So I told Franny Moore, "Thank you. I appreciate your help."

I didn't have a job until Bill Longmire took me on as his first appointee at UCLA in 1949. Harry Muller, Frank Spencer, John Beal, and I all reported for duty at Wadsworth VA Hospital, which was a clinical facility of the new UCLA Medical School, on July 1, 1949.

Dale: How many years did you have as a resident with Bill Longmire?

Barker: I had had a year and a half when suddenly I was promoted out of the residency to be chief of the General Surgical Section. They had to cheat a little bit to let me have enough time to qualify for the boards, but since part of it was listed as "chief of the General Surgical Section under William P. Longmire, Jr.," they allowed me to qualify.

Dale: Bill always struck me as a sort of gentle giant. What sort of service did he run?

Barker: It was a strict show. There were no tantrums or harsh words. In fact, when Dr. Longmire's voice softened, people began to get nervous. I worked with him for thirty-seven years, and I have never seen him lose his temper. The only time he was upset with me, I damn well deserved it.

Dale: So you and he got along well the entire time?

Barker: Exceedingly well. He was not only my beloved mentor but also one of my best friends.

Dale: Was he a good technical surgeon?

Barker: He was a good technical surgeon in the sense that he never looked as though he was doing much. You'd watch him picking at a massive scar around the biliary tract and an hour or so later he'd have carved the common duct out cleanly. He never seemed to get in trouble.

Dale: Did he do any vascular surgery?

Barker: Well, he started in vascular surgery in the sense that he was the intern on the first blue baby operation at Hopkins, by Dr. Blalock. I had been the resident on the first blue baby operation that Bob Gross did in Boston.

Longmire did several things early on in what we could today call vascular surgery; he was interested in congenital arteriovenous malformations and did some of the first renal artery reconstructions, the first truly successful coronary reconstructions, with Jack Cannon. While he was a consultant to the air force in Europe, he performed and published an account of an aortoiliac endarterectomy; when he finished the repair, the wall seemed so thin, he wrapped the thing with a dermis graft.

Dale: Let's go back to your experience with Bob Gross.

Barker: We'd heard about all those blue baby operations being done at Johns Hopkins in Baltimore. The cardiologists found a twenty-year-old woman with untreated pulmonic stenosis, who by that time had severe pulmonary insufficiency and terrible cyanosis. She lived only a day or two after the operation. We didn't know how to support such a patient in those days.

Dale: How did Gross accept that loss?

Barker: Bob Gross never showed much emotion about any battle that he had lost. But I know that he was deeply disturbed about it.

Dale: Let's return to California and learn how you became interested in vascular surgery.

Barker: John Homans had been my mentor at the Brigham Hospital in Boston. He was a fascinating character. Basically he was a general surgeon, because there were no vascular surgeons in those days. Homans's contribution to vascular surgery was largely in the field of veins, but he became interested in the arterial side and did sympathectomies in the years before arterial reconstruction was known.

One of the last things he did during his final hours, having been debilitated by a myocardial infarction, was to wish out loud that he could see his own arteries at autopsy! He was a fiery and cantankerous character with an immense number of stories of all sorts. He was a delightful person.

Dale: So Homans got you interested in vascular problems. What's the next part of that?

Barker: Bill Longmire knew that I'd worked with Homans. In 1950 he assigned Jack Cannon and me to run the Peripheral Vascular Clinic. I was still a resident and Jack had finished his training a few months before. After that, we ran the Peripheral Vascular Clinic at the Wadsworth VA Hospital. We made attempts at endarterectomies. We had not at first understood how to do the operation; we were not clearing the full length of the obstructed segment, especially distally. We were beginning the endarterectomy in the middle of the obstructed segment and trying to peel out the atherosclerotic lesion in fragments from that one spot. Our first six patients were thrombotic failures, but they were followed by a series of good results.

Dale: Did you know about João Cid dos Santos's work?

Barker: I had read it when it first came out in a limited translation, but I didn't appreciate the details of his technique. I had known Jack Wylie in medical school, and John Beal had known him at Cornell. We knew of his early work, and invited him to visit with us in the summer of 1951, shortly after he had presented his first work on thromboendarterectomy, before it was published. For the first time I understood the importance of tailoring the distal limit of

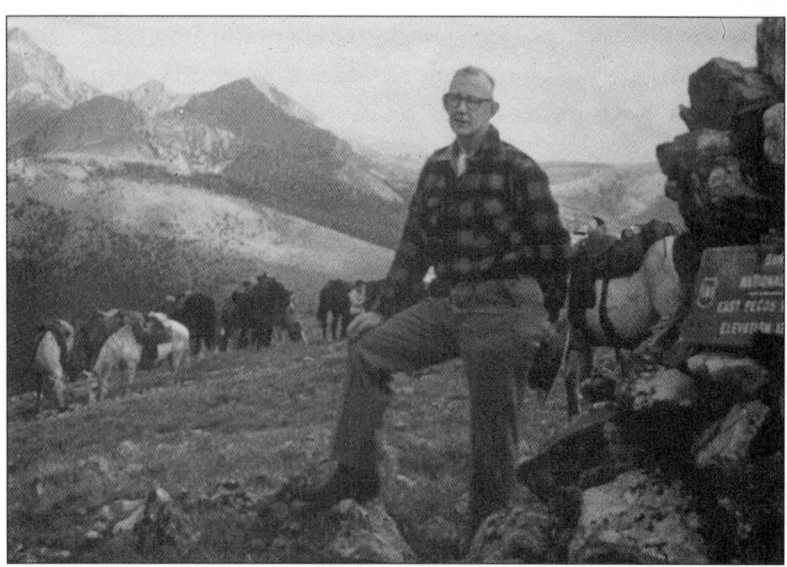

Wiley in the Pecos Wilderness

the dissection correctly. In October 1951 I did our first successful case, one that involved an endarterectomy of an abdominal aneurysm, tailoring it to size and wrapping it with fascia lata, then extending the endarterectomy in one incision all the way to the top of the right popliteal artery. The patient immediately had a good pulse, and she preserved that pulse for nine years—without any recurrence of her aneurysm, either—but she died of a cancer of the tongue at that late date.

Dale: How long did all that take you?

Barker: Well, I didn't get home for dinner that night. It was at least a twelve-hour operation.

Dale: When did you report those?

Barker: We presented these nineteen cases at the Western Surgical Meeting in Houston in 1952. My sponsor, Arnold Stevens, invited Mike DeBakey to discuss it, but he declined, telling Dr. Stevens he had had experience with only one arterial reconstruction at that time.

Dale: What else did you try?

Barker: Very early on, we repeated some work that Jean Kunlin had done in France, although I didn't know his paper at that time. It was a one-page paper that appeared in a discussion on the healing of endarterectomies in a French journal. René Leriche couldn't believe that blood flow would continue over a raw artery. But Kunlin showed that the flow allowed reconstitution of the endothelium very quickly if heparin was used. We did the same thing in the lab. If you give heparin to a dog, you see a good lining of endothelial cells very early. Within twenty-four to twenty-eight hours, there are sheets of endothelium growing all over the internal surface—maybe they grew from circulating cells.

Dale: Did you begin to use heparin regularly?

Barker: Yes, way back in the 1950s.

Dale: That was much sooner than the rest of us. Is this why you were getting such good results so early?

Barker: I think it was. It was also given after the operation for about ten days to two weeks, and almost all patients healed perfectly and did not have any recurrence. Soon however, some of our residents recognized heparin wasn't necessary to make the thing work initially, so they either gave no heparin postoperatively or maybe one dose. Within two years, seven patients had recurrence of atherosclerosis—most of them were reoperated in the endarterectomized site. I am still convinced that the early maturation of an endothelium in the endarterectomized segment under the protection of low-dose heparin protects the artery.

Dale: Did you always use heparin postoperatively?

Barker: In relatively low doses—5,000 units every six hours for a week or ten days.

Dale: Was there any trouble with bleeding due to heparin?

Barker: At one time we reported at a conference sponsored by Andy Dale several hundred consecutive arterial operations, some done with postoperative heparinization, some not. We had no more—in fact we had fewer—hematomas in heparinized patients than in the nonheparinized patients. That doesn't mean that heparin prevents hematomas. It just means that if you are going to heparinize the patient, you should be a bit more meticulous about hemostasis.

Dale: How long did Jack Cannon stay at UCLA with you?

Barker: Jack became disenchanted with UCLA and left about twenty years ago. At that point, I was substantially alone. Samuel

Marable, one of our very early residents, stayed on for a time before he went to Ohio State. Shortly after that, Herbert Machleder, one of our own residents, came back to us and began doing vascular surgery, and then Dennis Baker came along.

Dale: When did Denny join you?

Barker: About twelve years ago. He'd been trained by Emerick Szilagyi. Then another of our residents—Ronald Busuttil—began to show a real interest in vascular surgery. When I left as chief of the Division of Surgery and chief of the vascular service at UCLA, Wesley Moore came from Arizona to follow me. That was nine years ago.

Dale: To change the subject, when were you married?

Barker: We married in 1943 in the middle of my third year at Harvard Medical School. Nan and I had met in Santa Fe just after I graduated from college. We have three adopted children, none of whom are physicians.

Dale: How did you become interested in orchids?

Barker: That goes way back to my college days. In order to receive an honors degree in biochemistry, I had to write a thesis. My thesis consisted of synthesizing a series of the compounds of indolylacetic acid and its various salts, which had been demonstrated to be a plant growth hormone. I synthesized a series of these things, isolated the products, and then tested them on grape trimmings and oak seedlings. I was working in Harvard's botanical laboratory and came to know a man named Oakes Ames, who was an eminent taxonomist. People sent him orchids from all over the world to classify, and I became interested in his plants. He gave me tickets to a couple of orchid shows in Boston. When I moved to California, there was an orchid nursery about two blocks up the street. I bought a couple of plants in 1951 and I've been at it ever since.

Dale: How many do you have now?

Barker: About three thousand, including many small seedlings. We raise them commercially, selling the blossoms primarily. They come in many colors, sizes, and shapes, but for the most part I grow the flowers of the big "mink-coat" type—the *Cattleya* and associated species and their hybrids.

Dale: Does anyone help you?

Barker: My wife waters the orchids once in a while when I'm gone, but I don't have anybody else to help. We still raise the whites and purples that are the classic orchids, but I've focused on a collection of oranges, greens, blues, and other unusual colors. We finally found a florist who was interested in these unusual colors, which do make magnificent table decorations.

Dale: I associate you with horseback riding. Is that just a minor interest?

Barker: I acquired my father's attitude toward horseback riding, really the Texas attitude: You don't necessarily ride for fun—you ride only when you need a horse to get somewhere. My grandfather came from Virginia to Texas shortly after the Civil War and then in 1889 moved onto a ranch in northern New Mexico. I spent a modest amount of time on that ranch, but horses were used only when we had somewhere to go that we couldn't easily manage on foot. So I have always ridden, but not as one would ride in the English manner. About 1970 my wife and I began to take trail rides in the great wilderness areas of the Rockies. I can tell you exactly when it was, because my Uncle Elliott is ninety-nine and he came to my father's ninetieth birthday party but was late getting there because at eighty-one he had just led a trail ride through the mountains of New Mexico. He said, "That's my last ride," but I replied, "Uncle, I'd always hoped that Nancy and I someday would have time to get back into the real high country of New Mexico with you." He said, "All right, let's go again next fall." So he went on about seven more rides before he had to give it up. We went with him on our first ride when he was eighty-one.

Dale: Wiley, did a horse ever throw you?

Barker: I don't know whether they threw me or not, but I have fallen off horses. I once had my ear stabbed by a horse that took off through a spruce tree, but I was never seriously injured.

Dale: What is the outlook for a young man or woman going into medicine today?

Barker: The future is going to be quite different. Knowing what I know now about what's happened in the last forty years, I would be uncomfortable about entering the field, but if I were innocent of the experiences I have had during those years, I think that it would still be a challenging area. When we started doing vascular surgery, it amounted to a major vein ligation or an occasional embolectomy.

Heparin was not consistently available, and we didn't have good antibiotic coverage. There was penicillin, but it was expensive. We didn't have a flame photometer for potassium levels. Arteriography was a rare procedure done for cerebral lesions; neurosurgeons did cutdowns, sticking the needle into the artery to inject thorotrast. The x-ray equipment was primitive. The tools today offer an immense opportunity for diagnosis and treatment.

Dale: Surgery has progressed to the point now where it's doubtful that a surgeon can invade any more of the body or become much more skillful from a hands-on standpoint.

Barker: Of course, that's a dangerous thing to say. I think that we will see further advances in microsurgical techniques. We're still going to be faced with major vascular problems. Perhaps we'll all be put out of business by reversal of the atherosclerotic process chemically.

Dale: What do you see on the horizon for surgery?

Barker: There will always be a role for the surgeon. We will always find new things to do. I don't know what the future for vascular surgery will be, but the laser is going to have a role in it. That may put many of our current surgical procedures out of business.

Dale: Is it true that too many carotid operations are being performed?

Barker: In a sense, that is correct. There are areas in the country where if a patient has a carotid murmur and has a slight fainting spell at 100° on the golf course, he is very apt to have his carotid operated on the next day. That is not justified. On the other hand, the majority of patients with significant carotid atherosclerosis do need the operation. We need to be sure that patients are operated upon with the minimal mortality and morbidity rates: 10 percent combined morbidity and mortality rates is too high.

Dale: The same thing has been said about coronary bypass surgery. Are too many being done?

Barker: Possibly so, but this depends upon the point of view. How many times have you seen a cardiologist or a lay person who has been critical of the use of the operation rush to have an angiogram and an arterial repair at the first twinge of angina? How long does it take the critic to find someone to provide the definitive treatment?

Dale: What do you think about it being said that cardiac surgeons charge too much, that they are making enormous amounts of money because, although they do many cases, the fees haven't decreased?

Barker: All surgeons are charging more than is appropriate. I have an idea that we surgeons have been led astray philosophically by the governmental programs that allow an indigent patient to go to a doctor but not as a charity. My mentors—John Homans, David Cheever, Francis Newton, and Elliott Cutler—did about half their practice on charity patients. Then the philosophy developed that the beneficiary of such charity was not being treated in a dignified manner. The government introduced the pattern of payments, with extensive documentation and controls, and gradually the philosophic approach of the doctor has seemed to veer from the primary role as the one who cares for a patient into the role of a money maker. We have been seduced, but I also believe that many of us have been willing "seductees."

Dale: Is it true that younger doctors have such great costs now in going through medical school that they become money-hungry very early because they are in debt? Or is it simply a matter of we older fellows shooting at the younger ones and saying that they are bad and we weren't?

Barker: It's a bit of both. We must remember that the expenses of a medical education are in a completely different order of magnitude now. I received a full scholarship to Harvard for six years, but the most I ever received was $1,400 in one year. That included tuition, books, board, room, and a little spending money. The first few years of my residency were completely uncompensated. I received nothing at the Brigham as an intern, then $500 a year as a resident. And the Arthur Tracy Cabot Fellowship paid $1,000 a year.

Dale: At present, a sixth-year resident can make as much as $30,000, which leads me to believe that residents are not paupers.

Barker: I cannot find sympathy for a young man who complains bitterly about how much he's in debt and how much he's going to use that as a basis for charging high fees, when you find a third-year resident driving a Mercedes. Bill Longmire says that he doesn't mind them getting that level of payment, in comparison to what he received; he just wishes that they wouldn't gun the Mercedes when they pass him in the garage.

Dale: Of the 120 papers you've written, of which one are you the most proud?

Barker: I think probably there are a couple that I'm most proud of. One that I would choose would be an old study of the healing of the artery after endarterectomy, which I think has, by and large, been overlooked. Another series of papers that I think were important in my career were on a nonvascular subject, inflammatory bowel disease. I was responsible for the surgery of ulcerative colitis and Crohn's disease at UCLA and the veterans' hospitals here for many years, and I believe I participated in or performed nearly five hundred colectomies during those years.

Dale: In closing, if you had to do it over, is there anything that you would change in your career?

Barker: There are two things that I would change, one of which I couldn't have. I would have spent more time acquiring basic research skills, and the second thing, which I could not change, is the fact that a couple of times in my career, I've had an illness that knocked me out of step. One was hepatitis and the other one was tuberculosis.

Dale: Pulmonary tuberculosis?

Barker: Possibly. I had close contact with a destroyer skipper whom we had to relieve of his duties because of advanced pulmonary tuberculosis, but it is more likely that I contracted a variant, perhaps bovine tuberculosis, while in Italy. I developed a mild gastrointestinal upset and then a swollen liver, but never had any tests positive for liver dysfunction. Ten years later I developed a period of weight loss and was found to have some nodules in my liver that the pathologist failed to diagnose correctly at that time. Five years later I developed a series of convulsions and frightened my wife and neurologist into thinking I was done for. Fortunately, he was a good physician who went back over the record, went to the pathology department, looked at the slides of the liver biopsy, and found the acid-fast organisms the pathologist had missed. He treated me for tuberculosis rather than having my cranium cracked by the neurosurgeons. He was right, and I was back at full speed in about eight months.

William Blaisdell

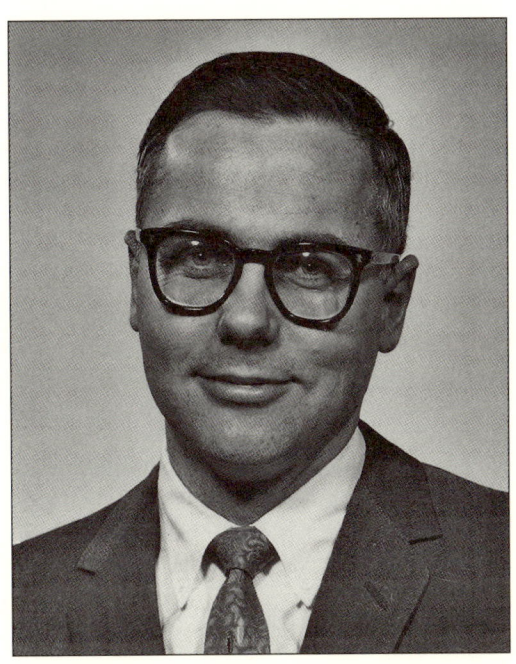

B ILL BLAISDELL represents the optimal result of a broad education in surgical training centers in San Francisco, Philadelphia, Boston, and Houston. At age thirty-three, he became chief of an important surgical service, and other chairmanships followed.

Blaisdell's analytic mind has already produced important, innovative therapeutic programs, among them the extra-anatomic grafting principle and high-dose heparin treatment for acute arterial problems. In 1979 his peers made him president of the prestigious Society for Vascular Surgery. He has been called to visiting professorships at forty-one different universities in North America and Europe. In addition to leadership in vascular surgery circles, he has also become a recognized expert in trauma surgery. In 1972 he was named Citizen of the Year by the San Francisco Police Department.

Blaisdell is, however, no dry academician. Good humor and quiet wit mark his bright personality. A wife, six children, and four grandchildren form his immediate family. His interest in Civil War history is generally unknown but attests to the variety of his interests. He was interviewed December 13, 1986.

Dale: Bill, tell me about your early years.

Blaisdell: I was influenced by my two grandfathers, both of whom were physicians. My paternal grandfather was a professor of surgery at Stanford University. He was primarily an anatomist, but in those days anatomy was part of surgery. He was on the faculty from 1906 to 1932.

My father was also a physician. He graduated from Stanford, having been taught by my grandfather, but he reacted against the academic life. He recognized that his father had a paltry income, and at home they were always trying to "make do."

Father embarked on a career in private practice, but I believe that he would have been far better off if he had stayed in academia. He would have been better as a teacher and professor than he was in private practice.

I was born on March 30, 1927, in Santa Barbara, but we soon moved to Watsonville, where my father joined my uncle, who had been a classmate, in practice. Father was an internist. I obtained more of my outlook on life from my uncle, who was a surgeon. Santa Barbara was hit very hard by the Depression, whereas Watsonville, on the coast about a hundred miles south of San Francisco, was doing very well, as was my uncle's practice. Subsequently, their clinic became a multidoctor one in the town where I was raised.

Dale: What about high school?

Blaisdell: I was in high school during World War II, and because the war was on, I finished in three years. I was a center on the basketball team. Although I didn't study particularly hard, I ended up as valedictorian of my class. My mother encouraged me to take extra courses and start at Stanford before I had graduated from high school, and, subsequently, a year later I returned to participate in my high school graduation in 1944.

Dale: Your college program was accelerated. Did that leave you any time for any nonacademic activities?

Blaisdell: I was class president and also was on something called the Rally Committee, which put on the razzle-dazzle for the football games. We organized the first activities when football resumed at Stanford after the war. I did two and a half years at Stanford before I started medical school there, just at the end of the war in 1945.

Dale: Why did you enter medical school?

Blaisdell: I had always wanted to be a doctor. I was not necessarily interested in surgery, but during the course of medical school it became apparent to me that I could do more if I studied a little surgery. That's the trap one gets into. You see that somebody explored for appendicitis and it turned out to be a perforated cancer, and you say, "I'd better go on a little further so I can master that as well."

Dale: So you call that a trap. Do you think people get trapped into a field?

Blaisdell: Yes, I think some do. If you had told me I was going to take seven years of training after medical school, I would have said you were crazy. But I did. I had a rotating internship at Philadelphia General Hospital. My teachers had warned against that, because it ordinarily didn't lead to becoming a surgeon. At Stanford, one entered a straight surgical internship program, which led to upward progression in a pyramidal system. Each year, one saw fewer rise up the ladder to become chief resident.

Dale: Was it a good experience?

Blaisdell: It was an extremely competitive two-year internship when I started. But by that time the Korean War had begun. The military did not recognize two-year internships and decimated the program by drafting young doctors after the first year. So it became apparent that I was going to have to go into the military after a year. With my roommate, I carefully reviewed the optimal service to go into, and we concluded that the best was the navy because it was in the larger cities.

I said, "I get seasick. What if I get onto a ship?" My roommate looked at the statistics and convinced me that the odds were overwhelming that I would get a shoreside job because the permanent military doctors were the ones who were stationed on the capital ships. The only thing left was destroyers.

Needless to say, my assignment was destroyers! I became a destroyer division medical officer, and I did get seasick!

Dale: What was the name of your ship?

Blaisdell: It was Destroyer Division 122, which consisted of four ships. We had a commodore who subsequently became head of Annapolis, by the name of Kaufman. His father had been an admiral and he was a captain, well on his way to becoming an admiral. He was a military strategist, and liked to discuss strategy with me as a listener. He couldn't do it with his ship captains on other vessels or with his first lieutenant, but I was a neutral who would listen.

Captain Kaufman would take me along with him to the officers' club, where he persuaded me to stop drinking Scotch and Coca-Cola; he said that was "no drink for anyone." That was fine, but there was one disconcerting thing. When we were in the Mediterranean at the height of the Cold War, he said, "Bill, wouldn't it be great if war with the Russians broke out right now?" When I asked why, he said, "Well, look. We'd go full tilt, flank speed, right into the Black Sea, where all their oil refineries are, swoop, and we'd wipe out all their oil!" I looked at the map and saw all the Russian installations around the mouth of the Black Sea, so I said, "Captain, how would we get out?" He replied, "Oh, we wouldn't get out, but we would be famous," and I thought, "My God." I prayed every night that the war wouldn't escalate. That was the military mind; just be fantastic, be a hero.

Dale: Well, tell me about your motion sickness. Was it a problem for you?

Blaisdell: I was in a position to do a very good study of motion

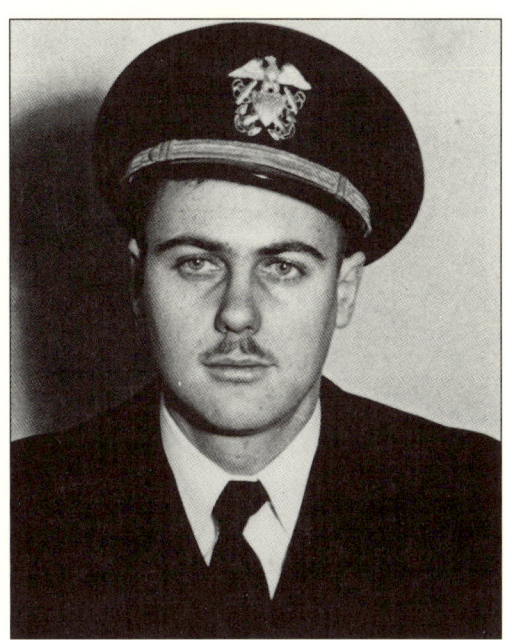

Bill in naval uniform, 1953.

sickness on destroyers. When I joined the destroyers, they were in the Mediterranean, which was like glass, relatively speaking, and I was not sick at all. So I thought, "Gee, I've mastered this," but then on the return trip, eight days across the Atlantic, it came. We left Gibraltar, and I didn't have anything solid to eat for eight days. I spent most of the time lying in my bunk.

One day I got a call, "Doctor to the bridge, doctor to the bridge," and I went up to the bridge, and there was this guy spread-eagled across the deck. I didn't know what the hell was going on. I felt lousy, but I asked that he be taken to sick bay. While examining him, I'd run over to the sink and vomit; then I'd go back and examine him some more. I concluded there was only one guy on that ship sicker than I was, and that was the fellow I was examining. He apparently had the same problem that I did; he was seasick. He had passed out; I was still viable.

I finally got over it. I learned where the exact balance point was on the destroyer, and when I didn't feel good, I'd go up and sit right on that balance point in the middle of the ship. I'd sit on a pail and look at the horizon to get over my seasickness. Later, I found out that the semicircular canals become immunized. The first day out I would feel nauseated, but if I managed to eat and go up on deck and sit in the appropriate place, I'd get over it.

I became an observer of how well people ate. Even the captain missed a meal when we first went out to sea. I noticed just about everybody missed meals, but most of them would not acknowledge it. I think all the senior officers had some degree of motion sickness.

Dale: What did you do after two years afloat?

Blaisdell: I started my surgery residency at Stanford. It was a very competitive pyramidal program in those days, so that you were always looking over your shoulder for the competition. There were six residents in the first year of training, of which only one would finish as chief resident.

Emile Holman was chief my first year of training; he had been a friend of my grandfather's, who had been godfather to one of Dr. Holman's children. He was a fine old gentleman; however, he had not impressed me when I was a medical student. He tended to be kind of a monotone type of speaker; our surgical clinics almost always were right after lunch, and in the large auditorium at least half my class would routinely go to sleep. When he caught somebody in the front row sleeping, he would explode and chew that person out. But he was a very nice gentleman, a real gentleman of the old school. As a matter of fact, I had determined that I would never come back to Stanford for training, but through the influence of my father and uncle I did. I thank God that I went into the service, because that gave me a hiatus during which I could think about the future and during which my father and uncle had the opportunity to work on me a bit.

Dale: Was Doctor Holman still operating?

Blaisdell: Yes. He was quite a good operator. He was William S. Halsted's last chief resident and he had the ultimate Halstedian approach to things. Everything had to be very meticulous; closures were meticulous and tissues were handled very gently.

Dale: Who came on then?

Blaisdell: Victor Richards was the bright young star at Stanford at that time. He was appointed chairman of the department of surgery during the second year of my residency. Vic is one of the brightest people I have ever met and is an absolutely fantastic technician. The two people that have impressed me most as superb technicians have been Denton Cooley and Victor Richards. Those two are really superstars from the standpoint of operating. Both of them have a similar characteristic: they have a tendency to grandstand from time to time in terms of their technical ability. But both are extremely good.

Dale: How did you happen to go to Boston?

Blaisdell: During my second year of surgical training, I received the happy news that I was the person designated to become chief resident later. In those days, the designee was sent to an eastern university program for a year preceding that. I was offered the opportunity of going to the Peter Bent Brigham Hospital in Boston.

Dale: Who was chief there?

Blaisdell: Francis Moore. He was an extremely interesting person. It is not a good thing to say, but I concluded in a month or two that I was the best operating surgeon in the Brigham Hospital. Everything was quite academic there. It was a very stimulating environment and the preoperative and postoperative care was out of this world, extremely well done. I learned a great deal about that and a great deal about managing complications, most of which I had never seen at Stanford. Stanford surgeons were polished technically, and quite clinically oriented, whereas at Harvard everything was academically oriented, and Franny Moore rarely operated. They were more committed at Harvard to the theoretical or academic aspects of surgery than to the technical apsects. The residents had far less clinical experience. Part of the Stanford program was situated at the county hospital. Early in a resident's career in the training program, the combination of university hospital with the county hospital resulted in a large volume of technical experience. At the Brigham I had occasion to work with a chief resident who had been in training for eleven years, and I led him through a number of operations that he had not seen or participated in.

Dale: So part of it was the volume of patients. Today we recognize that the volume of patients is more important than it was considered to be at that time.

Blaisdell: Harvard got a lot of mileage out of an individual patient; many people saw each case and discussed it in detail.

Dale: After your year there, what did you do?

Blaisdell: I returned to Stanford and finished my training at San Francisco General and University Hospital. My final year as chief resident was six months at the county hospital as chief resident and the same at the university hospital. I was the last chief resident in San Francisco before Stanford moved to Palo Alto in 1960.

Dale: When and why did you go to Houston?

Blaisdell: In the course of my time in Boston in 1955, I rotated to the West Roxbury Veterans' Hospital, where Dr. Richard Warren was chief of surgery. The residents at the Brigham found it hard to work with Dr. Warren, yet I found him fascinating. He was called "Itchy-twitchy-Richie." He was always complaining about his help and assistants. For whatever reason, perhaps because of my greater clinical experience relative to my years of training, he took a liking to me, and as a result I volunteered to stay on a second tour on his service. None of the residents wanted that service, so I stayed on.

Dale: Why did they not wish to be on that service?

Blaisdell: The amount of surgery one got to do on Dr. Warren's vascular service was negligible. There weren't any minor cases. But I didn't find it at all difficult. I was fascinated by the things he was doing, such as endarterectomies of the superficial femoral artery for occlusive disease. We used pressurized homografts that we obtained from the autopsy room.

I talked to Dr. Warren about a vascular career and asked him what I should do. His reaction was, "You should go to Houston. That's where vascular surgery is really flowering." When I got back to Stanford, I told my professors that I was interested in vascular surgery and that I'd like to go to Houston, and asked them if they would help me. Carl Mathewson knew Mike DeBakey quite well and said he would arrange it. During my fourth year I made a commitment to go to Houston in 1959 and 1960 for vascular training.

Dale: How did you find Houston?

Blaisdell: It was entirely different from Stanford. Stanford was kind of a gentleman's program; the surgeons might chew on you a bit, or get a little upset in the operating room, or occasionally fly off the handle, but one always knew that afterwards they would apologize and everything would be fine. I'd liken Houston to a jungle where it appeared to be survival of the fittest. They had two classes of fellows there: four who were recruited and paid by Baylor, and eight or ten who were paid by their own hospital or faculty and who were coming to spend a year at Houston. They were volunteers paid by their respective governments or their respective schools.

They were looked on as "second-string." Generally the "first-class" fellows were the first assistants and the "second-class" fellows were the retractor holders.

I was first assigned to Denton Cooley's service. I had been working with Frank Gerbode in San Francisco; he had helped place me in Houston. I think Denton was anxious to know what Frank was doing. The two were opposite kinds of personalities. Frank was a very meticulous surgeon, did things by the numbers, and worked on developing a disc oxygenator.

When I saw Denton's pump-oxygenator, I said, "Gee, Dr. Cooley, don't you have a lot of problems with this?"

He replied, "Why, no."

I came back with, "Well, what happens after you use it for more than fifteen or twenty minutes?"

He closed that conversation: "Hell, Bill, I can reconstruct the heart in five minutes!" I concluded the secret of Denton's success in the early days of cardiac surgery was simply that the patients could hold their breath long enough for Denton to correct something going on with blinding speed.

Dale: Was he using a bubble oxygenator?

Blaisdell: He was using a bubbler of his own design, modified from earlier ones. You actually could look right into the oxygenator. The blood that was exposed to the oxygen was also open to the room. We would simply wash up the oxygenator in the sink and autoclave it between cases. It looked like a series of tin cans, one piled on top of the other. But it worked, and Denton was doing remarkable things. He was repairing five hearts a day at that time, which was unheard of. In other words, he was an extremely rapid surgeon. He did most of the work himself. The fellows didn't place any critical stitches. Denton usually did the operation from skin to skin.

During my first four months, fellows began to accumulate on Cooley's service because they were being fired from Dr. DeBakey's service. We started off with a couple of us, and by the time I finished the four months, there were six or eight people all vying to participate in Denton's operations.

After four months with Cooley, I rotated to Stan Crawford's service and spent four months working with him. At that time Stan was an itinerant surgeon. When we operated at Methodist Hospital, he was the youngest member of the faculty and was picking up cases wherever he could, which meant we were operating all over Houston. We'd go with him and then when he went out of town we'd double back and make rounds for him at the respective hospitals. He was operating in three or four hospitals at that time, including helping at the VA. I concluded that he was unquestionably the finest peripheral vascular surgeon in the group.

If we had problems with an artery, Stan would actually take the whole repair down and redo it. It was obvious that his results were as close to 100 percent as one could possibly expect. He was just absolutely, extremely good. He was not quite the technician that Denton was, not as flashy, but I think a far better vascular surgeon.

Dale: What about Mike DeBakey?

Blaisdell: Perhaps I should not go into an analysis of the atmosphere there, but there was obvious resentment, at least on Cooley's part, of DeBakey. I never heard DeBakey say anything bad, but Denton was always putting Mike down. In fact, Denton had a dart board with Mike's picture on it, at which he would throw darts and comment sarcastically.

Mike was a perfectionist; the light had to be perfect, the retractors had to be properly placed, and the sutures had to be followed appropriately. He demanded a lot of his second and third assistants. I found it a challenge. I knew I was the best assistant that he had, and, rightly or wrongly, I could stand up to him a bit. So Mike would lay off me and pick on more junior members of the team. At that point I figured that I had it made. I realized that Mike did the finest aneurysm operation that I'd ever seen. It was a production line. We did as many as eight aneurysms in a day. Mike was extremely good; if we found something unusual, such as an acces-

sory renal artery or a left-sided vena cava, he would call for someone like Stanley Crawford to come in and help him. We were just
starting to do renal arteries. They were extremely difficult. George
Morris would sometimes come in and help.

Subsequently, Alton Ochsner of New Orleans said that before
Mike went to Houston, he couldn't get him out of the laboratory at
Tulane. If you go back and look at DeBakey's bibliography, it's
apparent that he had been productive academically in the laboratory and in clinical reviews. So I believe that Mike was an academic
surgeon up to the time he went to Houston. There he was joined by
this outstanding technician, innovator, and creator from Johns
Hopkins, Denton Cooley. They would go out to the county hospital
and find ten aneurysms, bring them in, and operate on them. In
their early days, Denton always helped Mike. After he stopped helping him, Mike adopted Stanley Crawford as his superassistant when
he encountered something different. Once the procedure was
devised, Mike kept it going and by repetition became expert.

Dale: DeBakey must have been a good administrator?

Blaisdell: Yes, he was. He also writes superbly and recruits good
people.

Everyone was a bit afraid of Mike. The residents never showed
him complications if they could possibly avoid it. It was rumored,
although perhaps apocryphally, that when Mike was about to make
rounds at the county hospital, all the complications were transferred to x-ray or to the basement, so that he found no complications on the service. Sometimes the patients were discharged and
readmitted if necessary to the rehabilitation unit in another building.

Dale: What else did you learn in Houston?

Blaisdell: Dr. DeBakey had just hired a technician to run a new
direct blood pressure monitor, which was installed between Mike's
two main operating rooms. I was fascinated by the machinery, so I
learned to operate it. Then something happened and Mike abruptly
fired the technician. That was okay, except for one thing. They had
sent an abstract to the Society of University Surgeons about pressure monitoring of one hundred carotid artery lesions, so at every
operation by Crawford or DeBakey, the monitor was used to build

the series to be reported. At the time the technician left, the abstract was accepted for publication, but they only had about sixty or seventy cases of the one hundred they had projected. No one could get the equipment working. They called me and said, "Hey, Bill, you know anything about this?" So I went in and did my best to get the equipment working, but I couldn't. Finally, I concluded that it had been sabotaged by the fired technician. He and I had become quite friendly, so I called him and said, "I've got to talk to you." He said, "I don't want to talk to anybody from that damn place." So I said, "Can I buy you a beer this evening? Where are you?" So he agreed and we arranged to meet. I bought him a beer, and I said after a few more, "What did you do to the equipment?" He said, "I'll be damned if I'll tell you." I told him my job was on the line, although it really wasn't. So then he said, "Bill, I'm not going to go back to that place, but I'll tell you what I did. I switched this wire and that wire." I went back and got the equipment working. They put me on the paper as an additional author. They did the last two cases on the morning that the plane was due to leave, so the numbers were literally put together on the plane going to Minnesota where the meeting was held. Stan went to the public stenographer and had the paper typed, and then presented it with my name on it. But we learned that pressure didn't always predict the result. We operated under local anesthesia on one patient who ended up comatose, despite a back pressure of sixty.

When I was with Denton Cooley, I also learned to run a cardiac pump. Mike started cardiac work when the crown prince of Belgium was referred to him with the diagnosis of aortic stenosis. Mike scheduled the case with the help of fellows like Sam Henley and John Ochsner, who had some experiece with cardiac problems. Mary Martin, the pump technician, had a full schedule of cases for that day, so he asked her if there was someone else who could run the pump. She said, "Yeah, Bill can." I was then working with Stan Crawford, so they drafted me from his service to run the pump for DeBakey's case. I went over and had a quick refresher on the pump, and then pushed it across the parking lot from Children's Hospital to Methodist Hospital. We all worked like hell to keep the guy alive, and he was sent back to Belgium, but he subsequently died there.

Dale: Where did you go next?

Blaisdell: When I had left for Houston, I had a firm offer to return to Stanford, having been told by all my professors that I would have a job there. But the medical school was moved to Palo Alto, a new dean was brought in, and the emphasis shifted to a strictly academic department of surgery. Victor Richards became a thorn in the side of the medical school.

Victor was asked to resign, and Garrett Allen was brought in as chairman. Just before I left Houston, I was assured by Roy Cohn that he had talked to Allen and that I had a job. However, about seven months later, when I visited Stanford to confirm my job, Allen didn't know who the hell I was. Far from having a job, I wasn't even in the picture.

When I was at the Brigham, I had met Englebert Dunphy, who had just moved to the University of Oregon. Several months later, around May, I still didn't have a job, but by that time I did have kids. So I went up and interviewed with Dr. Dunphy in Portland. The interview went well, and I suspect from later conversation with Dr. Dunphy that I would have had a job. However, on the way back I stopped in San Francisco and Dr. Mathewson, one of my professors, asked me if I knew that the job as chief of surgery at the VA in San Francisco was open.

The VA Hospital in San Francisco had been run by Stanford and the University of California equally, but that ended when Stanford went to Palo Alto. My friend and mentor Dr. Mathewson called Leon Goldman, who was chief, and told him that Bert Dunphy was about to make me chief of surgery at the VA in Portland. That was not true; he was perhaps about to take me on as a junior faculty member, but not as chief.

When Dr. Goldman interviewed me, thinking I was about to be chief in Portland, his jaw dropped and he exclaimed, "My God, you're awfully young!" Matty had warned me not to let on that the Oregon position was as an underling. Goldman went on, "So Dunphy has offered you the job in Portland. How do you feel about it?" I responded, "Well, I'm not from Oregon. If there were an equivalent here in San Francisco I would prefer that." Goldman repeated, "You're awfully young," so I wrote it off in my mind. A week later he called me and offered me the job, so I went to the VA in San Francisco.

Dale: How long were you there?

Blaisdell: Six years, beginning July 1960. That was probably my most productive time. I set up the vascular service there. I had learned to use angiography liberally. We were doing cerebral angiography, which the neurosurgeons at the University of California at San Francisco thought was terribly dangerous. We were injecting all the vessels and the aortic arch, which they thought would surely kill patients. I know I was much criticized by them and others on that, but we had no major complications. I published an article summarizing three hundred cases of panarteriography with a negligible complication rate.

Dale: Was it about that time that you developed the extra-anatomic bypass principle?

Blaisdell: That's correct. I had some experience with vascular infections at Baylor. Mike and the others had few complications, but when you're doing eight operations a day, even if your complication rate is half of one percent, you're going to see some. We had a number of graft infections that were admitted to the rehabilitation unit. I carefully nursed them along. I tried everything: antibiotics, local compresses, and iodine irrigations. If the anastomosis was exposed, eventually they ruptured, bled, and died. I became convinced that the only way to treat a graft infection was to remove the graft. Of course, if the graft involved the abdominal aorta, you couldn't remove it without a replacement to carry blood to the legs. I began to think of alternative possibilities.

On the first day that I took over as chief at the VA Hospital in San Francisco, I got a call stating that an aneurysm that had been resected and grafted a month before had been festering with infection in the hospital, and that the patient had suddenly gone into deep shock. We operated to remove it in that infected field. There was nothing else to do but to put another graft back in, so I did that. I knew as sure as anything that in spite of massive antibiotics and drainage, it would also become infected. Sure enough, the patient remained septic, but I had a month to think about what to do.

When that patient blew the next time, we were right on top of it. I went in and ligated the aorta and the iliacs, then opened the left chest and anastomosed a Dacron graft to the descending aorta, tunneled it out through the chest wall, down subcutaneously to the left groin, and then across to the right groin. That worked and we reported that case in 1961.

The chief problem with that technique was that it caused a terrible strain on the patient to have a thoracotomy. I'd done some work in Houston in the laboratory to find out how much blood flow was required to maintain patency of a vascular graft. It turned out that at least 30 cc per minute was needed for a Dacron graft. In the course of more experiments, I made some arteriovenous fistulas that caused a high rate of flow. Even with a rate approaching the total cardiac output, the dog's femoral artery could accommodate the increase. That meant that it wasn't necessary to use the aorta as the in-flow source, since a smaller artery could carry enough blood. That background allowed me to think that the subclavian artery could probably supply enough blood for a graft to the lower body and legs and still supply the arms.

In 1962 we operated on a man who had acute ischemia of his remaining leg, the other having been lost earlier by amputation. The plan was for an aortofemoral bypass to provide blood to that limb. Unfortunately, cardiac arrest occurred just after anesthesia began. Although massage restarted the heart, the EKG showed a massive infarct, so what to do?

To make a shorter story, we placed a graft from the subclavian artery to his femoral artery. It was successful. He died of another massive infarct two years later, and his wife insisted upon an autopsy, which showed the graft was patent.

Subsequently, Dr. DeBakey referred to me a fellow who had had a graft thrombosis three or four times. He lived somewhere in the Bay area but had been operated on in Houston. He obviously had a chronic graft infection.

Dr. DeBakey came to San Francisco for a meeting in 1963. The patient learned of it and camped outside his room in the hotel. DeBakey, in frustration, said, "Why don't you go see Bill Blaisdell?" We took his infected graft out and rerouted blood via an axillofemoral bypass. That fellow went on for ten years. He left a will stating that he must have an autopsy. The graft was patent.

Dale: When did you move to Sacramento?

Blaisdell: After six years at the VA, I became chief of surgery at San Francisco General, where I spent the next twelve years. I started a cardiac and vascular program in 1966.

The municipal ambulances brought all trauma patients there, so my interest began to shift to that. Surgeons skilled in vascular work easily handled trauma, so we mounted a large service. When I became chairman at the University of California at Davis, and was living in Sacramento, it was natural to build an even larger trauma center.

Dale: How did vascular surgical training programs evolve in California?

Blaisdell: Young surgeons graduating from the University of California programs always possessed a rich vascular experience. Malcolm Perry, currently in New York, really was the first fellow, in 1961–1962, and others such as Wes Moore, Jerry Goldstone, and Bob Lim followed, but they were a part of general surgery.

By 1970 the requirement for formal credentials in vascular surgery prevented some of them from doing that work. On that basis, Jack Wylie finally convinced the chief, Bert Dunphy, that a formal postgraduate vascular surgical program was needed.

Dale: Before we finish, tell me about your family.

Blaisdell: I met Marilyn Janeck during my second year at Stanford. I was running the Sophomore Carnival, in which she participated. We subsequently dated throughout college and my early years of medical school and were married during my senior year of medical school. We had our first child at Philadelphia General Hospital. She was the only white baby in the nursery, so we had no problem identifying her. We ended up with six children—four girls and two boys. There are four grandchildren presently.

Allan Callow

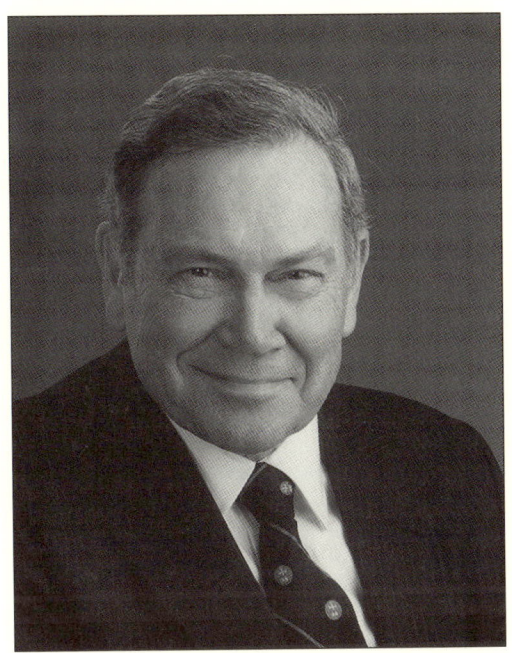

Aᴸᴸᴀɴ ᴄᴀʟʟᴏᴡ has affected everything he has touched. He rose to the top in the military in being promoted to admiral, and his achievements in vascular surgery were honored by his presidency of the prestigious Society of Vascular Surgery. His keen mind for discovery and research resulted in continuous funding for vascular surgery. He is a trustee of Tufts University and president of the International Society for Cardiovascular Surgery. He was interviewed December 8, 1986.

Dale: Tell me about your origins.

Callow: The family name originally was MacCallow. My Scottish ancestors backed the wrong side at the Battle of Bannockburn in 1314, and they had to flee. They traveled to Liverpool and later to the Isle of Man, where they dropped the "Mac" and then emigrated to Boston. My mother's family were Fowles from Wales, who came to this country several generations ago and settled in coastal Maine. My great-great-grandfather was master of a coastal sailing ship out of Wiscasset, Maine. He also had a saltwater farm, but it couldn't support three sons, so one of them inherited the ship, one received the farm, and the third came to Boston. Curiously, there is a village named Callow on the Welsh-English border.

I was born April 19, 1916. My father was a businessman and a good man. I became the first physician in the family, which both my parents encouraged. I wanted to become a doctor because I was given books to read when I was very young that supported that ideal, like *Yellow Jack* and *Arrowsmith*. For as long as I can remember, I intended to be a doctor, even before high school.

Dale: Did your parents support your aspiration?

Callow: Yes, but they couldn't support me much financially. I worked through college as a laboratory instructor.

Dale: Where did you go to college?

Callow: I went to Tufts. It was just around the corner, so I could live at home for a couple of years. I got a job on the campus as a laboratory instructor in biology. I'd take the freshmen out to the saltwater pools, the tidewater pools, and show them things from the sea.

One of the influential men in my life was Paul Warren, a botanist and geneticist, who was chairman of the Department of Biology. He didn't want me to be a doctor, but to be a botanist like himself. I was to go to the University of Maryland, from which he had graduated, and get a Ph.D. in botany. All of this was to be subsidized by the Burpee Seed Company.

Dale: Frequently, a teacher who recognizes a good pupil wants that pupil to go into his own field.

Callow: I suppose so. When young research fellows or residents come along, I think they should be in academic medicine, even though they may wish to do clinical practice. So I'm guilty of trying to influence people in the same way.

Dale: Then you entered Harvard Medical School?

Callow: Yes. For a time Dr. Warren wouldn't write a good letter to them for me. But he did eventually help me to enter the Class of 1942.

Dale: Did you find the medical school agreeable?

Callow: It was an exciting place because of the stimulating people. I think all of them could have done outstanding things if they had so chosen. It was a good mix.

We were encouraged to consider academic careers. They told us the first day, "You will not flunk out; you have been carefully selected. This is not like the law school; if you're not here next year, it will be because you don't wish to be here." The failure rate was almost zero.

Dale: There were some schools where the students were warned that half the class would be gone the next year.

Callow: Not at Harvard. We had a reception with the dean the evening of the first day. He said, "You are here because we believe that you will do well, and if you don't do well, we look upon that as our mistake. Now relax and go to work, and you will work very hard." But it was a collaborative effort. The challenge there was an intellectual one. You were challenged to work, but you were not challenged to do something or else fail.

There was one exception, a young instructor. He went on to be a professor and chairman of his department at Hopkins. He took me aside and asked me where I thought I stood in my class of 125. Being modest, I told him that I probably was in the middle to upper third. He took out a little notebook and said, "No, out of 125, you are 124th. Now, the final exam is coming up in two weeks." So I went to my room and studied unceasingly. I put the sun to bed and got it up in the morning. I received an A in his course.

Dale: So that was just a ploy.

Callow: I later discovered that the largest number of honor grades were in his section. When I saw him several years later and told him about this, he denied it, but did so laughingly.

Dale: How did you decide to go into surgery?

Callow: As is so often the case, it was probably because of the influence of several individuals. Without always knowing it, one develops role models. One of mine was Elliott Cutler—a dynamic and dramatic man. I can recall being in the operating room with him one day at the Peter Bent Brigham Hospital. The patient was to have a craniotomy. Cutler made a bone flap and placed a biopsy needle in the brain. He did it dramatically, with a great flourish, withdrew his hand, and pointed out that the needle was moving. He turned quickly to me and said, "Did the patient have a bruit? Did you listen with a stethoscope?" I replied, "No." Then he said, "Well, we may kill this patient when we biopsy his brain. He may bleed to death right in front of us." Dramatically, he put his hand up in the air and then pushed one finger down on the biopsy needle and withdrew the stylus. We expected a geyser of blood, of course, but there was none. I don't know how many times he had done this, but we all thought what a great person he was to have that courage.

Dale: Was he chief at Brigham?

Callow: Yes, and Soma Weiss was chief of medicine.

Dale: And what was Robert Zollinger doing then?

Callow: He was a young staff man. Bert Dunphy was there. Bert was regarded as the friend of the students and the house staff. He and Zolly were both considered to be "doctor's doctors."

Dale: Did you know John Homans?

Callow: Homans was there also. There are many stories about him. One of his friends was a slow, meticulous operator. They used to operate two cases simultaneously in a large operating room, with only portable cotton curtains between them. John Homans would complete a cholecystectomy, a simple mastectomy, and strip a varicose vein of the leg, three cases, while his friend was doing one radical mastectomy. Homans looked at us, winked, put his head around the curtain, and said, "It will have metastasized before you get it out." That sort of thing went on all the time.

Dale: What happened after you graduated in 1942?

Callow: I was uncertain about what to do. I felt I should train at the Massachusetts General Hospital or the Brigham. I adored the Brigham because I had spent so much time there. It had excellent teaching, but its volume was not large. The General was larger but was less personal.

Two of my classmates were going to Boston City Hospital, where the patient volume was huge. In those old municipal hospitals for the poor, you could obtain enormous experience. What I didn't appreciate, at the time, was that the surgical instruction might derive from a staff who were not as well trained, at least not as compared to the staff at the Brigham or the General. Nevertheless, I had a great year there before I was called to military service.

The navy sent me to a training camp in Fort Pierce, Florida, where we practiced with guns and bayonets and tried to learn how to protect ourselves. We were to join a combat landing unit to care for casualties on the beaches of North Africa, but our assignment was changed to the Pacific, where the war was going badly.

Our landing team included communications, boat repair, and medical personnel. We were to accompany the assault troops of an invasion. My job was to get the casualties off the beach. My team made seven invasions. We got shot at a lot. It was one of the most profound experiences of my life. I survived, but I also lost a lot of friends. We were all convinced we could not survive the war. Having fought the Japanese in so many places for three years, we all felt that when we attacked Japan itself, although we might eventually win, it would be at a terrible price. I had given up hope of returning, as had most of my companions.

Dale: Did your unit transport marines to the beaches?

Callow: I was in the navy, but I was assigned to a combat landing unit. We worked with both army troops and marines. From Pearl Harbor we went to New Zealand and from there invaded Tarawa with the marines. Our landing party was in the third wave of boats, because the military thought that the chances of surviving the ride into the beach were better. But the hydrographic maps were old and the tides were not predicted correctly, so the landing was delayed and difficult. The low tide and the fierce Japanese defense created havoc among the invading boats.

My boat ran onto a coral projection and hung there in the midst of the firing for hours before the tide freed it so that we could land. Battleships, cruisers, and destroyers had shelled the beach very heavily, and strafing planes were helpful, but the defenders would duck into holes and defensive positions until the shelling and strafing ended and then come right back.

Dale: What was your job on the beach?

Callow: It was to sort out the wounded and get them ready for the boats to go back to the ship. It might be a plasma transfusion, a morphine injection, or bandages and splints. The doctor stayed on the beach while the boats came and went.

Dale: Were you glad to hear about the atomic bomb that ended the war?

Callow: Yes! Most of my friends didn't believe it. We thought it was propaganda. Most of us believed we survived the war because of the atomic bomb.

Dale: What did you do after the service?

Callow: I was discharged six months later. I returned to the Boston City Hospital for a year, but found that the best people had left. I was disillusioned.

At a class reunion I learned that the Pratt Diagnostic Clinic was building a new medical center, and that Dr. Stuart Welch was looking for someone to start a research laboratory. I saw him and he accepted me, so I designed the lab with him.

When Welch asked me what I wanted to work on, I said, "Well, since I saw so many arms, legs, and lives lost in the war, I think I'd like to do something with arterial surgery." He was discouraging: "Read about it. There isn't any. There aren't many people who stab themselves with a knife. Are you serious about this?" I answered yes, and he said, "You'd better learn something about blood vessels and vascular disease." He sent me to the Mayo Clinic, where Allen, Barker, and Hines were running a vascular service. After a year he called me back to fill a resident vacancy caused by illness.

Dale: What were you working on in the dog lab at that time?

Callow: Sewing arteries together. To keep the lumen open, I was using a dried albumin shunt. I also did some reversal of circulation experiments.

Dale: When did you actually finish your training?

Callow: After the war I started as an intern at Boston City Hospital, and then went to the New England Medical Center at the Pratt

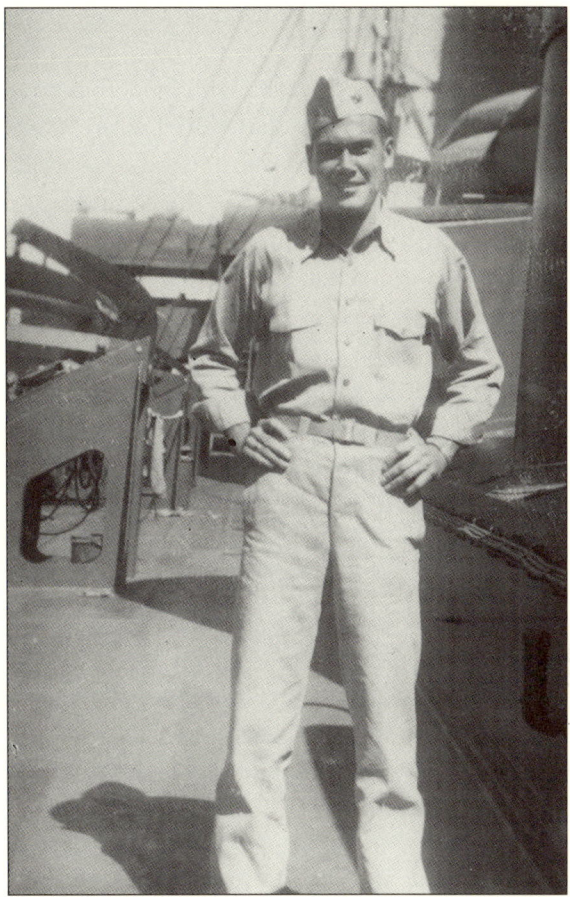

Lt.(j.g.) Callow in the Pacific, aboard the USS Harry Lee, 1943.

Diagnostic Clinic, which was Tufts University Teaching Hospital. I finished training in 1952 and was at Tufts from then on.

Dale: Vascular surgery really started in the early 1950s. Do you remember when you did your first vascular case?

Callow: The first aneurysm I did was in 1951. I simply ligated the aorta and excised the aneurysm. It had been bleeding for two to three days and the patient was in severe pain. After surgery I put him under wet sheets and had a fan blowing across him to try to reduce his metabolism. But my patient developed gangrene, as one would have expected, and died.

Soon after came a man in his fifties with Leriche's syndrome. His aorta was blocked. I took a sheet of fascia lata from his leg to make a tube graft to replace the distal aorta, for there were no synthetic grafts available at that time. We had a graft bank, but a very limited number of grafts and sizes. I would travel to any institution to obtain vessels, usually from victims of motor vehicle accidents, keep them refrigerated with dry ice, and then, having teamed up with a postdoc electrical engineering student at MIT, I would take them over there, where we would radiate them with a two-million-volt electron beam. These were kept in dry ice until used, when they were reconstituted in saline at room temperature. As you know, these ultimately developed aneurysmal dilatations, and it was fortunate that synthetic grafts came along when they did. The patient with the fascia lata tube graft came back ten years later because of claudication in one leg. His iliac artery had occluded on that side, but his aorta was patent and could be barely detected when we did the iliac femoral graft using a synthetic at that time.

In those early days, there was not much volume in vascular surgery; no one talked about it very much. Practical physicians said vascular surgery was a waste of time: Everybody has arteriosclerosis, and there is nothing you can do about it.

Dale: When did you do your first carotid repair?

Callow: That was about 1955. I did about a half a dozen of them. They were all completely occluded, the only ones a neurologist would refer. Later, when the patients began to come directly to me, and in larger numbers, the chief of neurology asked if I would share these patients with the neurology fellows. I said, "Of course." I built my practice on a private referral basis, not from within the hospital, a fact that stood me in good stead years later as I negotiated for better conditions as a full-time academic surgeon.

Dale: Ralph Deterling also gave impetus to the vascular program.

Callow: Yes, he followed Gardner Child as chairman until Dick Cleveland came in 1976. They both stabilized the situation.

Dale: Did you continue to do general surgery?

Callow: I stopped doing general surgery about 1972. Vascular practice had become so big that I could not do both.

Dale: Who was on the team with you?

Callow: No one else was doing vascular surgery at the medical center in those early years. I rarely did anything but care for patients. I did not take vacation, and when I did it was usually at home.

Dale: What if you needed to go to a vascular meeting?

Callow: I stopped operating for two or three days beforehand and would not stay for the entire meeting. We rarely went out of town, and what travel we did was in association with a meeting. In time, Ralph Deterling joined the staff and could cover for me.

Dale: How did you happen to stay in the naval reserve?

Callow: I had no intention of doing so. Initially I stayed in the reserve because it paid a little during the nonsalaried residency years. We received no pay in training except during the last year, the seventh year, when the medical school gave us $1,000 in return for teaching. We did have board, room, and laundry, and most everything else. We worked every other night and every other weekend. The pay for the reserve was $10 a night for a couple of hours. That was a sizable amount then. When I became a member of the full-time staff in 1952, my entering wage was $6,000 a year.

Dale: Were you allowed to keep your fees for patient care?

Callow: No, everything went into a common pool. We had just our salary, but it was a busy and satisfying life. Quite accidentally, I was asked to do some particular things from time to time, and I agreed often because I liked the particular person, the naval officer who made the request, or the task. Once I was asked to set up a school to teach hospital corpsmen after the dreadful morbidity and mortality they suffered during Korea. I went to Vietnam, and they wanted me to go as a professor, but in uniform, saying I would have more weight with civilians as an officer and more weight with the regular navy personnel as a professor.

That proved to be an interesting experience. The air force wanted to build a super hospital plane to transport casualties from Cam Ranh Bay and Da Nang, which would have meant a continuous nonstop flight from Vietnam to one of three bases in the United States. The army, navy, and marine people opposed the proposal, as it was thought it would be far too stressful on the casualties. I was sent to evaluate the problem and the possible consequences.

I flew back and forth, with a helicopter at my disposal. I would stay with wounded soldiers, get them loaded onto the plane, and fly with them to the destination. We'd land at Elmendorf in Alaska, where the crew would change, but, of course, the severely wounded couldn't get off the plane.

I wrote a report saying that the most advanced airplane in the world would not be a hospital and could never be made into one and that a plane ambulance is merely an up-to-date, sophisticated version of the horse-drawn ambulance used in Flanders in World War I. That caught the eye of some people in Congress and was published in the *Congressional Record*. The money was not appropriated, and the plan for that type of evacuation to the States was ended.

I wrote notes to the parents of some of these casualties, to reassure them that their sons were getting the best possible care, and I became tremendously depressed about that war. What was so heartwrenching was that I had been through the same thing twenty-five years earlier—bodies broken by explosives, burned, sometimes beyond saving—terrible things happening to fine young people, and twenty-five years later it was happening again. Vietnam was a terrible, dreadful mistake.

Dale: You've been influential in the International Society for Cardiovascular Surgery. When did you first become active in that?

Callow: In 1952 or so, Cuth Owens and I were walking on the boardwalk in Atlantic City, where we were attending a meeting. He offered to propose me to the International Society. At that time Ralph Deterling was secretary. When he moved to Boston, he needed some help and I was made assistant secretary general. Our offices shared the work and the expenses.

Dale: Looking back at the many scientific papers you've written, can you select one or one group of which you are particularly proud?

Callow: Undoubtedly the papers on surgery of the carotid arteries to prevent strokes.

Dale: What is your reaction to the current suggestion that too many carotid operations are being performed?

Callow: On the surface the statement is true. Unfortunately, it condemns the innocent more than the guilty. Possibly too many carotid arteries are being operated on, but that doesn't mean carotid endarterectomy is a worthless operation that should be discarded. Thousands of patients need it and benefit from it every year. But it has become overused in some places.

Dale: Is there a parallel with the coronary bypass operation, which also may be overdone?

Callow: I can't speak to that. I am aware of it, but not on the basis of personal knowledge.

Dale: Is a medical career attractive to young people in the same way it was to you as a young man?

Callow: Yes, definitely. We are living in troubled times, but every generation has its own troubles. It is unfortunate that cost plays such a determining role for medical care today. I believe that we face the rationing of medical care, as has occurred in so many countries.

Dale: So, Allan, can we continue to operate on an eighty-five-year-old man with a ruptured aneurysm? It is costly to save such a nonproductive person. Neither the Russians nor the British would allow it!

Callow: First, I would say he is not necessarily nonproductive! However, I think we cannot continue our present generous policies. Physicians are going to be seriously challenged on the benefits we contribute to our society rather than the benefits to the individual alone.

Dale: It is a philosophic question that James Michener illustrated in one of his *Tales of the South Pacific,* when he wrote of the cost of rescuing a single fighter pilot in World War II. How will such a decision be made?

Callow: It will be made by society, which will say, "We've gone far enough with the elderly." But it is naive to think that the cost of health care will not increase. It is our fastest-growing industry. The health industry is a huge employer. With rationing, there will be tragedies, and many more disappointments. If cost is a major factor, will operations to save Siamese twins be permitted, when we know that at best only one of the twins can survive and, even then, only for a few years? As experts we must be more objective in evaluating priorities. We must also become patient-centered and treatment outcome–oriented.

Dale: What do we do? The old man with the ruptured aneurysm is likely to cost $50,000. How can he pay it, either in money or productivity?

Callow: I can't answer that. We spend untold millions on cancer therapy. The amount is incredible, yet the survival figures for breast cancer today are little better than when I was a resident forty years ago.

Dale: What about the future of surgery? Is there anything more that the surgeon can do with his hands than he is doing today?

Callow: It will be less. The skilled, manipulative side of surgery, once so highly prized, will become less so as it is standardized and popularized.

Dale: Is it correct to say that a few years ago there was so much "art" in operating on an aortic aneurysm or a carotid artery that some surgeons were much superior to others, but that today the standardization of technique and of training has produced many surgeons who are approximately equal in their ability?

Callow: That is correct. There's no longer just one outstanding person in this or that field.

Dale: I've been interested in a question which has never been discussed. In most fields of endeavor, when a young man finishes his training, he still has to rise through the ranks—he is still considered junior. Today in surgery we have the attitude that when a man finishes his training he is a polished, finished practitioner, and he is turned loose to operate on anyone he chooses. Will that continue?

Callow: The young surgeon who has just finished a residency program is full of confidence that he has a great technique and that he is a capable person. But he needs a period of maturation. The transition is often too abrupt. The real training and judgment development come only with years of one's own practice.

Dale: Do you wish to make any further comments?

Callow: I would like to comment on private medical education. There are only twenty or twenty-one private medical schools in our country. They need financial and personal support. I am not opposed in any way to our state-supported schools and universities, but we must have more than one system for education. So I plead for the support of our private schools.

Jack Cannon

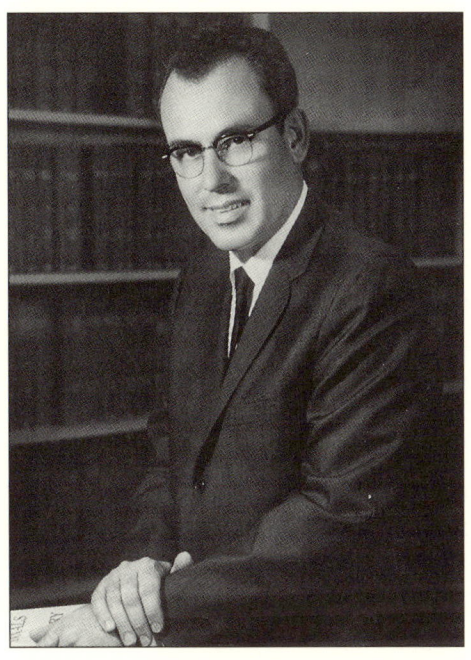

J ACK CANNON was one of the early technical innovators in vascular surgery. Arthur Allen's early influence made him a compassionate doctor and a good surgeon, and his association with Jack Wylie stimulated him to develop instruments to facilitate endarterectomy. Cannon's almost single-minded commitment to improving the technical components of vascular surgery led him to reach new horizons in the treatment of diseases of the vascular system. It is appropriate that he has lately used his expertise to work with industry in product improvement.

Cannon was interviewed December 3, 1990.

Johnson: Jack, tell me about your parents and where you were born.

Cannon: I was born in a town called Salina, Kansas, on July 17, 1919. My father was an athletics coach at St. John's Military School. He later taught general science and finally became a junior high school principal.

We lived briefly in Lucas, Kansas, then in St. Francis, Kansas, and then for seven years in the tiny town of Bird City in northwest Kansas. My mother taught in the high school and coached the girls' basketball team. As an only child, I don't think I would have succeeded as well as I have if it hadn't been for their love, their pride in me, their encouragement, and their very real financial sacrifices made on my behalf.

As the Depression of 1929 hit the country, my folks lost most of their savings in a bank crash. We moved to Klamath Falls, Oregon, where my father tried building houses. We lost everything and ended up with mortgages we could not handle on three very nice, brand-new, unsalable houses. My father loaded everything we had onto a four-wheel trailer towed behind the trusty Hudson, and we fled to Los Angeles.

Luckily, my father landed a position in Redondo Beach teaching a junior high school class of "problem boys." Later he obtained a position as principal of the home school for sick children in Glendale, California. Many of the children had congenital heart disease. I remember becoming friends with a cyanotic, dyspneic boy and another with tuberculosis who had had numerous thoracoplasty operations.

Johnson: Do you think this school had any influence on your becoming a surgeon?

Cannon: Not specifically. My father had always wanted to be a doctor, but said he was not smart enough and did not have money enough to try for medical school.

I entered as a premed student at UCLA but majored in zoology and stayed the full four years to earn my B.A. degree. I was quite flabbergasted to learn that I had been accepted by Harvard Medical School, to begin in September 1940.

Johnson: What made you decide to go into surgery?

Cannon: Two courses turned me on to surgery. One was called "Introduction to Clinical Medicine," which included having the class observe its first surgical operation. We gathered in the observation dome of an operating room at the Peter Bent Brigham Hospital. Dr. Elliott Cutler, assisted by Dr. Robert Zollinger, performed a sigmoid resection for cancer. The entire procedure went perfectly, with both surgeons constantly explaining and describing exactly what they were doing. Zollinger was at his usual humorous best, even getting away at times with chiding Dr. Cutler. I was enthralled. Here was an example of truly doing something positive to battle disease. From then on I was hooked.

The other course was an innovative experience in the animal lab at the Brigham in which the students were instructed in the performance of several operations. The course was run by Dr. Carl Walter, who was very tough and frightening in his supervision and instructions to the burgeoning "surgeons." I was assigned to perform a splenectomy. I found it rather easy and certainly a satisfying experience and became further hooked on surgery as my future specialty.

My experiences rotating on the surgical services at the Massachusetts General Hospital became the clincher. The war was still going on, all but the senior surgeons had gone into service, the caseload was tremendous and the house staff extremely overworked. There was always something challenging and fascinating to do. I remember my agony of frustration at being left on my own in the outpatient clinic to remove a large wen from under the scalp of a patient. I was sure he was going to bleed to death before I managed to excise the miserable lesion. I remember the Coconut Grove fire and the frantic effort expended in dealing with the problem of the sudden influx of scores of severely burned patients.

I applied for and was accepted in a straight surgical internship at the Massachusetts General Hospital. I served on Dr. Arthur Allen's East Surgical Service, and in addition to a fine group of senior residents, I worked with and for many of the fine and famous senior surgeons of the MGH, both in the clinic and on their private services.

During my internship and residency (1943–1946), I believe, the surgical service at the MGH was possibly the only institution in the country which recognized peripheral vascular disease as a separate surgical interest. Peripheral vascular rounds were made every Friday throughout the hospital, mostly on the surgical services. These rounds were attended by the house staff and all interested attending staff surgeons. The cases consisted mainly of patients with lower extremity ischemic problems such as diabetic feet, atherosclerotic gangrene, arterial emboli, Buerger's disease, and Raynaud's disease. There were also varicose veins, and deep venous thrombosis in all its manifestations.

Surgical management of ischemic extremities consisted of amputations. Dr. Leland McKittrick taught us how to select and perform transmetatarsal amputation successfully. At that time, below-the-knee amputations were frowned upon. We were taught the safest and simplest way to perform supracondylar above-the-knee amputations. I am sure many lives were saved by using Dr. McKittrick's simple pillowcase closure above-the-knee amputation technique. Other "vascular" surgery consisted of lumbar and dorsal sympathectomies, embolectomies, vein ligation and stripping, and treatment of stasis ulcers.

At the time, Dr. Allen became intensely interested in the problem of pulmonary embolism. He initiated a study to determine whether bilateral prophylactic interruption of the common femoral veins would be helpful in lowering the postsurgical mortality from pulmonary embolism. Patients were selected on the basis of swelling in a lower extremity, a positive Homans' sign, and chest symptoms suggestive of pulmonary embolism. A great many of these operations were performed.

Once a large-enough series had been accumulated, they were compared with matched controls. Dr. Ben Roe, then a resident on the West Surgical Service, examined the entire case material and found no reduction in the incidence of pulmonary embolism (a diagnosis which at that time was very hard to make with certainty). I am sure Dr. Allen never forgave Dr. Roe for torpedoing his series. Undaunted, Dr. Allen then developed a series using prophylactic dicumarol versus placebo controls on patients having major general surgical operations and proved conclusively the benefit of this method.

Johnson: What about Dr. Robert Linton?

Cannon: Linton was an early believer in the prophylactic merit of elastic stockings. He was a very bold surgeon. He would chew you out thoroughly if you, as his assistant, didn't perform exactly as he demanded. He was patient, persistent, and never a quitter. I can remember a man with bad mitral heart disease who threw a large saddle embolism to his terminal aorta. Linton operated immediately and successfully. Within a few hours, at about 2:00 a.m., another embolus lodged in the common femoral artery on one side. Linton returned and operated immediately. He would have returned again if needed.

During that time, Dr. Reginald Smithwick, along with Dr. James C. White, chief of neurosurgery, had been studying the anatomy, physiology, and function of the sympathetic nervous system. Dr. Smithwick developed the operative procedure and proved that lumbodorsal sympathectomy combined with splanchnic nerve resection was effective in the treatment of essential hypertension. He used to run two operating rooms, and would start the first case in the morning and the second in another room about a half hour later. Jesse Thompson was resident on Dr. Smithwick's service. He would start the second case, and we would race to see if we could remove the sympathetic and splanchnic nerve chains before the boss finished the first case.

Along with Jesse Thompson and other MGH trainees, I remained an advocate of lumbar sympathectomy, in spite of the work of Eugene Strandness, which purportedly proved the operation to have no value. I have seen too many real improvements in rest pain, healing of gangrenous toe lesions, healing of ischemic ulcers, and even improvement in intermittent claudication to totally condemn the procedure. The death knell of lumbar sympathectomy, in my opinion, occurred because too few surgeons understood the anatomy of the lumbar sympathetic nervous system. Too often, using lumbar sympathectomy was much like sending a boy to do a man's job.

A fascinating reflection for me, when I look back to the time when I was a fourth-year medical student, is the status at that time of abdominal aortic aneurysms. On ward rounds an occasional patient would be presented whose only complaint was the presence of a pulsating abdominal mass. If someone asked about therapy at the bedside, he would be "shushed" and we would gather in the hall to be told that the patient was doomed to death from rupture of the aneurysm in the near future.

At the time, Bob Linton was experimenting with stuffing aneurysms with hundreds of feet of fine stainless-steel wire. The night before such an operation, a hapless house officer would be assigned the task of abrading a few hundred feet of wire off a spool. The wire was soaked in ether, respooled, and later autoclaved. At the operation, Dr. Linton would patiently insert a fine cannula into the aneurysm and stuff in as much wire as possible.

Postsurgical x-rays would show a great mass of wire in the aneurysm with loops sometimes extending up into the heart and down peripheral arteries. Linton would treat luetic thoracic aneurysms as well as abdominal aneurysms. I do not remember any cases of limb loss resulting, nor instances of proven distal thrombosis.

Johnson: What was your involvement in World War II?

Cannon: My class at Harvard graduated six months ahead of time, becoming the Class of 1943B. Mine was among the classes allowed a maximum of three nine-month periods of residency training. By the time I finished my twenty-seven-month training period, the war ended. I was sent to the Philippines as a replacement for those who were due for discharge. I stayed for eighteen months as chief of surgery at the Fourth General Hospital in Manila.

When I got out of the service, I elected to remain a Californian. Through luck and a mandatory six months of service in the admitting room at the Los Angeles County General Hospital, I then joined the fourth-year resident group and completed my fifth year as senior resident there in 1950.

After completing my residency, I opted for an academic career and was fortunate to be taken on by Bill Longmire, the newly appointed chairman of the Department of Surgery at the UCLA School of Medicine, which started its first class in 1950 using temporary barracks-type buildings as classrooms and the Wadsworth VA Hospital for clinical and residency experience.

Johnson: Who was on the faculty when you joined the UCLA Department of Surgery?

Cannon: Harry Muller had finished his residency about six months earlier and had joined the department as chief of the Division of Thoracic and Cardiac Surgery. Willard Goodwin also left Hopkins to join the department as chief of urology. John Dillon left the Los Angeles County General Hospital as chief of anesthesia to become chief of anesthesia at UCLA. Joel Pressman, who had been in the private practice of otorhinolaryngology, joined on the stipulation that he become chief of head and neck surgery. The other divisions were gradually added in subsequent years, with not infrequent changes of chiefs. Wiley Barker joined the Division of General Surgery after he finished his residency at the Wadsworth VA Hospital, about six months after I arrived.

Dr. Longmire frequently quoted his former chairman, Al Blalock, as stating, "Of all the problems left in surgery, the transplantation problem is the one that absolutely must be solved." Longmire, as a consequence, established a transplantation laboratory for which he obtained NIH funding.

I gained an interest in homotransplantation and began attempting organ transplants between canine models, which included kidney, lung, bone marrow, and three or four abortive attempts at liver homotransplantation. I was flattered and amazed when Tom Starzl told me that he believed I was the first person to attempt a liver transplantation. I had never published formally on the subject of liver transplantation, but had discussed my attempts during a transplantation panel, the transactions of which were published under the sponsorship of a drug company. Tom honored me by including my picture and mention of my work in the introduction to his book on liver transplantation. The honor was hardly deserved, because all my attempts resulted in immediate postoperative failure from gangrene of the small bowel in the host animals. My subsequent emphasis on vascular surgical research led me away from transplantation endeavors, but I have always maintained an interest in the field.

Johnson: How did the surgical group at UCLA let you concentrate more on vascular surgery?

Cannon: At the time my clinical experience was limited to the small number of private general surgical patients I could attract, plus my participation on the clinical staff of the Wadsworth VA Hospital. Longmire suggested that I take over the peripheral vascular clinic at the Wadsworth VA. The load was quite great and subsequently Wiley Barker also came on as a co-attending.

Leading up to this time, René Leriche had begun publishing papers reflecting his interest in obstructive atherosclerosis and its treatment by endarterectomy. The results did not seem very impressive, but the concept was, of course, attractive. I explored a few patients with terminal aortic obstructive disease and attempted some primitive "disobliterations," with no real resultant improvement. At this time, 1950–1951, Jack Wylie was serving in the army in Europe. He obtained a temporary duty assignment to spend some time with Leriche. They operated together, and Wylie had the genius to realize that in order for endarterectomy to be effective, it was necessary to start above the top of the lesion and extend the endarterectomy procedure to a level below the lesion. He also recognized the importance of finding and staying in the cleavage plane in the arterial media that exists between the atherosclerotic plaque and normal smooth muscle. At first, because of the rather frightening thinness of the residual aortic arterial wall, he wrapped the endarterectomized aorta with fascia lata. His paper reporting the first successful cases was published in 1951. The method was proven spectacularly repeatable by many subsequent operators. This clinical research, in my opinion, basically laid the groundwork for successful major arterial reconstructive surgery. He had the vision, foresight, and nerve to accomplish the procedure.

In our vascular clinic and hospital, femoropopliteal disease was more common than aortoiliac disease, in a ratio of about four to one. Femoropopliteal disease was not at the time amenable to direct

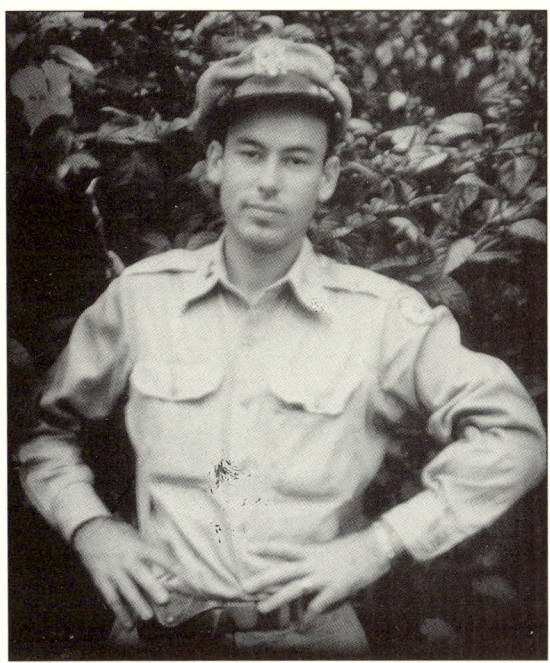

Jack in Luzon, Philippine Islands, 1946.

arterial surgery. Barker and I both concluded that something should be tried to improve the situation. We realized that Wylie's principles of endarterectomy must be applied if there was to be any chance of success. We also learned that the more symptomatic the extremity, the longer the involvement of the femoropopliteal segment was apt to be. Endarterectomy therefore would involve very long arteriotomies, the closure of which would be time-consuming and tedious. Nevertheless, we achieved some excellent results, Barker more so than I because of his enviable patience. I became disenchanted with the hours required to complete these operations.

In my earlier years, I enjoyed making model airplanes and had learned how to bend and shape piano wire. I fashioned some crude loops of variable diameters on the end of stiff piano wire shafts, and fitted the shaft end into a jeweler's pin vise, thereby fashioning the first "Cannon Endarterectomy Stripping Loops." The method worked in the absence of extensive calcification or arterial tortuosity. I found it best to start just below the lower extent of the lesion and proceed to the upper end, which was most often in the common femoral artery. Two, or at the most three, short arteriotomies were involved. The favorable cases with little calcification or tortuosity and with lesions of a firm, rubbery consistency yielded to the procedure with the most gratifying long-term results. Unlike bypass grafting, in which the graft feeds the distal tree only, endarterectomy can additionally open proximally occluded collateral. Along with Barker and Kawakami, we reported our first fifty-nine cases of femoropopliteal endarterectomy in 1958.

Johnson: How did you become involved in the surgery of coronary atherosclerosis?

Cannon: In the course of our work with femoropopliteal endarterectomy, Barker and I began to expose the distal popliteal bifurcation into the anterior and posterior tibial arteries. It occurred to me that the distal popliteal was only a modest amount larger than the left main coronary artery, and that the anterior and posterior tibials were only slightly larger than the left anterior descending and left circumflex arteries, respectively. Likewise, the right main coronary is in the size range of the peroneal artery. The atherosclerotic lesions encountered in the coronary tree are typical of such lesions elsewhere in the arterial tree—segmental, characterized by a discernible top and bottom delineation, and tending to occur at or in the regions of arterial bifurcations.

I did a series of coronary artery dissections on the cadavers of VA Hospital patients who had died of coronary artery disease, and confirmed that the above description was true of lesions of these vessels. I also noted that the primary atherosclerotic lesion tended to be segmental and relatively short. I found in these dissections that the lesions were subject to successful endarterectomy using Wylie's technique if one used fine instruments, supplemented with optical magnification. I had developed a coronary-sized set of endarterectomy stripping loops and ancillary instruments for coronary endarterectomy.

It happened that the first patient with severe, intractable angina pectoris deemed suitable for exploration by the referring cardiologist was referred to the departmental office. The departmental chairman notified me of the referral, saying he planned to do the operating with me assisting and showing him how I would do the operation. Although the patient, a man in his thirties, had extensive bilateral coronary atherosclerosis, we elected to perform an endarterectomy of the right main coronary only. In spite of the necessity of operating on the beating heart and a cumbersome bilateral fifth intercostal approach (median sternotomy was not yet being used at that time), the procedure went well. The patient was angina-free and able to be physically active for the next three years until his angina recurred and he died of a massive myocardial infarction. Autopsy showed complete occlusion of the endarterectomized segment of the right main coronary. It was filled with cellular material, which we subsequently identified as typical of neointimal hyperplasia.

Longmire developed a coronary endarterectomy series at UCLA that was published extensively. Rodney Smith, Jim McEachen, and I developed a series at St. John's Hospital. We soon were doing all cases with the aid of cardiopulmonary bypass. By this time, Mason Sones had perfected his technique of transbrachial artery coronary arteriography, so we now could diagnose the nature and location of the lesions with good accuracy. The results were encouraging but marred by the fact that only the most severe cases of angina, for which there was no other possible treatment, were subjected to operation.

One of the patients treated at St. John's Hospital was a blind man in his forties, who was totally incapacitated by angina. He had a very successful result with right main coronary endarterectomy for many months but then suffered recurrence. We reexplored him and found that the endarterectomized segment was nothing but thick scar tissue. In the course of the exploratory dissection, the distal right main coronary was transected. The distal tree was still open. We could think of nothing else to try but a reversed autologous saphenous vein bypass. The operation was performed on February 18, 1964, at St. John's Hospital in Santa Monica, California. The patient remained angina-free for another two or three years. One evening, during a violent altercation with his wife, he suddenly died. To our later amazement, Mason Sones told us that, as far as he knew, ours was the first case of successful coronary artery vein graft bypass.

Johnson: How many endarterectomies did you and Wiley perform together while the two of you were at UCLA?

Cannon: Even though we worked at the same institution and were both interested in vascular surgery, it quickly evolved that Wiley was doing his own thing and I was doing mine. We did collaborate on most of our vascular surgical papers. I think we actually operated together on vascular cases only four or five times, and that was early on.

Johnson: How many endarterectomies do you think you did?

Cannon: I doubt if it was more than 350 of all types, including the cases on which I acted in a supervisory and teaching capacity, as a first assistant to the senior residents.

Johnson: What was your early experience in the repair of abdominal aortic aneurysms?

Cannon: We had a problem with the availability of the essential spare part, the replacement graft. During his senior residency at UCLA, Rodney Smith, in spite of his very heavy caseload, decided that it was time to develop freeze-dried preservation of arterial homograft. He did so almost single-handedly, and his product was immediately in great demand.

My first aneurysm case was at Santa Monica Hospital. The patient was an elderly man with a large asymptomatic aneurysm. His general condition was good. Rod brought his one set of lyophylized arterial homografts to the operating room. He opened the vacuum-sealed glass vial containing the graft and reconstituted it in sterile distilled water. We proceeded with the resection and called for the graft, but there was silence from Rod, for he discovered that his reconstituted graft was not an abdominal aortic bifurcated graft, but a large graft consisting of the ascending aorta and the aortic arch with its branches. Undaunted, he suggested that we transect and close off the distal aortic arch and transfer the descending aorta to the proximal ascending aorta with an end-to-end anastomosis. The result was a trifurcated graft. We anastomosed the innominate to one common iliac and the carotid and subclavian branches to the opposite external iliac and hypogastric arteries, respectively. The patient recovered rapidly, suffering no complications. He lived six or seven more years and then died of a massive stroke.

We soon found that the postimplantation structural integrity of arterial homografts was not very satisfactory. The search was quickly on for a synthetic graft, stimulated by the original work of Arthur Voorhees. Along with others, I inserted a few nylon bifurcated grafts, which I sewed by hand the night before the operation. Nylon also had to be discarded because of its lack of long-term structural integrity. We quickly switched to Dacron grafts when they were available.

Johnson: When and why did you leave UCLA?

Cannon: I left in 1969. In the preceding few years my feeling of discontent had been building. For a long time Wiley Barker and I had hoped to be allowed to establish a Section of Vascular Surgery within the Division of General Surgery. We hoped to begin by starting to hold weekly vascular rounds in the medical school hospital. We tried repeatedly, even on our knees, to obtain approval from the chairman. He always stated in a most adamant fashion that our proposal could only be put in effect "over his dead body" and that he would be damned if he would tolerate any further fragmentation in his department.

I thought I had a good chance of becoming director of the surgical residency training program at a hospital in Phoenix. I pulled up stakes and departed UCLA after nearly twenty years of endeavor there. It almost cost me my sanity and indeed my family, for I soon realized that I was trying to leave the "gown" and join the "town."

My practice soon consisted of about 80 percent vascular surgery and 20 percent general surgery. Initially, I was referred cases of coronary artery disease, and I performed the first aortocoronary bypass to be done in the state of Arizona. Soon the chest surgeons took that over, without engendering much feeling of regret on my part. Being one of the most incapable of businessmen, I belatedly and painfully discovered that, over the course of about six years, I had been embezzled by my office nurse. And, to my great misery and frustration, I also allowed myself to become involved in a difficult medical-political wrangle over closed staff versus open staff appointments at one of the hospitals.

One of my main joys has always been in the teaching of residents. In 1976, I was offered the position of chief of surgery at the Phoenix

VA Hospital, and in the next two years, I had the satisfaction of resurrecting a dying residency program and building a vascular surgery service of which anyone could be proud. At the end of the two-year tenure, it became obvious that I was no bureaucrat. I could not go along with the standards and policies which obtain in non-university-affiliated VA hospitals. I resigned, and we moved to Flagstaff, where I intended to take time off and loaf for a year to compensate for the sabbatical year I was always afraid to take while at UCLA for fear that my laboratory and office space would be allocated to someone else during my absence.

After only a few months into my loafing period in Flagstaff, I was contacted by John Giovale, the plant manager of the Medical Products Division of W. L. Gore & Associates. At that time, the use of the Gore-Tex vascular graft was coming into increasing clinical acceptance. He told me that the company's directors had come to the conclusion that there was a need for authoritative vascular surgical consultation with regard to the increasing use of the graft. He had been told of my work in vascular surgery and that I had moved to Flagstaff. The result was that he offered me a desk and a telephone in an office at the plant with no assignment other than to "see what would happen."

It has been a real privilege to work with Gore Associates, and I have found this affiliation to be a most satisfying way in which to complete my professional career.

Johnson: Who do you think probably has had the most influence on your professional life?

Cannon: I would say that Arthur Allen influenced me the most, although in a general sense I remain in awe of many of the teachers both at Harvard Medical School and in my residency training periods for what beneficial molding of my surgical entity they were able to accomplish.

Arthur Allen stands out because he was a fine teacher, a most excellent surgeon possessed of an admirable scientific mind. But he was a doctor above all, in the real sense of the word; his patients came first, and his aim was constantly to improve the care he rendered them. He once told me that he tended to forget the patients who did well, but those who did not forever preyed upon his mind, causing him to wonder what he could have done differently and better. I always wanted to emulate him.

Johnson: You have been part of the beginnings of vascular surgery. Can you sum up what you think has happened in the last twenty to thirty years of your involvement?

Cannon: I believe that the concern of Longmire and his confreres about fragmentation has turned out to be ill founded. I still consider myself a general surgeon. I agree with the decision to keep recognizing this area of endeavor by the awarding of a certificate of special competence rather than the creation of another surgical board. I find it reprehensible to hear of surgeons devoting themselves exclusively to the practice of vascular surgery, referring their abdominal wound dehiscences to a general surgeon and their unsalvagable limbs to an orthopedist for definitive care. I agree thoroughly with Isadore Ravdin, who once stated something to the effect that any surgeon considered to be qualified should be capable of the total management of any problem encountered in an incision he makes, regardless of its location.

I dislike the burgeoning tendency of the so-called interventional cardiologist. I believe that freestanding vascular laboratories have gained acceptance largely because they give referring doctors some hard copy to look at. I agree with Gene Strandness, who used to say that anyone who understands vascular disease can evaluate it adequately with a history, a physical examination, a stethoscope, and perhaps a pocket Doppler blood velocity meter. I was impressed that one of Wes Moore's courses in endovascular surgery was attended by a class of about four hundred doctors, of whom 85 percent were surgeons.

I doubt that arterial bypass grafting will ever become totally archaic, and I believe that research into the fundamental nature of the "blood-seeing" surface should be intensified. I am not inspired by the frenetic search for usable autologous grafting material. This philosophy denies the fact that the disease is progressive and carries a mortality approaching 50 to 70 percent at five years after a given operative intervention.

On the other hand, there is a tremendous amount of research endeavor addressed to the potential of endovascular surgery. Reducing the invasiveness of surgical therapy has an appeal that cannot be denied. Endovascular surgical treatment may become even more competitive with standard surgery if breakthroughs in the techniques now being investigated occur. Results posting only a 30 percent short-term improvement are simply not tolerated by operating surgeons. Nevertheless, when the procedures are performed by non-surgeons, such results are considered highly acceptable, since at least the 30 percent of patients who are improved are saved from the morbidity, mortality, pain, and suffering of a standard invasive operation which more often than not has merely been put off! Any patient is eager to opt for a relatively noninvasive procedure if the big one can be delayed.

I hope that the increasing attention to the treatment of atherosclerosis will be fruitful. Breakthroughs in treatment are here, more will come, and one result of such progress will be that the practice of vascular surgery may well become smaller.

I feel very honored to have been included by Andy as one of his "brothers." His untimely death is a very great tragedy. He was a true southern gentleman in every sense of the word; was kind, caring, and charitable; and obviously loved his fellow men and was loved by them. He was a fine surgeon and doctor, and his contributions to the practice and teaching of vascular surgery have been major. His book on autologous vein grafting is a classic, and is one of the few medical texts which will never require significant revision. He is sorely missed.

John Connolly

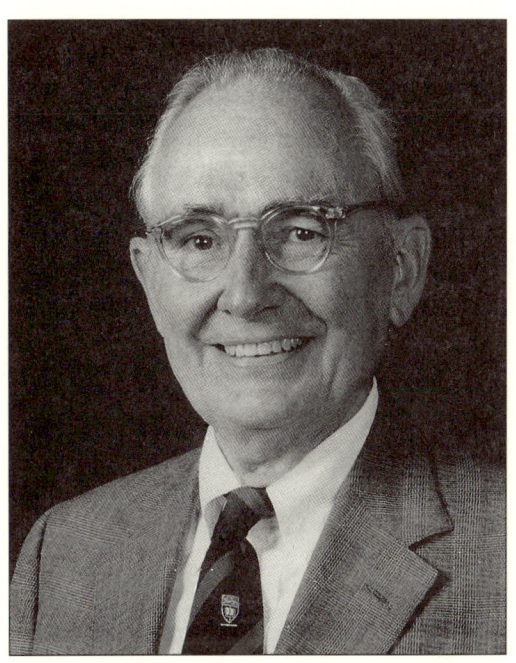

J ACK CONNOLLY has been a major contributor to vascular
surgery. His impetuous smile and innumerable friends have
carried him well through these important years. In addition to
being a superb surgeon, he is a scratch golfer. His leadership of
the *Journal of Cardiovascular Surgery* during its years of struggle was
significant. He was interviewed December 8, 1986.

Dale: How did you become interested in medicine as a career?

Connolly: My father was professor of surgery at Creighton University in Omaha, Nebraska. He was a general surgeon in the true sense of the word at that time—he did all kinds of surgery, including thoracic and neurosurgery. I remember that he even presented a paper concerning a brain tumor that he had removed. From the time I started school—I was born May 21, 1923—I would go with him on hospital rounds on the weekends, and I even watched him do an autopsy when I was eight years old. When I first became interested in medicine, the American Board of Surgery had not even been formed. My father became a Fellow of the American College of Surgeons in 1930, and he religiously attended all of its annual clinical congresses. He usually took the whole family along, so I was exposed to the postgraduate aspects of surgery. My father was one of the first to be certified in general surgery. It was in 1937, I believe, that he took the orals in surgery. His examiner was Allen Kanavel, the famous hand surgeon. My father was asked to examine a couple of patients as a prelude to questioning. The first one had a supracondylar fracture and his arm was up in a cast. My father could not find a pulse, so he sent for the examiner to return at once. Of course, a Volkman's contracture was avoided and the examination was over quickly. Needless to say, he passed.

Dale: Where did you go to college?

Connolly: I went on to Harvard College and then on to Harvard Medical School. My father had always wanted me to go to Harvard Medical School. He was very impressed with Edward Churchill, who was a professor of surgery there at the time and also chief of surgery at the Massachusetts General Hospital, and he thought that the best way to get into Harvard Medical School would be to go to Harvard College. That proved not to be the case. The medical school wanted to admit students from colleges around the country, and they had many applicants from Harvard College. Dr. Worth Hale was the assistant dean who chaired the admissions committee. When I interviewed with him, he asked why I had not attended the University of Nebraska. I told him that my father thought it would be better if I went to Harvard. He said, "Well, your father was dead wrong. It would be easier to get in if you were a graduate of the University of Nebraska!" Things looked bleak to me after I heard this, but, fortunately, I later learned that I was accepted. It was my intention to stay in Boston for surgical residency training, but I also applied to several good programs around the country. When internship notification day came, the only one that I didn't get was the Massachusetts General Hospital internship.

Dale: Weren't you lucky, because so many young men's careers were stunted by their necessity to remain in Boston.

Connolly: I was considering the Brigham, but they didn't have a chief at the time. That was 1948, a year before Francis Moore was appointed as chief. I called my father and he said, "Why don't you go to Stanford, because San Francisco is the best city in the world." We had played golf on a beautiful day at Pebble Beach just before my scheduled interview at the University of California the previous summer. I liked their program, but I didn't think I would come to the West Coast, so I had canceled the interview and application. However, I had already interviewed at Stanford. My decision to go to Stanford, of course, has affected the location of my career ever since. Dr. Emile Holman, who was the chairman of surgery, had been taking six interns each year, all from Stanford. My appointment changed their system because I was the first person he took from the outside.

Dale: Why did he limit his men to Stanford graduates?

Connolly: I don't know whether he had thought much about it. It was probably just convenient, since he knew more about his own students. Dr. Holman was very interested in running a service similar to what he had experienced under Dr. William Halsted at Hopkins, where an active experimental lab was an important part of the training program. In the Stanford program, there was only one chief resident at the top of a pyramidal system in which only two of the six interns became assistant residents, one of whom ultimately became chief resident. Dr. Holman did something new with me. Around April of my internship year, which was earlier than he ordinarily announced what was going to happen to the six interns, he called me in and said, "Next year you are going to work in the dog lab." I was terribly depressed because I thought I was being sent to Siberia. But it turned out that it was the signal that he had earmarked me to ultimately be his chief resident. So I worked in the dog lab with him for a year.

Dale: What do you mean "with him"? Did he actively work in the lab himself?

Connolly: Yes, he came into the dog lab and actually operated there at least twice a week.

Dale: Are there chairmen of departments now who do that? Or is that gone?

Connolly: I don't think there is as much of that today. There are chairmen who go to the dog lab to see what's happening—they meet with the residents but I don't think they actively perform animal operations like Dr. Holman did. The tendency, unfortunately, has been for schools to want their chairmen to be administrators who are at the beck and call of the dean to attend committee meetings. Many chairmen rarely even operate on patients themselves; they assist residents, but never do a case themselves from beginning to end. If I only did that, I would miss a great deal of the fun and satisfaction of surgery.

Dale: Let me ask about Dr. Holman. I believe that he was one of the few department chairmen who actively participated in World War II in the combat field rather than sitting in an administrative office.

Connolly: That's true. Although he was a distinguished professor and several of his contemporaries were generals or admirals, Dr. Holman entered the navy as a lieutenant commander and served in the South Pacific. He wanted to get out where the action was.

Dale: Did he ever tell you anything about Churchill?

Connolly: No, I don't recall him talking about Churchill. He had worked under Cushing in Boston at the Brigham and came to the West Coast before Churchill became chief at the Massachusetts General Hospital.

Dale: What did Holman believe? Why did he want to join the service instead of being a big wheel, as were some others?

Connolly: He was an idealist. He didn't believe in war, although if war occurred he thought he ought to do his part. Interestingly

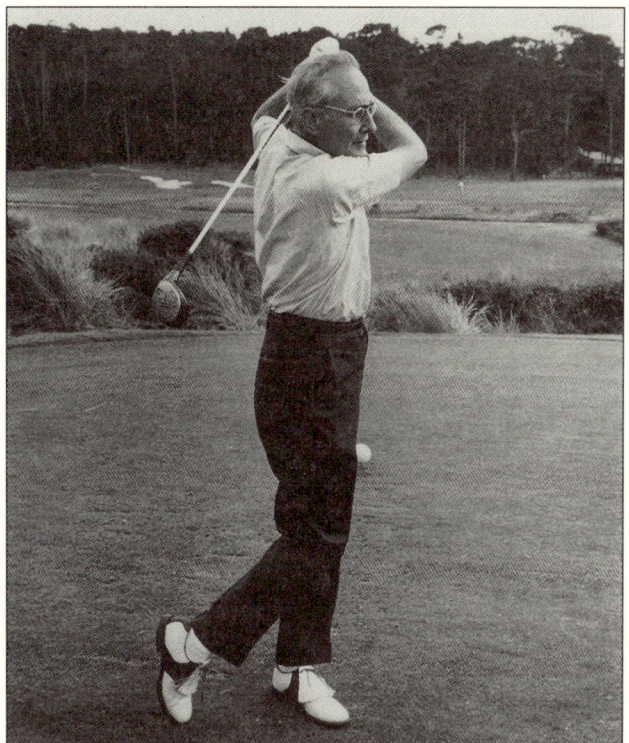

Jack at the Cypress Point Club, Pebble Beach, California, 1986.

enough, after the war he had a lot of contact with Russian surgeons. He also had some fondness for Mao, the Chinese leader. He had an unusual mixture of beliefs. His wife was a strong liberal influence on him.

Dale: Who was she?

Connolly: Dr. Ann Purdy. She was a Canadian whom he met at the Johns Hopkins Medical School, where they both obtained their medical degrees. She became a pediatric cardiologist and practiced at Stanford. As a matter of fact, she was the referring doctor for all of his pediatric cardiac surgical cases. She told him exactly when to operate and when not to operate!

Dale: Was Dr. Holman a good technician in the operating room? And was he a good teacher?

Connolly: Yes, he was both. The Stanford programs were designed after those at Hopkins where grand rounds were conducted at the bedside once a week. Dr. Bloomfield, who had also come from Hopkins, was the professor of medicine, and his rounds were even more sought after than Dr. Holman's. Holman would always come to Bloomfield's rounds, which would be so crowded you could hardly get into the ward. They would gather around the patient, the history was presented, and then Dr. Bloomfield would examine the patient. Then the group would kick it around and anybody who was present could interject, discuss, or ask a question.

Dale: Did they call the roll or did you sign your name as we must do today?

Connolly: No, they had no idea who attended. People went because of academic interest and the splendid teaching.

Dale: What do you think of this present business of signing in for every conference?

Connolly: It is ridiculous! But we do it also. The authorities demand evidence of continuing education.

Dale: Who are the authorities? Did Halsted do it?

Connolly: Of course not; they didn't have all the bureaucracy that we have now. If a teaching conference is worthwhile, people will find time to come. That's better than trying to force it by writing letters regarding absences, threatening to kick people off the staff, and other such petty matters.

Dale: Dr. Holman was a first generation disciple of William S. Halsted, who unlike most, went west. What was his greatest contribution to surgery?

Connolly: His laboratory and clinical studies of arteriovenous fistulas rank as classic contributions. Another was the pathophysiology and treatment of constrictive pericarditis. He was also a pioneer in cardiac surgery. He performed the first ligation of a patent ductus on the West Coast.

Dale: Was Holman a man who inspired the residents? Did you love this man like a father, or was he a cold figure?

Connolly: We respected him. We also feared him to some extent, so he wasn't exactly a father figure. He had quite a temper and could get very upset with us. He ran a good surgical service and teaching program.

I wanted to go abroad for a year during my residency, preferably to England, and he said, "No, I'm going to send you to Memorial Hospital in New York City, because we need someone to learn head and neck surgery. I am going to make you the head and neck surgeon in our department." I said, "No sir, I don't want that."

Dale: So that proposal was bad news to you?

Connolly: It was certainly not good news. I persisted and he finally agreed with my request to go to England, saying, "I'm going to send you to St. Bartholomew's Hospital in London to work with Sir James Patterson Ross." So I went there for a year. Patterson Ross had been knighted for performing a lumbar sympathectomy on the king. He also became the president of the Royal College of Surgeons of England, and I had a wonderful broadening experience that year.

Dale: Tell me about Frank Gerbode.

Connolly: Frank Gerbode had a great influence on me. He was a member of the staff when I became in intern at Stanford. Because of Emile Holman, Frank developed an interest in cardiovascular surgery, and he helped Holman a great deal. Frank was a good technician and he was a little more aggressive and secure in trying new things than the chief. It developed that Emile would never operate on a new or difficult problem without Frank, so Gerbode soon became the foremost cardiovascular surgeon on the West Coast.

Dale: Well, that's right, but you were saying that perhaps Dr. Holman might have been different if he had married a different person. Well, Gerbode's wife was a different person. What was her influence?

Connolly: He was married to Martha Alexander, whom I liked a great deal. Martha had a strong personality also, and was not involved in medicine. She was the daughter of Wallace Alexander of the Alexander and Baldwin Company of the Hawaiian islands. He managed the sugar interests of the company from the San Francisco Bay Area.

Dale: Did Frank's marriage to an heiress affect him?

Connolly: I think it was a plus and a minus. Frank was able to meet and entertain many people that he might not have met otherwise, and he was free of financial demands. On the other hand, there were some people, particularly in the medical school, who were very jealous of him, who thought he was getting ahead because of that. I don't think that was entirely true, but jealousy was a handicap to him in my estimation.

Dale: Did you know Norman Freeman?

Connolly: Yes. I think Norman Freeman was one of the real pioneers in vascular surgery. He was stationed near San Francisco during the war as chief of one of the three national vascular centers. The California Academy of Medicine had a distinguished lecturer who at the last minute canceled, and Freeman was substituted to speak in his place. His topic concerned the physiology of arteriovenous fistulas. Dr. Howard Naffziger, who was then the chairman of surgery at the University of California, heard it, and was very impressed, and subsequently offered Freeman a job after he left the service. Freeman thus became the first vascular surgeon at the University of California San Francisco Medical Center. In fact, in 1938, while still at the University of Pennsylvania, Freeman was the first surgeon in the country to limit his practice to vascular surgery.

Dale: What did he do?

Connolly: Freeman developed an early interest in the physiology of the vascular system while working several years in the laboratory of the famous Harvard physiologist Eugene Landis. During that time he developed his lifelong interest in the sympathetic nervous system. He was also aware of the innovative vascular procedures that the French were doing. Jacques Oudot performed the first aortoiliac endarterectomy in the early 1950s, soon after João Cid dos Santos had reported the first femoral endarterectomy. Freeman was one of the first in our country to employ endarterectomy, particularly of the abdominal aorta. He also performed the first femorofemoral arterial bypass. He used an endarterectomized occluded superficial femoral artery in a crossover fashion to the opposite groin ten years before Vetto described femorofemoral bypass with a prosthetic graft. Freeman also described the use of the translocated splenic artery to bypass the occluded abdominal aorta to the iliac artery as another type of extra-anatomic bypass. Both of these original procedures were published in *California Medicine* ten years before Vetto, but that was a rather obscure journal and it wasn't widely seen.

Dale: Before we conclude, what was his relationship with Jack Wylie?

Connolly: I understand that Freeman first interested Jack in vascular surgery. Jack worked with him after World War II at the University of California. Later they disagreed and separated. I'm not certain of the details. But Freeman left the University of California and went to the Franklin Hospital, which was a private hospital affiliated with the University of California, and was joined in practice by Frank Leeds and Rud Gilfillan. Leeds was also one of the first surgeons in the world to specialize in vascular surgery. Leeds and Freeman wrote a number of papers together. Finally, Freeman left the practice with Leeds and moved to Children's Hospital, which, in spite of its name, is another general hospital in San Francisco. He was practicing there when he retired.

Perhaps Freeman's most significant surgical first was the first surgical correction of renovascular hypertension. The year was 1952, at which time he was introducing aortoiliac endarterectomy in this country. He had a patient with an occluded abdominal aorta who also had hypertension and renal artery stenosis. He speculated that the renal artery stenosis could be causing the hypertension via a Goldblatt phenomenon, which he was familiar with because of his interest in physiology. Sam Roland, a urologist friend, was consulted, and he suggested that Freeman try to remove the proximal renal artery stenosis through the open aorta at the time of the aortic endarterectomy. He did so, apparently with a right-angle clamp, and cured the hypertension. This classic article appeared in the *Journal of the American Medical Association* in 1953, and the coauthors with Freeman are Leeds, Gilfillan, and Roland.

Denton Cooley

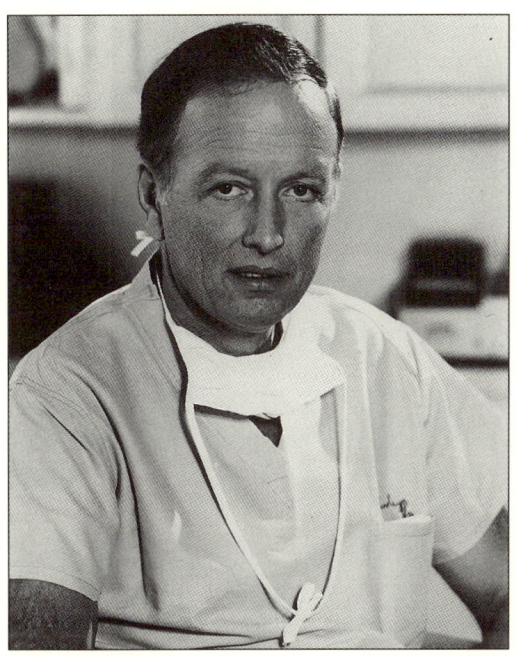

ACCORDING to the *American Heritage Dictionary,* an entrepreneur is "a person who organizes, operates, and assumes the risk for a . . . venture." Although the term is usually applied to a businessperson, it summarizes Denton Cooley, the surgeon who built the Texas Heart Institute in Houston virtually single-handedly.

Many contemporary surgeons believe Cooley to be presently the most technically skillful surgeon in the world. His dexterity, backed by wide knowledge and vast experience during the past forty-five years, has led him to perform procedures that are swift and sure—the mark of a surgeon's skill. A quick operation by such a master results not from hurried glances at a clock, but from thorough preparation for any eventuality, rapid choice of options, avoidance of trouble, and the help of an experienced veteran team.

Denton Cooley has always been a superior person, physically and intellectually. He played forward on the championship University of Texas basketball team while maintaining a scholarly academic record. His surgical training under Blalock at Johns Hopkins in Baltimore, plus another year in England, laid the solid foundation for his medical success. He has survived the difficulties that often beset talented entrepreneurs. The Texas Heart Institute is a monument to his imaginative talent.

Repeatedly, he stuns us with reports of large series of new techniques; the results are usually remarkably good. A well-known surgeon once told me, "I showed Denton the first of a new procedure, but before I could report it, he had accumulated and published ten!"

As yet, he has no thought of slowing his pace. He was interviewed December 12, 1986.

Dale: Denton, you are a native of Houston. Who were your parents?

Cooley: My grandparents moved there in 1890. My father, Ralph Clarkson Cooley, became a prominent dentist. Mother, Mary Fraley Cooley, was also a Texan, so I'm a third-generation Texan. I was born August 22, 1920. Father wanted both my brother, Ralph, and me to become dentists, but I changed to medicine and Ralph to business.

Dale: What was your early education?

Cooley: I attended the Houston public schools and graduated from a large public school called Jacinto High. There were 750 graduates in my class, so it wasn't a selective, individualized education. I went on to the University of Texas, where the enrollment at the time was 14,000.

Dale: Did you make a good scholastic record at Texas?

Cooley: I was a good student, or at least my grades were good. During the four years I made only two B's, even though I was playing varsity basketball—the rest were A's.

Dale: What position did you play?

Cooley: Forward and center. I was 6 feet 3½ inches tall. We had one fellow who was 6 feet 4½, so when he was available he jumped center; the rest of the time, I did. We didn't have those big 7-foot players prevalent today. I played semi-pro, city league–type ball when I was at Johns Hopkins in Baltimore.

Dale: What else did you do in college?

Cooley: I was a member of the Kappa Sigma fraternity. I participated in campus activities and politics to some extent.

Dale: How many basketball games did you have each year while in college?

Cooley: We played preseason games with the five other conference teams, and then I played in the National Invitational Tournament in Madison Square Garden one year and in the NCAA quarterfinals in San Francisco. Every year we went to Oklahoma City to play in a tournament during the Christmas holidays. So I had some good times playing basketball.

Dale: How did you find time to do your schoolwork along with the basketball?

Cooley: It was difficult. You had to steal time. You didn't want your fraternity brothers or your classmates to think that you were a bookworm, for, among peers, that was the worst. I would sneak off to the library when the fraternity boys were all playing pool and get my work done.

Dale: What about on the road—how did you study then?

Cooley: At first, when I was a sophomore, I'd take books, but after a while I realized that I couldn't really study on the road, so I didn't take any books along.

Dale: How did you first become interested in medicine?

Cooley: I had gone down to San Antonio on a dove hunt. On that Saturday night, a friend of my host took me to visit his friend who was an intern at the City-County Hospital. He was busy sewing up lacerated Latin Americans. He told me, "Pick out one of those fellows over there and sew him up." I watched him suture one fellow, and then I got a needle and thread and was inspired to sew up another fellow. I liked that. It was more fun than I thought I'd ever had.

Dale: How did you happen to go to Johns Hopkins Medical School?

Cooley: I went to the University of Texas Medical Branch at Galveston for my first two years of medicine, entering in 1941. Then Pearl Harbor came along in December. All sorts of anti-German political strife followed. The Texas legislature sent a committee down to investigate our faculty in connection with this. I saw Texas Rangers questioning my highly respected professors. Those Rangers put their boots and spurs up on the desks while our professors of medicine and surgery were sniping at each other. I thought that was bad and that the school might be placed on academic probation. So I decided to go elsewhere.

Dale: That was unusual.

Cooley: It sure was unusual for Texas. There were a lot of two-year medical schools at the time, but ours was a respectable four-year school. Anyway, I applied to five different medical schools and was accepted at four but turned down at Harvard. I chose Johns Hopkins, where I graduated in August 1944. It was really a three-year experience in medical school because of the war.

Harvard had rigid requirements and courses which were taught in the East but not everywhere. All who were enrolled in medical school when the friendly Japs bombed our naval base at Pearl Harbor attended classes on a year-round basis during World War II. The same had occurred during World War I. It raises a question as to why the same program is not used regularly. The medical program is so long that any decrease would be welcome. But the academic faculty are accustomed to lengthy vacations, and the clinicians who teach the final two years have not cried for change.

Dale: Where did your military service take you?

Cooley: Two years later, in 1946, I went on active duty in Linz, Austria, at the 124th Station Hospital, where I stayed for two years as chief of surgery. Incidentally, Linz was Adolph Hitler's birthplace.

Dale: Let's return to your time as a resident at Hopkins. Was Alfred Blalock chief? What did you think of him?

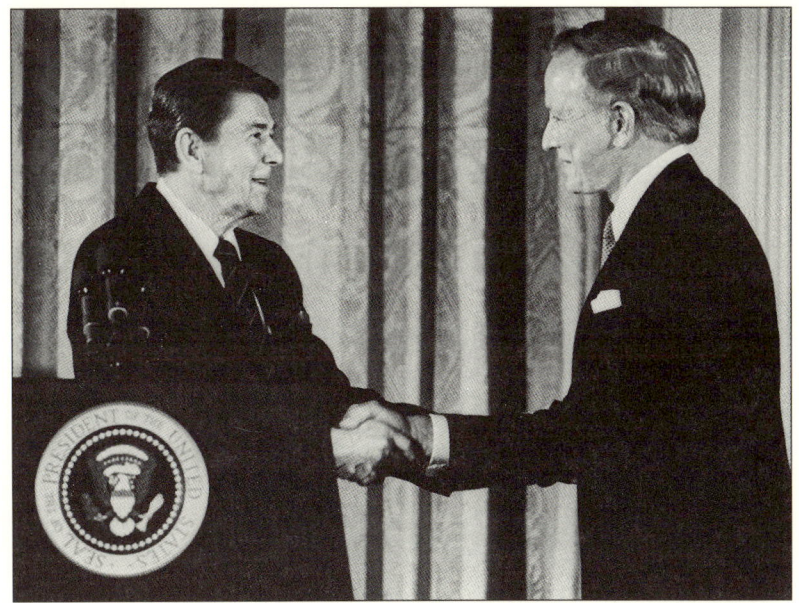

Dr. Cooley receives the Medal of Freedom, the highest civilian award in the United States, from President Ronald Reagan at a White House ceremony on March 26, 1984.

Cooley: I respected him highly. I had ended up either first or second in my graduating class. I applied to go to the University of Michigan to work under Dr. Coller in a rotating internship. Dr. Blalock called me into his office, though, and asked, "Mr. Cooley, aren't you going to even apply for my program?" I told him that I had learned about as much as Hopkins could offer. But I did apply for his internship and was accepted.

Dale: Who else in your residency class did well?

Cooley: Of course, Hank Bahnson stands out. He stayed on the full-time faculty at Hopkins and later became chairman of surgery at Pittsburgh.

Dale: He was always outstanding. He and I were in the Class of 1941 at Davidson College. What happened after you finished your residency?

Cooley: I finished the residency in 1950. Mr. Russell Brock, who later became Lord Brock, came to visit from London. In Britain, surgeons are called "Mr."—an appellation of which they are proud. I was infatuated with the man. I went to London and spent a year with him as his senior registrar at the Brompton Hospital. Then I went back to Houston.

Dale: What sort of person was Lord Brock?

Cooley: He was a quite severe and stern man. He had a lot of pride, perhaps with a bit of pomp. He was a difficult taskmaster in the operating room, but he knew that I was an American and he tried to show me a more relaxed attitude so I wouldn't think he was a stuffed shirt. He realized that things were more relaxed back in Baltimore than they were in London.

There was a lot of tuberculosis at the time. My principal reason for going with him was because I wanted to see his treatment of it and also to see how he was attacking pulmonary stenosis by a direct operation. At the time, the surgical treatment of tuberculosis was a big challenge. It was a wonderful opportunity to learn about it at a place like the Brompton Hospital.

Dale: Most of our contemporaries also wanted to learn tuberculosis surgery. I wished to learn it and worked at the Iola Sanitaria for that purpose. You and I both know that it wasn't important later on, because chemotherapy appeared and made surgical operation unnecessary.

Cooley: That's right. I did a few cases at the Veterans' Hospital in Houston. But then the anti-tuberculosis drugs replaced surgery.

Dale: Tell me about Dr. Blalock. He was one of the most important American surgeons; in fact, he was internationally recognized. Did you know that he was also a fine tennis player? He was doubles champion of Nashville in 1925, along with Dr. Tinsley Harrison. He also made a hole in one at the sixteenth hole of the Belle Meade Club, which is still recalled by a little silver inscription there.

Cooley: He was a great sports enthusiast. That was one thing that attracted me. The first time I met Dr. Blalock, I was cutting his class. I had just arrived in Baltimore from Texas. It was in February and for some reason the sun came out, which is unusual in Baltimore at that time of year, so a friend of mine, Lester Persky, and I went out to play tennis. Lester had played football at Michigan; he substituted for Tom Harmon so he didn't get to play much, but he was a good athlete anyway. He and I were out playing tennis during the time of Dr. Blalock's Friday clinic. Here came Dr. Blalock and Mark Ravitch and the whole crowd, parading across the grounds there at Hopkins, to the place where Persky and I were playing tennis. I said to Lester, "Look, we're going to really get sacked, the professor seeing us out here playing tennis." He must have had a conference with Dr. Helen Taussig over in the children's unit. When he came back out of the building, he brought the whole group over. They sat on the lawn and watched us play half a set of tennis. Then he came up to me and said, "You're Mr. Cooley, the new transfer." I replied, "Yes, sir." He said, "You play a good game of tennis, Mr. Cooley. Do you know how to play ping-pong?" I said, "Yes, sir. I can play a credible game." He then said, "Dr. Rienhoff has loaned us his summer house down on Gibson Island. I'm taking the family down, and I need somebody to play ping-pong with me. Will you come?" So that's the way I got to know Dr. Blalock, on a weekend trip with him and his family down at Gibson Island.

Dale: I only knew him obliquely because he had left Vanderbilt by the time I arrived there, but he seemed a very kind person.

Cooley: He was a kind, humble, and honest man.

Dale: What do you know of the development of the Blalock operation for blue babies? It's been said around Nashville that Vivian Thomas actually worked it out and then showed Dr. Blalock how to do it. Is that true?

Cooley: Yes. There is a good measure of truth in that. There is also another operation called the Blalock-Hanlon that was really Vivian's invention, but as for the Blalock-Taussig, I'm sure Dr. Blalock directed the thinking on that. While he was at Vanderbilt, he told Vivian that he wanted to study pulmonary hypertension and suggested that they produce it by creating a shunt to deliver arterial blood to the lung. Vivian worked out a lot of the technical details, but Dr. Blalock set up the experiments. So you can't give the credit to the "doer."

Dale: How was it to work with Blalock? When you assisted him, did he do everything or did he turn some of it over to you?

Cooley: I assisted as the lowest man on the totem pole on the first Blalock-Taussig operation, so it's rather vivid in my memory. I was an intern. It was about the first week in November 1944. That first one went very well. I remember so well when he opened the anastomosis to flow, Dr. Taussig said, "Al, he has a wonderful color; his fingernails have turned pink!"

Sometimes he was a little difficult. He had a demeanor in the operating room that I thought was unbecoming. He whined and complained a lot, and talked in a little voice at times—"Why doesn't someone help me?"—that sort of thing. That was just his demeanor, but I determined at the time that I was going to develop a different one in my career.

Dale: You went from the year with Brock in England to Houston. How did that occur? Did Mike DeBakey recruit you, or did you recruit him?

Cooley: It was a little of both. I wanted to stay in academic medicine permanently, but when I was about to finish, Dr. Blalock said, "Well, Denton, I don't know what you're going to do with your career. You'll probably go back to Houston and get to be the biggest society surgeon in town. But I hope you'll write a paper or two during your career." But I wanted to stay in academic medicine and had talked to Dr. DeBakey the year I finished at Hopkins about going to England for a year. He thought that was a good idea. Then I would come back and join the faculty at Baylor and take on a job as an instructor. I did that in 1951 and stayed full time at Baylor for eighteen years.

Dale: Were you there before Oscar Creech?

Cooley: No, Oscar was there at the time I arrived, but he was down with tuberculosis. He had to spend a year in bed, so he lost about a year in there, and I moved into his favored position. About 1956, Oscar left Houston for New Orleans as chairman of the department at Tulane. He died a few years later, not of tuberculosis but lymphoma.

Dale: What sort of person was Oscar?

Cooley: Oscar was a fine person. Everybody liked him. I think he always felt a little jealous of me because I had the good fortune of coming into his place while he was tied up with illness.

Dale: Who else came to Baylor in the early years of the fifties?

Cooley: There was B. W. Haynes, who is now in Richmond, and John Howard, who is in Toledo.

Dale: What year did you leave Baylor? What happened?

Cooley: It was 1969. There had been slow growth and some annoying feelings. When I went to Houston I was branded a heart surgeon. I remember one day after I had been there about a month, I posted five cases on the same day. I don't think that sat very well with Dr. DeBakey. I know it wouldn't set too well with me if I were in the same position. Anyway, there was a certain bit of rivalry growing up, so I withdrew from Methodist Hospital because Mike dominated the place, and I was always second fiddle to him. I thought if I was going to establish myself, I ought to move. I was interested in pediatric surgery, so I really confined my work after about ten years in Houston to St. Luke's Episcopal and Texas Children's Hospital. I remained on the full-time faculty and even got St. Luke's Hospital to convert from the University of Texas program to Baylor so I could develop a cardiovascular program.

Dale: Were you still doing peripheral vascular?

Cooley: Yes, I've always done peripheral, still do.

Dale: Still do, even though that's not widely known?

Cooley: Well, perhaps not.

Dale: What percentage of cardiac is your personal practice?

Cooley: Well, if you call abdominal aneurysms peripheral vascular, I think maybe 20 percent.

Dale: When did the Texas Heart Institute come along?

Cooley: I thought that we needed one institution that had a designated purpose. We had already gained a reputation in cardiovascular surgery, but in all those different hospitals like St. Luke's Hospital, Methodist Hospital, and Herman Hospital, nothing was designated as a heart program. So on my own I asked my lawyer to draw up a charter for the Texas Heart Institute, which I hoped to establish at St. Luke's and Texas Children's Hospital. I knew if I put it before the Baylor faculty they would say no, that it would have to go to Methodist, so I went ahead and did it on my own and just announced in the newspaper that we were building. My wife and I were celebrating our twenty-fifth anniversary, so it was 1962.

Dale: How many beds do you have now?

Cooley: I modeled it after Johns Hopkins, where they have all those different programs, such as the Halsted Clinic, the Harriet Lane Clinic, and the Brady Urological Institute, which are all part of the Johns Hopkins complex. It seemed to me you could place the cap of the institute over all. We've designated 300 beds in our 1,000-bed complex now, but that's sort of token. We could have 500 or we could have 100.

Dale: How many surgeons are associated with you?

Cooley: Right now there are seven other board-certified surgeons who work together. We also have six residents. It's one of the largest residency programs. There are also an average of twenty to twenty-five fellows.

Dale: How many cases are there annually?

Cooley: It has varied through the years. Right now the oil recession is affecting the medical profession in Texas, but this year we'll do 3,000 open-heart operations. Five years ago we did 5,000 in one year, in addition to twice that many other types of cases, including vascular and nonopen, or closed cardiac surgery.

Dale: How do you work the program for Belgians to come over on a package plan?

Cooley: We started with Belgian patients, mostly congenital heart disease. Twenty years ago we were approached by the Dutch and had what we called a Dutch airlift. We operated on some 1,200 patients from the Netherlands who would be airlifted over to us, spend two weeks, and go back. Their government supported it but now has discontinued it and takes care of its own patients. I understand that a few of them still go to the UK, which is just across the Channel and more accessible.

Dale: Last year at the international cardiovascular meeting in Monaco, it was said that you might soon have an affiliation in Monaco. Is that correct?

Cooley: They are building a heart institute there. Charles Hahn has invited me to come there and spend a month or something like that and do some operations. It's not a formal arrangement.

Dale: So that may occur in the future. Let me have your opinion regarding some other things of current interest. It's been said that the day of the surgical entrepreneur is past, that the younger surgeons are going to be a different sort of people. Will you comment on the next generation?

Cooley: It's a sign of age when you say that all good things have passed and that we're going to see average-type personalities without the prima donna surgeons that we have known in the last fifty years. It is true that much of the glamour of surgery, especially heart surgery, has disappeared. At the turn of the century, appendectomy was quite a thing; then abdominal intestinal surgery reached a zenith. Later, the neurosurgeon came along—brain surgery was all the thing. Then came heart surgery, but now that seems to be tapering off, so perhaps there's not going to be any great new opportunity.

Look at those of us who were involved in the early days of heart surgery. We took advantage of the cardiopulmonary bypass, which opened up a whole new era. We were explorers like explorers of the sixteenth century. The whole world was at our feet. Almost every case was a reportable one. A hole in the heart got headlines in the newspaper. But now that the heart has been transplanted and artificial hearts have been used, the field is hardly as newsworthy as it used to be.

Dale: How is your heart transplant program coming along?

Cooley: We are active. We've done 158 heart transplants. I think we did the first successful one in the United States in 1968.

Dale: What's your current one-year survival rate?

Cooley: We claim 80 percent survival at one year. We've been characterized as being loose in our selection of patients. Some groups have age restrictions on patients for acceptance. We haven't had any age restrictions. We've operated on people with active bacterial endocarditis, or diabetes, and on little children. We had an eight-month-old child who's a wonderful success two years later. So I've never tried to protect our mortality figures by selecting only the most favorable cases, but have been more inclined to push back the frontier. I've always believed that, in an institution like ours, we have an obligation to do that.

Dale: What's the average cost of a heart transplant?

Cooley: If everything goes well, and the patient is in the hospital for two weeks, the total cost runs around $50 thousand to $75 thousand. Some insurance programs will pay for parts of it. Medicare may soon designate ten or twenty centers where they will pay.

Dale: It's being said that too many carotid arteries are being operated on. Some people say too many hearts are having bypass surgery. We have a report that in southern California ten times as many carotids are done per unit of population than in the Southeast.

Cooley: There is some truth to it. But I can't vouch for what other people are doing around the country. I do know that no one has ever been able to say what the indications or contraindications to any surgery are, whether it be gallbladder, stomach, or heart. They all can be overused.

Dale: What are your interests besides surgery? Do you have any time to fish or play tennis or whatever you like to do?

Cooley: I still like to play games. Golf and tennis are my favorites, but I have a large family that needs time. I have five daughters and eleven grandchildren. Ten of them live on my block in Houston, and one of them will move there when her father finishes his residency at John Hopkins.

Dale: It sounds like the Kennedys. I had the impression that you gave up golf a while back for tennis.

Cooley: Actually, I gave up golf for a while because all my children were playing tennis.

Dale: Did you tell me one time that you played a good golf game against Jack Burke, Jr., the professional?

Cooley: Yes, I did. It was funny. I've always been a golfer who would shoot about 80 or 85. I'd had a hernia operation done on July 4th, and on Labor Day I was playing so well I just couldn't miss. He said, "If you par in from here you're going to have a 69." So I bogeyed the last two holes for a 71, which wasn't a bad score. He took me to the Bing Crosby Pro-Am tournament in California the next year. I sure didn't shoot a 69 or a 71 there!

Dale: What's your golf handicap now?

Cooley: I'm working with a 16 at present. I fell about three years ago playing tennis. I was going for an overhead on my backhand. I put my head up, and I guess my vertebral arteries must have closed off. I went blank and fell backwards on my left hand and got the worst Colles fracture that you can imagine in my left hand. You can see it.

Dale: You do have an abnormality. Did you forget to get it reduced?

Cooley: Well, I had six operations to do the next day, so I told the orthopedic man to just wrap it up, that I had to operate the next morning. And he said, "I'll do that, Denton, but I don't want you to tell anybody that I was your orthopedist." I said, "I'll go one further. I'll tell them another fellow was my orthopedist." He said, "You've got a deal." Three days later I got on a plane, went to Holland, and did three operations there. The whole thing was a real character builder.

Dale: It sounds to me as if you belong in the NFL. How much sleep do you require a night?

Cooley: It's creeping up all the time, it seems. I usually look for five or six hours at night. I sometimes steal a half hour after lunch also.

Dale: In the middle of your surgical schedule?

Cooley: Yes, I do that. I have a good team. I just lie down on the couch. A fifteen-minute nap sort of does something to help my brain.

Dale: What about your relationship with Mike DeBakey now? Both of you are world famous. I've interviewed him, and he's spoken fairly of you.

Cooley: I don't have any personal problems with Dr. DeBakey. I think in a way it was unfortunate that it became a worldwide piece of information that we were having this rivalry or conflict. I have a debt of gratitude to Mike because he gave me a job when I went to Houston, but I think that the best thing I could have done was to resign, to develop my own career and my own institution, go my separate way.

Dale: That's a fair statement. Thanks for this interview. I hope you're not going to shoot 71 when we play golf this afternoon.

Cooley: Probably, I won't.

John Cranley

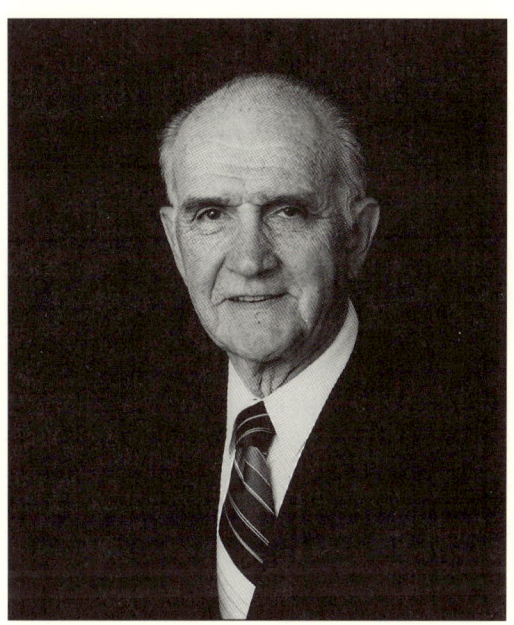

J ACK CRANLEY'S monographs on arterial and venous disease
became the standards for future books on vascular surgery and
have had a major influence on surgical management of vascular disease. He runs a superb vascular fellow training program,
and his contributions to the physiology and diagnosis of venous disease have greatly influenced therapy in this area. The initial evolution
of the Doppler ultrasound technique in combination with real time
ultrasound was another of his significant contributions. A pleasure
to have as a golf companion, he was interviewed December 11, 1986.

Dale: Jack, how did you start? Tell me about your parents and your early education.

Cranley: I was born in Brooklyn on September 23, 1918. My parents were poor immigrant Irish people. Father's mother died when he was quite young, so he was in an orphanage for several years until his father remarried. My father began taking odd jobs at six years of age and was working full time at twelve. He finished the eighth grade, but that was all of his formal education. He eventually worked in a place where they made comptometers. After that he obtained a job with G. Schirmer Music Company in New York. A little later, Mr. Schirmer bought the Boston Music Company and placed my father in charge of it. A year after that, he bought the Willis Music Company in Cincinnati and put my father in charge of that. During most of my youth, my father was commuting between Boston, New York, and Cincinnati. He ended up as owner of the Willis Music Company. He also became the sole trustee of the Schirmer estate. The reason he didn't own the Boston Music Company was that he had to sell it to the highest bidder, as trustee. My father and mother had five children—three boys and two girls. I am the second child, the oldest boy.

Dale: Where did you first attend school?

Cranley: My education included the public schools in Boston, Malden Catholic High School for three years, and Medford High School, from which I graduated in 1936.

Dale: And what were you interested in, besides lessons?

Cranley: I played trumpet in the band. At that time, it was all band music, but now I sometimes fill in with other types of bands when I'm friendly with the band leader.

Dale: What else did you do in high school?

Cranley: I spent a year in bed. I had a back problem that was thought to be an injury, but much later I learned that it was dorsal epiphysitis. I had eight different doctors and four operations. I ended up going to the YMCA for almost a year, exercising and things like that, so I did lose a whole year of school work. It left me a year behind my contemporaries.

Dale: Where did you go to college?

Cranley: Boston College. There I took the liberal arts honors course, which was difficult. I already had finished six years of Latin, four years of French, two years of German, and three years of Greek.

Dale: Did all those language courses help you? What do they mean to you today?

Cranley: I have since thought that the best thing would have been an in-depth course in English to specifically learn the derivation of all words that come from Greek, French, and Latin. That would have been a better course, I think, than all the years of Latin that I studied.

Dale: Would it have been better to study some philosophy and history?

Cranley: I did that, too. I had a very in-depth course in philosophy. It was a Jesuit course; they still give it today. It occurred every day.

Actually, my father gave me the opportunity to work my way through college. He provided me with the funds to lease a gasoline station. So I had Jack Cranley's Texaco station, where I worked nights and had someone else work during the day. When the first draft occurred, just before World War II, I lost my day worker, so I got rid of the gas station. That year I did play in the band and also made the debating team during my last year in college, which was 1941.

Dale: How did you become interested in medicine?

Cranley: From my childhood, I wanted to be a doctor. Perhaps it was because I was treated by so many of them.

Dale: You entered medical school the same year I did, 1941, just prior to World War II.

Cranley: I was in the first year at Columbia Medical School when Pearl Harbor occurred. The government told us all to stay put. No one was supposed to drop out at that time, although I believe one man did. They recruited us all into the army or the navy. I became a midshipman in the navy—the V-12 program. That was done to ensure a continuing supply of young doctors. We graduated in 1944, after a compacted program in three years. I went right on to Boston City Hospital for a straight surgical internship of nine months' duration. Then I went into the service in the navy.

Dale: And what did your service time consist of?

Cranley: My first tour of duty was for three months at the San Diego Naval Hospital. Then I waited about nine months on shore at San Francisco for a ship which was decommissioned as soon as it arrived. So I applied for and was accepted on the animal research team that shipped out to Bikini, where an A-bomb was exploded.

Dale: That was after the war ended?

Cranley: The war had ended. But President Truman delayed the test for several months, so we didn't leave until June 1, 1945. It was a great experience. On our ship were all the medical research teams from Bethesda, as well as the animals, so I got to know a number of these people. Among the most eminent was the head of the medical expedition, Shields Warren, a pathologist from New England Deaconess Hospital. We became good friends and played chess all the way out.

Dale: He was the man who arranged for several people from the University of Rochester to attend the test. Among them was my old chief, John J. Morton, Jr. He was quite interested in the A-bomb test and in Japan.

Cranley: While we were there, our ship was second only to the admiral's ship, so we were able to see the explosion. Perhaps it was fifteen miles away. We could see it plainly.

During the trip out to Bikini I had helped the research team by doing blood counts on some of the animals. So although I was assigned as the ship's medical officer, I had been accepted as a member of the research team, which was composed of ten physicians from Bethesda.

When the firing was imminent, the sailors were ordered to curl up with their heads between their knees, because no one knew exactly what was going to happen. The doctors had quite thick, dark glasses, but the men had none, so they couldn't look.

As soon as the bomb went off, we could hear the stateside radio describing the shock wave. But I didn't feel a thing. I jokingly held

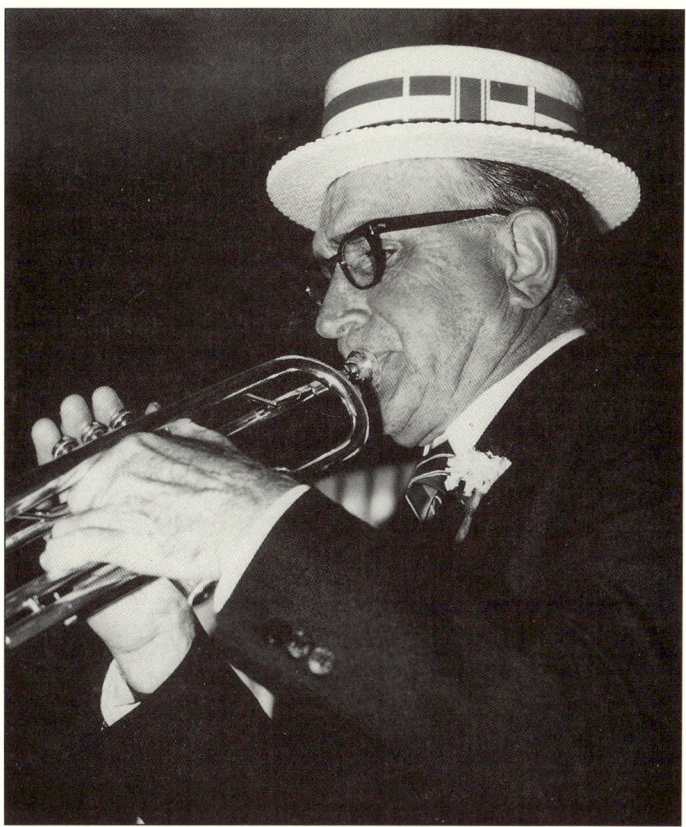

Jack the music man.

up a wet finger, and felt nothing. No one else felt a shock wave either.

The next day, as a part of the medical team, I went on board the ship with a Geiger counter and helped with the measurements of radioactivity.

Dale: What happened after the test shot?

Cranley: The navy put out the word that they would send all reserves home by September, but no one believed it. However, I put my name in. One of the men from Bethesda said, "Jack, if you are relieved, I'll be the ship's medical officer for you so you can go home." But after the last ship departed I was still stuck out there in the mid-Pacific with everyone laughing about my request. One day Dr. Warren came back to the ship and handed me a little slip of paper, with one word on it: "Tare." It was a tare priority, which was the second priority of the navy. The next day a seaplane taxied to our ship, asked for me, and flew me to Kwajalein. That night I was put on another plane to Hawaii, then on to San Francisco. I was home within five days or so.

Dale: What did you do then?

Cranley: I thought I would take a vacation, so I went back to see my former chief and told him I had been discharged and that I was going to take a vacation. He replied, "No, you're not. You're going to work tomorrow." So I again became a surgical resident.

Dale: Who was your chief?

Cranley: He was a man named T. K. Richards, who was in those days a well-known general and orthopedic surgeon who was the team doctor for Harvard for years. He was head of the Fifth Surgical Service of Boston City Hospital. I completed my residency there.

Dale: What happened after you finished your residency?

Cranley: I finished in 1949, after which I began as the second vascular fellow at Massachusetts General Hospital. Dr. Robert Linton had provided by donations the money that he saved during the war. Dr. Simeone was chief of the vascular service and Davitt Felder became the first fellow. I followed him for a two-year period. By then my wife and I had five children. I worked nights during my residency.

During the early part of the war, when I was in medical school, there was such a shortage of physicians that somehow or another I learned to give anesthesia under Virginia Apgar, who became well known later as the author of the Apgar scores for babies. Since I was the only resident who could give general anesthesia, and there was only one anesthesiologist in the hospital, I was called to give anesthesia a great deal. When I moonlighted I would also give anesthesia at one of the local hospitals. I'd send out cards telling them when I would be off from the hospital for after-midnight calls.

Dale: Did Simeone do much clinical work or was he chiefly a laboratory man?

Cranley: Simeone was more or less in line to be the next chief of urology when the war came. He was in for the whole thing—he worked with Mike DeBakey a good deal. During the war he studied shock and blood vessel injuries, and when he came back he set up a vascular laboratory. At the time, Simeone was doing clinical practice and also running that laboratory. A year and a half later, he left for Cleveland and Dr. Linton asked me to take over the vascular laboratory. I stayed three years. It was actually a two-year fellowship, but shortly after I ended my first year I was in charge of the lab and also worked with Dr. Linton clinically, so I stayed an extra year before moving to Cincinnati in 1952. An anesthesiologist, Gillies, came over from Scotland and taught us hypotensive anesthesia. It is rarely used today, but is a perfect technique to use in portal hypertensive cases. A year later he sent his son over for a residency in anesthesia, so we then had his services. I well remember doing portal hypertensive cases without using any blood. At the end there would be only ten or twelve gauze sponges that were blood-soaked.

Dale: What were you using to produce the hypotension? A chemical or spinal anesthesia?

Cranley: High spinal, supplemented with pentothal and nitrous oxide via an endotracheal tube.

Dale: Why isn't that technique used today?

Cranley: Today people are afraid to lower the blood pressure that much. Nowadays low pressure anesthesia means 70 or 80 mm of mercury. Gillies taught that it takes 40 mm of pressure for blood to cross a normal arteriole, but if you paralyze the arteriole, then the blood would flow across at 10 or 15 mm of mercury. So when we operated with Dr. Gillies, or his son, the pressure would be below 40 systolic. Those patients didn't bleed when the pressure was later returned to a normal level; they'd be fine.

Dale: Now tell me about Robert Linton. I knew him and respected him a great deal. Unfortunately, he died before I was able to interview him for this book.

Cranley: He was a wonderful person. He was basically shy, so sometimes he came across as an arrogant person. He was knowledgeable and quite precise—very precise. He was a good teacher and I worked with him for two and a half years.

Dale: Did you scrub with him? Was he a slow operator or just meticulous?

Cranley: Later he had a reputation for being slow, because he would work all day on one case. Actually, I didn't think that he was slow. When I came aboard, he was doing a number of portal hypertension cases. Dr. Linton had his own instruments, his own nurse, his own needles for the skin. He took a tremendous amount of time with an arterial anastomosis. Of course, he didn't have prolene or modern suture then; we used silk. But his anastomoses were things of beauty. I had an opportunity to see a splenorenal some twelve years later at autopsy and still have a picture of that anastomosis. You wouldn't believe how good it was. It looked like the splenic vein just grew there.

Dale: How long would he take to make an anastomosis?

Cranley: I can't recall now. The point is that he made the anastomosis the most important part of the operation. He would split the body cavity open from near the spinal column, through the tenth rib, all the way around across the mid-line. It would take a long while to obtain that exposure, but while he was doing the anastomosis everything was so well exposed that he could comfortably do a perfect anastomosis. That splenorenal operation would take about four hours.

Dale: Did Linton do any general surgery or was it all vascular?

Cranley: At that time, at Massachusetts General Hospital, most of the famous specialists were doing general surgery (but not writing about it). Because Dr. Linton had started out in the thyroid clinic and gynecological clinic, he still had thyroid and gynecological patients to operate on, so he did do general surgery all the time.

Dale: Robert Linton never became a full professor. Why was it that he never advanced in his academic rank?

Cranley: Two reasons come to mind. First is that the Massachusetts General Hospital had a tradition of many famous men who didn't have academic rank. I was first appointed as clinical assistant in surgery, and then was made assistant in surgery and later, as an inducement to stay (presumably a big deal), I was made associate in surgery. They were minor ranks. They didn't give out big academic ranks. The second thing is that there had been competition with Dr. Churchill. A famous surgeon, E. P. Richardson, who was dead long before I arrived on the scene, was the chief. Dr. Linton was his closest associate. It was generally believed that, if Dr. Richardson had lived,

Linton would have followed him as chief. But Dr. Richardson died prematurely. He had a stroke when he was only about forty-five years old. The trustees of the hospital appointed Dr. Churchill as chief.

Dale: What other vascular surgeons were there?

Cranley: At that time, of course, many of our friends were in Boston. Stan Crawford was a resident when I was a fellow. I didn't work with him, but I have always thought that he was not only a skilled surgeon but the funniest human being I ever knew. It got so that as soon as he stood up, people started to laugh, because he would present the case in such a humorous way that nobody could hold themselves in.

Dale: I do agree with you. Stanley uses a lot of colloquialisms, and he not only is a brilliant surgeon but could become a star as a stand-up comedian.

Cranley: Sterling Edwards was an intern when I was there. He had asked Dr. Churchill what he should do about entering the developing field of vascular surgery. Churchill advised him to take a year of physiology, so Sterling went to Cleveland under Wiggins for a year.

Dale: My own time occurred after completion of the residency program—three years with Dr. Hermann Rahn in pulmonary physiology. Bill Scott and John Sawyers, the previous and present chairmen of surgery at Vanderbilt, also support that policy of laboratory experience.

All right; so you left Boston for the west—to Cincinnati. How did you choose Cincinnati?

Cranley: My father had just become head of the music company. I knew that he and my brothers would end up there, and I wanted to be near them. It was just at the time that Dr. Noland Carter was leaving. He had invited me to come there, but then he left. Dr. Bill Altemeier became the chairman at the University of Cincinnati. Dr. Carter introduced me to Dr. Louis Hermann, and I worked with him for two years.

Dale: What sort of man was Louis Hermann?

Cranley: He was the same age as Dr. Linton, but physiologically much older. He had become world famous when he had worked with René Leriche, and then he invented the Pavaex method to aid circulation. He was a magnificent speaker, and at one time he had a whole floor of the hospital for his patients.

Dale: Was that [Pavaex] intermittent air pressure?

Cranley: Yes. I never used it personally, but I did learn that gangrenous legs had been returned to life. I was interested in that, so I tracked it down and learned that it was actually frostbite, so that the skin was black but the tissues were viable. I couldn't find any ischemic patient who was helped. Perhaps some embolism patients were helped, but you don't know whether that was natural or due to the treatment.

Dale: What was your relation to Bill Altemeier?

Cranley: Dr. Altemeier and I became quite close over the years, but he did not want a vascular surgeon. I had been there two years and was running a vascular clinic. Some of the residents had asked me to have vascular rounds, so I asked him about that. One Sunday morning he told me that he didn't want a vascular service. He thought that subspecialization was a problem in most universities. In fact, he gave me the best compliment of my life. He said that as he traveled around it appeared that the worst thing for universities were giants in a specialty. I thanked him for telling me frankly. Shortly afterwards, I left the university and opened my own private office.

Dale: That was certainly a bad call of his. Did it delay the development of vascular surgery at the University of Cincinnati Hospital?

Cranley: For ten or fifteen years I was the only one in Cincinnati doing primarily vascular surgery. I had been on the staff of Good Samaritan Hospital. When I came to Cincinnati in 1952, you could be refused from hospital staffs without any explanation. I applied to several and was turned down from every hospital in Cincinnati and in northern Kentucky except Good Samaritan. It was years before I obtained privileges on staffs.

Dale: So that's been your home base ever since?

Cranley: Yes. I took my first associate, Ray Krause, in 1954, and then Edward Strasser in 1955 and Donald Hafner in 1960, and I continued to grow, with five others in the group.

Dale: Tell me of your association with Tom Fogarty.

Cranley: I had been in practice for a couple of years when I met Tom. Tom was a poor boy who had worked his way through high school and then college, helping to support his mother at the same time. When I first knew him, he had three jobs. He was an operating room nurse at Good Samaritan Hospital, an x-ray technician at St. Francis Hospital, and a night orderly at St. Luke's Hospital across the river. Our chief of surgery at that time, Lloyd Johnson, had told him he would put him through medical school. But the year that Tom was to go to medical school, Lloyd dropped dead in the operating room, and it was too late for Tom to get any help from the school, so he had a tough problem. During his four years of medical school, he worked for us whenever he was free. Otherwise, we advanced him whatever money he needed to pay his tuition and to live. He worked with us all through medical school as a scrub nurse and as a handyman. He did any work which came along. Anything! He even babysat my children. For his internship, under Engelbert Dunphy, he went to Portland. At the end of his first year, he asked Dunphy if he could have a year off to come back with us. He was allowed that, so he returned and worked with us as a fellow, although he had only one year of internship. One day he asked me if I thought a balloon at the end of a ureteral catheter would pull out clots from an artery. I told him it was worth trying, so he made one—the first of the now well-known Fogarty catheters. He also made his own vascular clamps. He stayed with us a year and also did a little study to learn if in some instances bloodletting would help a patient. Some patients of advanced age also have emphysema and hemoglobin of about 20, and bleeding those patients seemed to help them a great deal. I asked Tom if we could demonstrate it in the laboratory by skin temperatures and digital pulses. He found that we could actually increase the pulse pressure in the toe by reducing the hemoglobin from 20 or 21 to 16 or so. After that, for many years, our elderly patients who had emphysema and atherosclerosis came to the office regularly for bleeding. Their emphysema and their toes would improve.

Dale: How did you become associated with the Grass people?

Cranley: Mr. Grass was a graduate of MIT who did part-time work for Walter B. Cannon in Boston. His wife had been one of Cannon's Ph.D. physiology students. Dr. Simeone had also been a student of Cannon while he was in medical school. That's where Simmie and Al Grass became good friends. When I had the fellowship at Massachusetts General, the only instrument available was the Burch-Winsor plethysmograph. It cost $1,400, which was tremendous in those days. Also, it was photographic, so if you made an error in developing the film, everything was lost. It was a single channel recorder. When we asked them to make multiple channels, they told us to buy multiple machines. Simeone asked Al Grass to make us a multiple channel, and the first thing he needed for it was a low-pressure transducer. My job was to help develop and calibrate the low-pressure transducer, which they still have. So that's how I came to know Al Grass.

Dale: What is the history of the phleborrheograph that you developed with Grass?

Cranley: That is a longer story. A man named Nils Kachelmacher was an entrepreneur in a little town in northern Ohio; he died in 1917. He left a handwritten will, the end result of which was that after all of his bequests were completed, and ten years after his sister died, all the residual money would go to research and treatment of varicose veins in South Logan, Ohio. The sister died in 1959, so ten years later, in 1969, they started to look for someone to fulfill that. It went to the courts because South Logan, Ohio, probably doesn't have fifteen or twenty families, but Logan, Ohio, is a larger town of about five thousand. It's in Appalachia and has a nice little hospital. The judge said that if they could get somebody who would take care of varicose veins, they could do it in Logan, Ohio. They started looking around for somebody to do research in varicose veins. They tried at Ohio State in Columbus, then the University of Virginia. Finally they went to the Mayo Clinic, which said they would send a man down every six weeks to hold a clinic, but they wanted a lot of money. It didn't seem to be going forward. One of the Lofgren brothers, Eric or Karl, told them, "We really can't do it; you ought to get hold of Dr. Cranley in Cincinnati." So they called me. The upshot was that we have run the clinic since then, every week.

Dale: How far away is it?

Cranley: Driving, it's 163 miles each way. But I usually fly.

Dale: Do you fly your own plane?

Cranley: Yes, usually with an instructor because the airport is foggy in the morning and I'm not instrument-rated yet. At any rate, we run the clinic over there and they provide the money.

Back in 1949, Dr. Linton had asked me to determine whether or not to buy a Grass recorder for impedance plethysmography; that is, to measure volume by changes in electrical resistance. Al Grass said, "Forget it. Impedance is a bad way to measure anything." He had spent a year of his life learning that. He said that we needed to measure volume or pressure but not impedance.

Twenty years later, I again discussed with Simeone and Grass why we couldn't use impedance. They had the same opinion, although Brownie Wheeler was using it as a crude measure of volume. Al Grass, however, said he would construct a miniature direct volume recorder. Six months later we had it and were making clinical measurements with the phleborrheograph.

Dale: When did you begin to use the duplex scanner to look inside veins?

Cranley: In 1979 Tom Fogarty and Frank Burt of Detroit and I looked at several Doppler scan devices. We also sought advice from Eugene Strandness in Seattle. First we used the duplex scanner to study carotid arteries, and then after two years began to look at veins. We had agreed to do research in the field of venous disease, so I started looking around for something related to phlebitis.

The B-mode scanner immediately became the most important thing in our vascular laboratory. The veins of the entire extremities may be studied noninvasively. You can see a clot in the vein, you can see the blood flow in the vein, you can see that a vein won't compress if it has a clot in it.

Dale: Now let's switch to a more personal query—Helen, and how you met her.

Cranley: We were both invited to a New Year's Eve party. We'd have never met otherwise, because we lived in totally different areas of Boston. But while we were in college, I decided that night that she was the one I wanted to marry. But it took four years to convince her.

Dale: And how many children?

Cranley: Eight, and working on ten grandchildren.

Dale: When did you take up golf?

Cranley: When I was forty-five, kind of late. I was told then that I could never be good, but I didn't believe it. I thought that I could learn it.

Dale: When did you learn to fly?

Cranley: Last year. My youngest daughter had taken it up. She and I were talking about it and I sort of fell in love with one plane and thought I could learn to fly that plane. It is a very high performance plane and actually I'm not allowed to fly it. The insurance companies won't accept it unless you have a great deal of experience. It's a Piper Malibu. So I fly smaller planes that I rent.

Dale: But you fly to the clinic?

Cranley: Yes, that is fun. Since our town is fogged over every week, I made a deal where I fly up blindly with a teacher and my daughter flies back. And then she flies up and I fly back. So we get lessons at the same time.

Dale: Is there anything to the report that the mortality rate is higher among doctor-pilots than any other group?

Cranley: I've heard that also. I will say two things. At this point in my life, it really doesn't matter; secondly, I try to be careful. I don't intend to fly alone. To pass the exam, I flew alone, but I fly with my daughter or with another pilot.

Dale: What do you do if the weather is bad and you are supposed to go to the clinic?

Cranley: Twice we have had to come in under instruments, but we made it.

Dale: What if the weather is bad at the start? Do you go ahead and force it?

Cranley: Actually, the weather is usually only bad for the first three or four hundred feet, and then you get out of the clouds and it's all right. The landing is a problem. It's a small airport, and if we couldn't get in we'd have to go to Columbus, and that would be bad because I'd have to rent a car and it's forty miles away.

Dale: How do you view the future of vascular surgery for a young person?

Cranley: The vascular surgeon now is going to have to concentrate on vascular surgery alone. When I started, Dr. Hermann insisted that I limit my practice to vascular, and I agreed to that. But none of my junior associates have. I've told them all to do what they want, so they've done general as well as vascular. But we're to a point that you're going to have to limit yourself to vascular.

Dale: What of the future of the vascular laboratory?

Cranley: The duplex scanner is revolutionary. It makes all other tests that we ever had for venous disease obsolete, although they are still used because of cost-effectiveness.

Dale: What does a duplex scanner cost?

Cranley: Too much! $100,000 to $150,000. The maintenance contracts on a scanner are $10,000 or $12,000 per year. They are very expensive, but it depends on what you compare them with.

Dale: What do you intend to do with the rest of your life?

Cranley: I am continuing to run the laboratory. I continue to practice a bit, but not nearly as much as before. I run the clinic. I go up to Logan myself now and I enjoy it. It's a free clinic. I see about thirty patients and intend to do that for a few more years.

I have a place in Naples, Florida. I could retire there, except I don't want to yet. We're working on so many things. For example, we need a practical way to measure swelling of the legs. It can be done by water displacement, but the problem is that the usual methods are not very accurate. We have been able to find a technique which permits us to measure the leg repeatedly, with an error of less than .5 percent. All other methods that I have tried, and I have tried them all, are inaccurate.

Stanley Crawford

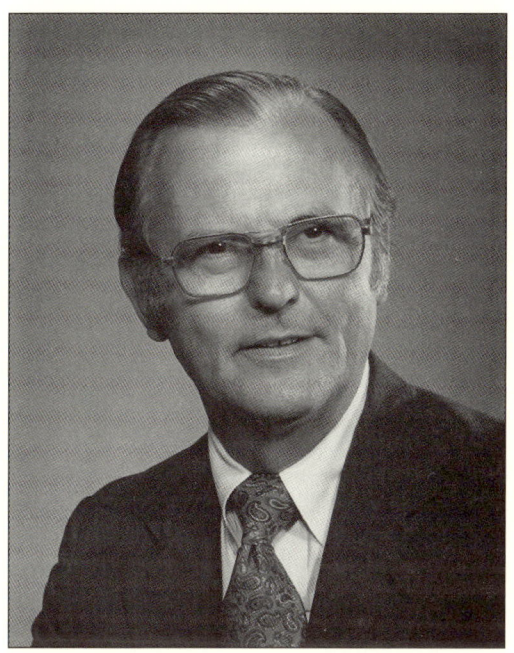

THE EPITOME of a true surgeon, Stanley Crawford skillfully managed a great variety of diseases during his surgical career. He could perform a carotid endarterectomy, a thoracoabdominal aneurysm, a cholecystectomy, and an aortofemoral bypass in rapid succession, all in a day's work—and have a similar schedule the next day—all the while taking the time to speak with a referring doctor. His long-term follow-up of cases was the highlight of many vascular surgery meetings, and his discussions were a southern gentleman's one-upmanship. Crawford died on October 27, 1992.

He was interviewed December 8, 1986.

Dale: Like the song says, did you "come from Alabama?"

Crawford: I was born on May 12, 1922, in Conecuh County, Alabama. Conecuh is an Indian name meaning "cane break." A cane break is a place where sugarcane grows very thick, making it difficult for both humans and animals to get through. The county seat is Evergreen, and my home was on a farm about ten miles from there. It took about a day to go and come from Evergreen to shop for groceries or whatever was needed. My father, John Lloyd Crawford, was a farmer who raised everything we needed to eat: turkeys, chickens, guineas, goats, sheep, and cows, as well as all kinds of foodstuffs. He would only buy things like clothes, salt, coffee, and gasoline. He had very little education but was extremely talented; for example, he was an excellent cabinetmaker who could look at a piece of furniture and make an exact copy. He made extra money that way, and he furnished our home with elegant furniture that he made himself. He was also a gifted musician—not of the classical sort, but of the hillbilly type. He was an expert fiddler and could play the guitar. In fact, he could do everything but sing. He was a happy man even under extreme adversity; he could always see the good in everybody and everything.

Dale: What about your mother?

Crawford: Like my father, my mother, Myrtle, came from a family of twelve siblings. She was next to the oldest and had helped to raise the other children. She herself had only two children. They were good citizens, hardworking and God-fearing, but my mother was different from my father because she saw the bad in everything. She was a crepehanger type, but a wonderful woman.

The Great Depression affected our situation a great deal. My father was very successful in his farming operation—he had a lot of land and a lot of help. But he was always in debt. He kept up with the payments, but during the crash he lost everything except the homestead of about thirty acres. He had Scottish instincts, so he had already paid for that in case something bad happened. After the loss of the farm, things were tough for a number of years.

It was a tradition in that section of the country to recognize the importance of education. Today some people get out of poverty by becoming athletes or entertainers. But the average person in that time in the South realized the value of education. It was the ambition of my mother and father from the start that their children would have every advantage as far as education was concerned. No matter how difficult things might be, they would never interfere with schooling. I was not taken out of school to help cultivate or to harvest the crop. It was mandatory that I go to school.

Dale: Did you go to the local high school?

Crawford: The first seven or eight years I went to a school in a rural community. There was one teacher for about six or seven students in each grade. We were all in the same room and she would teach first one grade, then another.

Dale: Then you went on to high school?

Crawford: I went on to Evergreen High School. I worked in a drugstore during high school. The pharmacist planned to give me an interest in it if I delayed going away to college, but I knew we were going to get into a war and I wanted at least two years of college so that I could qualify for officers' training school, preferably in the air corps.

Dale: Were you a good student in high school?

Crawford: I was a fairly good student. I didn't win any honors, but I was in the upper ten of the fifty-six students who graduated. I was interested in sports, but I was awkward. When I played baseball they usually put me in center field, and the fly balls would come out there, hit my palm, and bounce out. I was not very good in sports.

Dale: Stanley, could you hit the curveball?

Crawford: No, I couldn't hit the curveball. But I still like baseball. I like all sports. My favorites among the traditional sports are ice hockey and basketball.

Dale: But you didn't see ice hockey in Alabama, did you?

Crawford: No, we didn't have it there. That came from the time I spent in Boston. In the modern era, there is a team in Houston.

Dale: Where did you attend college?

Crawford: I went to the University of Alabama at Tuscaloosa. At that time, the first two years of medical school were taught there.

Dale: What were you doing on Pearl Harbor Day—December 7, 1941?

Crawford: My roommate and I were studying on that Sunday. He liked to carry a radio around and always had the thing playing. We had a big desk and he'd put the damn radio in between us and keep it on. I got so that I could study and concentrate with that thing blaring away. On December 7, 1941, news of Pearl Harbor came to us on the radio. Of course, all studies ceased and everyone gathered around the radio to hear more.

The disc jockey gave the names and addresses of various recruiting stations. The students were very patriotic. We all wanted to get into the war; it was like an athletic contest at that period of time. All the students who lived in our dormitory decided exactly what they were going to do. I wanted to be a flyer.

The day after Pearl Harbor, I went with a group of friends to the air corps recruiting station. I only weighed 129 pounds, so they told me that if I weighed ten pounds more I could qualify to go into the army air corps. I was given ten days to fatten up. That meant I would have to gain a pound a day. The recruiting officer suggested that I eat bananas and drink cream, but I couldn't gain the ten pounds, so I didn't get in.

I had finished two years of ROTC and had won the prize for being the best soldier, so I thought that it was going to be a simple matter to go over to see the colonel who was the head of ROTC and get lined up for advanced ROTC. He had me examined and everything was fine, but they wanted ten more pounds. I couldn't gain the weight, so I thought that was that: I'd be drafted and would have to be a foot soldier or plain sailor, which wasn't the worst thing in the world; at least I'd do my part in beating Hitler and Hirohito.

However, about four weeks later the navy sent a recruiting outfit to the university looking for officer-type candidates, and I went for that idea. Much to my surprise, they thought I was a good physical

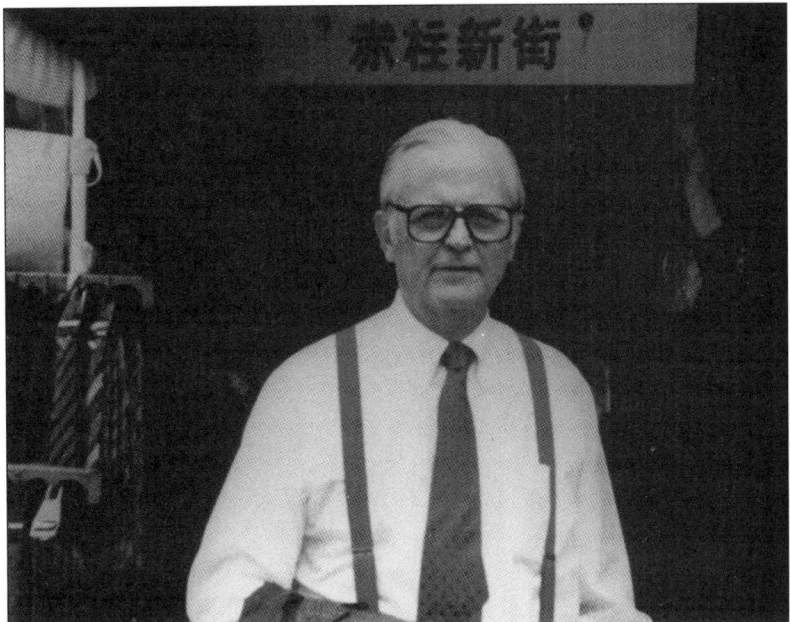

Stanley in Kyoto.

specimen and I was accepted. They gave me an ensign's commission as a hospital administrator; this was the first knowledge I had that there was such a beast.

My peers will remember that mobilization took place so rapidly that it was impossible to receive all those who were given commissions because there was no place to put them. New soldiers who were drafted didn't have guns to drill with; they used pieces of pipe or wood to learn the manual of arms. So I stayed in school; there was nothing else to do.

I went one semester with this commission on an inactive status. In July 1942, the Department of Defense decided that they were going to need doctors, so they subsidized medical students for obligatory service later on, and the V-12 and the Army Specialized Training programs were organized. I became a member of V-12, my commission was changed, and I became an apprentice seaman. The navy paid my tuition, bought my books, and paid me thirty dollars a month. I then transferred to Harvard Medical School and graduated from there.

Dale: How many transfers did Harvard take at that time?

Crawford: It was something like thirteen. I was 1 of 136 who graduated from Harvard Medical School in March 1946.

Dale: Later you went in the navy on active duty as a physician. What year was that?

Crawford: I had finished medical school and had had eighteen months of training in surgery. On July 1, 1947, I started active duty at a navy hospital in Portsmouth, New Hampshire. I stayed there for two years of active duty.

Dale: That interrupted your surgical training, but afterwards you went back to the Massachusetts General Hospital and completed it. Who was the chief of surgery there?

Crawford: When I started at the Massachusetts General Hospital, there were two surgical services, East and West. Dr. Arthur Allen was chief of the East Surgical Service and Dr. Edward Churchill was chief of the West. I was on the East.

Dale: What kind of man was Dr. Arthur Allen?

Crawford: Dr. Allen was a wonderful man. He was from Kentucky and had many of the traits that were consistent with my concept of a Kentuckian. He liked racehorses and was a very gallant sort of man. He was also a good teacher.

Dale: He was one of the early vascular surgeons, wasn't he?

Crawford: Dr. Allen was a general surgeon, but he did no surgery in the chest; actually, nobody did much then. He was interested in vascular surgery, particularly the thrombophlebitis problem. He was the first president of the Society for Vascular Surgery.

Somehow, Dr. Allen was impressed with my performance in medical school. Perhaps he was more familiar with the potential of the southerners than others at MGH. We talked slowly, in general were more conservative, and were not always as noticeable as our northern colleagues. Dr. Allen gave me a chance and, fortunately, things worked out very well for me.

Dale: Was he still there when you came back from the navy?

Crawford: Yes, but he was quite ill and he had retired. Dr. Churchill became chief of all the services, and thus for the major part of my training Dr. Churchill was the chief.

Dale: How was he?

Crawford: Dr. Churchill was the opposite of Dr. Allen. He was a reserved person, rather private, and much more difficult to relate to, but he was quite a scholarly person. His method of teaching was different from Dr. Allen's, and I think Dr. Churchill's method was better. Dr. Churchill used the Socratic method. Dr. Allen had taken the stance that the senior surgeons at MGH, particularly himself, knew how to treat things. Of course, he admitted there were some things that could not be treated by surgery, but he believed the surgeons should be the ones to determine that. Those things that were currently being treated surgically could best be treated by the senior surgeons at MGH; the objective in our training was to learn how to emulate them. Thus, the richness of the training experience was that we could come into contact with many clinicians of that caliber, combine the better qualities of each, and end up as a superior individual. Dr. Churchill agreed but also thought we should question everything. He thought we shouldn't blindly try to copy someone else. Every operation should be considered a laboratory exercise, and we could see what happened after each.

Dr. Churchill was famous because of his contribution to the fields of parathyroid surgery and surgery of the heart, particularly constrictive pericarditis and pulmonary resection. He was the senior consultant in the Mediterranean theater during World War II, with the rank of colonel. He maintained contact with many of his European friends. I didn't know Dr. Churchill until he came back from the war. He was there when I came back from my service, and I found him to be a fine man. He was loyal to the idea of teaching. He was good to those who performed well, and I was certainly grateful that he gave me the opportunity to be a chief resident. I'm also grateful that he offered me a position to stay at MGH.

Dale: Why didn't you stay?

Crawford: There were a number of reasons I didn't. First, I was a little impatient. By that time I was a trained surgeon and, like a lot of young people at that age, I felt that I should get about the business of doing surgery. I noticed that the junior people on the staff of MGH were getting to do very little surgery. The lines of referral were well developed. There were senior people, not-so-senior, medium-senior, and junior. Starting at the bottom of that hierarchy meant that it would be a long time before I would make the grade, either by discovering some important thing from research or developing a referral practice. Usually those two things went hand in hand.

Being from the southern part of the country, I thought the renaissance of the South was just getting started. There were not a large number of well-trained people in the South, but the cities were growing in size, and money was becoming available to build hospitals. Everybody was trying to improve the situation and make some contribution. I saw that I could shorten that period of self-sacrifice.

Second, and probably much more important, was the fact that at the beginning of my senior residency I developed an acute illness that lasted about three weeks. I had persistent casts and blood cells in my urine and was pronounced as having chronic Bright's disease, with a life expectancy from three years to an outside chance of ten years. I was married and had two children and was in debt, so I felt that it wasn't fair to get into a situation where I would not be able to leave anything for my wife and two children.

Dale: How did you and Dr. Mike DeBakey get together?

Crawford: As I said, Dr. Churchill suggested that I might stay at Massachusetts General. I thanked him for his generous offer but told him candidly that I wanted to return to the South. In applying to Harvard Medical School, I had stated that I wanted to go there because I wanted to obtain the best possible education and then come back to the South. I thought that region was about to bloom. Whatever contribution I had to make, I wanted amongst my southern people. My inclination was still the same. Even though I loved the New Englanders, I still had a hankering to go back where I came from. But I told him I certainly would appreciate his counsel, particularly in regard to people worth associating with, and he immediately suggested Dr. DeBakey, who had recently started in Houston. Both Churchill and DeBakey had been consultants to the Surgeon General during the war and were good friends.

I went to Houston seeking an opportunity, which did become available and turned out to be a good choice. I went there without telling anybody about my infirmity, because, as you know, a sick doctor is not much in demand. I was in Houston about a year and a half with protein and all kinds of casts in my urine, but my blood pressure was still normal and I felt alright.

That fall, I had an exhibit at the American College of Surgeons in Chicago. It was cold there, and I got sick and had to come home. I was not certain exactly what was wrong. I checked my urine and it had 4-plus protein and all kinds of damn things in the sediment, so I decided I just had to give up and turn myself in, so to speak. By that time I had made friends with a nephrologist in Houston, who became my doctor. He examined everything, did detailed renal function studies, and found that my renal function was normal despite the fact that my urine looked terrible. He thought that was unusual for a chronic glomerulonephritis. So he had urine cultures done every day for a month and found that the organism cultured was present in every urine.

I obtained my record from MGH and saw that the one culture that they had done on my urine had the same bug in it. The infectious disease expert in Houston, who was also a friend of mine, told me that there was a new drug, specific to this organism, called ilosone, which was the precursor to erythromycin. He gave me a gallon container of what was an experimental drug. I took it four times a day until I had taken the entire gallon. Within two weeks my urine was perfectly negative. I started taking it in October and continued until the latter part of April, at which time I became jaundiced with nausea and loss of appetite. They decided that I had an unusual form of hepatitis. I was advised to do the usual things for hepatitis, but on my own I stopped the medicine because every time I tried to take it I'd have to puke. Promptly, my jaundice disappeared. Later on, it became common knowledge that the drug could produce a form of hepatitis. I've been well ever since.

Dale: Who were the members of Dr. DeBakey's team at the time?

Crawford: Oscar Creech went with him to Houston from New Orleans; John Howard, B. W. Haynes, and Denton Cooley also joined his staff. By the time I arrived, these men had done many things. By guess and by gosh, with strength of character and productivity, they had developed a good surgical service. I didn't do it, because they had already won most of the battles.

Oscar Creech returned to New Orleans to be chief at Tulane. He later died of a tumor. B. W. Haynes returned to Virginia. He was interested in burns, surgical metabolism, and electrolytes. John Howard moved about—to Emory in Atlanta, and to Philadelphia and Toledo. He did a good job of surgical research in the Korean War. Denton Cooley founded the Texas Heart Institute in Houston, where he is today.

Dale: And you stayed on with Mike DeBakey, becoming a friend and close associate. How did Denton Cooley happen to leave?

Crawford: The entire story is not clear to me. Denton's operation activities and the location of his activities did not change; the only thing that changed was that he became disassociated with Baylor and later became associated with the University of Texas. He just left one medical school appointment and took up an appointment with another. I really don't know all the ins and outs of why he did this. He's extremely competent. He also had a lot of vision and foresight. He was in some sense an entrepreneur; I mean to use that term politely. He's a man of vision, imaginative. At Baylor the administration didn't have that kind of vision. They didn't know what they had, and they couldn't think in those terms, so opportunities could not be provided to a man like Cooley. This always was a constraint placed upon him. And, of course, he was second to Dr. DeBakey. There were not enough beds for everybody. In the operating rooms it was the same, and due to conservatism on the part of the administration, nothing was being done about it. About the only way Cooley could survive within the realm of his anticipated needs was to become independent.

Dale: It is sometimes said currently that the surgeons of your and my generation were often entrepreneurs, but that the surgeons of the next generation will not be. Do you think things are changing to that extent?

Crawford: There are certain things taking place that will be a burden to a young surgeon's development that did not exist in my time. On the other hand, the opportunities will be even greater; I think it's sad to hear young surgeons bemoan their lot. To be sure, many things have been discovered that won't have to be found again, but, on the other hand, there are great opportunities to improve on what has been done. With all the new technology, we can do things much better than we could, and that is opening new opportunities.

Dale: It is being said by some that too many operations are being done, such as in the field of carotid surgery.

Crawford: The great problem for the surgeon in the future will be the rules and regulations that are being imposed either directly or indirectly on the surgeon. When I came along, what a surgeon did was based solely on a decision between the surgeon and the patient. His peers by and large respected it, provided that the surgeon was competent, and that he made knowledge of what he was going to do available before he did it and the results available after he did it. Today there are many things that stymie the boldness of the surgeon. There are too many ineffective committees, there are doctors willing to testify against doctors at the drop of a hat just for the money or because of jealousy, and so on.

Andrew Dale

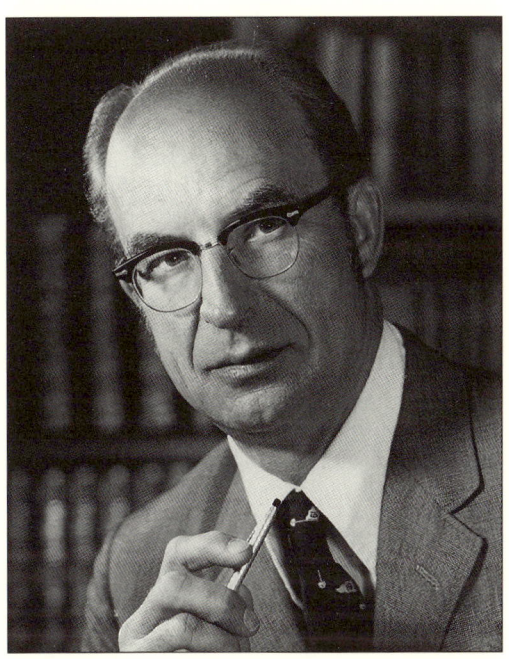

ANDREW DALE was a complete person, not just a vascular surgeon or a physician. He had the highest of principles, a strong ethical and moral code, and high standards of excellence in all that he undertook—traits apparent whether he was in the hospital, at home, on the golf course, or in the Swiss Alps. He was a superb physician devoted to his patients and sensitive to their needs, a superb diagnostician, and a skilled technician. And he was a scholar—an academician who searched for the truth, a historian, and a prodigious reader of the world's great works. Dale's honesty was legendary: He would "call a spade a spade," even if it was in reference to present company. His early passing on September 22, 1990, of acute myelogenous leukemia, is not a loss just to the surgical world, but to those who strive to leave this world a better place than they found it.

He was interviewed September 8, 1990.

Johnson: Andy, tell me about your heritage.

Dale: I had exceptionally good role models as parents; both were strong Presbyterians with a sense of the importance of the individual as well as the place of God in our lives. My father had a flour mill and was a businessman in Columbia, Tennessee, where I was born on March 13, 1920. Columbia was a nice little town. It had eight thousand people then, and still does.

My mother was a prolific reader, and she also taught me a love of reading. She was a person who believed that everyone ought to fulfill whatever potential he had, and she figured that I had more potential than I thought I did. My mother set almost impossibly high goals in the sense that a B on a report card would restrict me to the house on Saturday mornings so that I couldn't play football or baseball with my friends.

My father died when I was twelve, so I don't really know whether he read a lot or not. He was not college educated; he just had a high school education, but he made it on his own.

Johnson: How about your siblings?

Dale: Well, my brother Will is a lawyer. I had one sister who died as a baby.

My life as a child was easy, because my father, while not wealthy, was well off. I attended five schools, and from each of them I obtained different things. During my elementary schooling, I got a good background in the three Rs and learned to love reading. I started at Columbia Military Academy in the seventh grade, so I would have been thirteen. My military experience began with CMA, where I first learned to walk in the rear rank, which may be one of the most important lessons of my life: Walk in the rear rank until you deserve to be in the front rank. I can promise you that at every step I took in that rear rank I was promising myself that I'd be in the front rank someday, because I didn't like it back there. I was in the junior school two years.

For the last two years of high school, I attended Darlington Preparatory School in Rome, Georgia. It was there that I made my first entrance into the real world and received the inspiration to try to do better. The discipline there was not emotional, as it had been at home, but was dealt out on a fair basis. For example, after my roommate and I set the alarm bell to go off in the middle of the night, the headmaster called all the students in the following day to come by his desk and state, while looking him in the eye, "I did not ring the bell." Then the student was allowed to go into town. At the end of this, there were the two of us left seated. The headmaster said to us, "I gather that you have decided that you'd rather write three thousand words in the dictionary than go to town." We got the message.

I went to Davidson College, which to me somehow resembles an English boys' undergraduate school. There were approximately 750 students without any female influence, either as pupils or teachers, but we learned the rough camaraderie that occurs among young males. While the college lacked many physical facilities, it had a wonderful spirit and stressed high ideals and character as being considerably more important than any amount of scholarship.

After I graduated from Davidson, I was accepted at Hopkins, Pennsylvania, and Vanderbilt medical schools. It turned out that it was economically wiser for me to go to Vanderbilt, because my mother would be maintaining an apartment in Nashville to house my brother and there would be an extra room for me. Furthermore, I think my mother didn't want me to head off into the unknown regions of the country alone. Being a simple country boy, I went on to Vanderbilt.

When I arrived there, I was in for a shock, because I very quickly learned that the teachers there seemed to dislike the students and put them down at every occasion. For example, in my freshman year, one particular teacher apparently told everybody in the class that he or she was failing, in an effort to stimulate activity. Well, I couldn't be stimulated further, because I was going all out already, so I just figured that I would be one of those that flunked. Later on I found out what the true story was. In Rochester there were teachers and professors who looked kindly upon the students as friends, not as inferiors, and tried to help them accumulate knowledge. That was a big difference.

In medical school our class started in September 1941; the Japanese attacked in December and the war came along. Everybody had a draft number, and that was very unsatisfactory because they were always pulling the medical students out to draft them and send them here, there, or yonder. Then the authorities would have to grab them and bring them back, because higher up they knew we would need doctors later, but lower down they didn't. So maybe a year later they made us second lieutenants, Medical Administrative Corps, inactive duty. So we rocked along that way for a while. Then they decided they wanted more control over us, so they had us resign that commission and inducted us into the active army at Fort Oglethorpe, where we became privates. For some reason, the next day they made us privates first class. So we went back to medical school as privates first class with our little slash on the uniform and all that, and finished medical school that way. As soon as we finished medical school, we were given an honorable discharge from the army and made first lieutenants on inactive duty. I stayed on that through my internship, which was nine months. The arrangement was that a third of the intern class would be kept for a second nine months, and I was one of the third that was kept. I stayed eighteen months, and at the end of that time I was ordered to Maxwell Field as a first lieutenant in the air force.

I got to Maxwell Field, and it happened that I stayed there the whole time and never left. We never had any basic training or any paperwork. The day we got there, two young surgeons got out, because by that time the bomb had been dropped, and we took their places. I was so scared that I'd be moved from Maxwell Field, which was a good surgical job, that I laid low and didn't even take any leave. When active duty was finished, I ran into the field commander at a Christmas party. He noticed I had a Davidson ring with Phi

Delta Theta letters. He asked, "Are you a Phi Delta Theta?" "Yessir." He said, "At Davidson?" "Yessir." "Well, I went to Davidson." I said I thought he had probably gone to West Point, and he said he had gone to Davidson for two years and then to the Point. So I said, "Well, I'm sure glad to meet you," and he said, "You going to make a career of the service?" "No sir," I answered. "What are you going to do?" I answered that I hadn't finished my training and I very much needed to get back to civilian life and my residency. He said, "Well, when would you like to go?" and I said, "Well, I don't mean to be flip, sir, but I'd like to go tomorrow." He said "Tomorrow is Sunday, so that won't work, but you come by my office Monday and I'll see what I can do." So I rushed home and told Corinne about it. I went over there Monday morning and the sergeant said (I had become a captain by then), "I guess you're the captain we're looking for." They processed me out, and I think we left on Wednesday.

So that was my military career. Some funny things happened during that time. Once I was on a flight without a copilot. The pilot and I were sitting in a twin engine plane and got into a hell of a fog, couldn't see, and the pilot kept calling the ground saying, "I want to land . . . I can't see and don't know where I am." They kept saying, "No, you go on, you're going to be fine." That made me a little itchy. Anyway, we got on over toward Augusta, where we were headed, and he dropped the plane down through the clouds and he told me, "You watch over that right motor; look for the airstrip. We've got to find that thing." I knew that, so I was looking as hard as I could. We dropped on down and pretty soon we saw an airstrip through those wisps of cloud, so he put it down, and when we got closer, we saw big potholes in the runway. We taxied on up to operations and it said "Operations Closed." It was an abandoned airfield, and we were in the wrong place. The pilot said, "Well, I tell you what we're going to do," and he wheeled that plane around and took right off on the same runway, flew up over the city, and radioed, "We're lost up here in the clouds, help us get down." So we got over there and he swore us and the people in the back to secrecy and landed.

One time I took to Augusta a guy who had a knee that was locked—it wasn't just busted, it was locked. We had given him anesthesia and tried to shake it loose, but we couldn't. So the colonel wrote orders for him and for me to accompany him over there for orthopedic consultation. They said, "Well, after lunch the board meets, and that would be a good place." We ate lunch with him on his crutches. When we got into the clinic, a young doctor was there, younger than I was, even. He said, "I think what you need to do is take him back and give him some physical therapy." And I said, "Well, hell . . ." So we forced him into the hospital.

Another funny story in the same place concerned my classmate Lindsey Nelson Bishop, who was in the public health service and therefore entitled to air force care. He had a car accident on the outskirts of Montgomery, and they brought him to our hospital. I put him in a cast and called the orthopedic man at Nashville, Pop Regent, to ask him what to do. Pop was guiding my hand on every move and finally said, "Well, he's been in that cast long enough. You'd better get him a Taylor back brace." I found that we didn't have any, so the only thing we could do was to go back over to Augusta. When we got there, they sent us in to the orthopedic board. There was a fellow called Lt. Col. Dehne on the board; I saluted him, told him who I was, and said I had Captain Bishop with me. I said, "As you can see, he's in a cast, and here are the x-rays. We came over to get a Taylor back brace." When I said that, he hit the table with his fist and said, "Goddamn it, don't tell me how to treat patients." And I said, "Sir, I wasn't trying to tell you. I am just following my instructions, which were to bring Captain Bishop over here and obtain a Taylor back brace." It turned out that Colonel Dehne was a big physical therapy man. He banged his fist a few more times and said, "If you want this man treated, admit him to the hospital and I'll treat him." Finally he said to me, "What is your name, rank, and serial number?" I gave it to him, but that set my mind working and I said, "Colonel, I'd like to have your name, rank, and serial number also, please sir." I got out my little notebook, and he said, "Where'd you come from?" "Maxwell Field," I responded. He said, "Who's your commanding officer?" I said, "Colonel Dan Ogle." He said, "What kind of colonel is he?" I said, "Sir, he's a bird colonel." He thought about that for about five seconds, banged his fist down, and said, "Goddamn it, whatever the guy's name was, take this man and get him a Taylor back brace. I don't ever want to see him again." When I

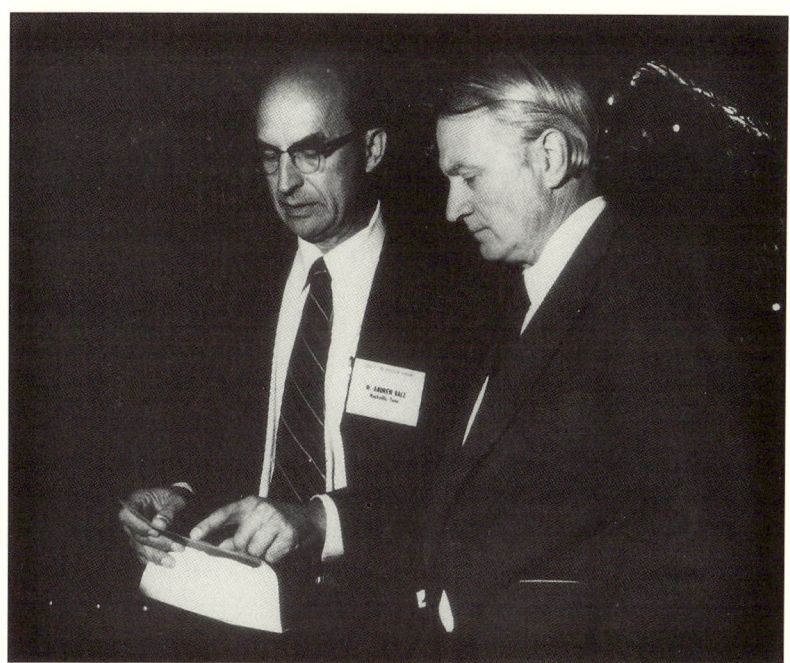

Andy with Jim DeWeese in Rochester, New York, June 1977.

told Colonel Ogle about this, he thought it was a scream. He said, "You outranked him with me, did you?" and I said, "Yes, sir, I did."

The war influenced my life first in a surgical sense, because I had a good position that made it possible for me to do a lot of operations while I was still young and certainly incompletely trained. Second, it introduced me to people from all over the United States whom I would not otherwise have met. Third, it allowed me time to think about the broader issues of life. Finally, it showed me that since I had done so much ordinary cut-and-dried everyday surgery, I wanted something better. This meant that I needed full university training and probably more than that, because I wished to become one of the better surgeons in the United States, not just an average one.

Johnson: After you finished Vanderbilt, why did you go on to Rochester? Why didn't you stay at Vanderbilt?

Dale: When I was at Vanderbilt, it became obvious to me that I didn't want to stay on the surgery service because the chief, Barney

Brooks, was a real despot, and I didn't ever want to work with a person like him. Second, I thought all my education had been in the South, and I badly needed to go to another part of the country. So when I talked to my intern advisor, I simply omitted the first reason, and told him I thought it would be good for me to go to another part of the country and learn about something else, with which he agreed.

Johnson: Had you decided to be a surgeon then?

Dale: I decided to be a surgeon at that time, and I'm not sure why. I guess one reason was that it was held up to me as being top of the line, or king of the hill, and I was stubborn enough to want to put myself there. So I suppose my stubbornness got me into that position. However, I have never had the slightest desire to be anything but a surgeon. If I were not a surgeon, I would simply get out of medicine and do something else. I have always thought since then how fortunate I am to be in a position where somebody pays me to do what I would do for free.

After I finished my residency at Rochester in 1950, I still had the strong urge to participate in academic medicine, because that had been pushed at me as the best. I looked around among the southern medical schools and there didn't seem to be much opportunity there. I would like to have gone to the University of North Carolina at Chapel Hill, but their medical school was still being set up and was not ready to go, so there wasn't any position there. I didn't find an outstanding position except at Birmingham, where Champ Lyons was chairman of the Department of Surgery, in a school which obviously was coming along because it had been funded properly. The mistake I made was not investigating Champ Lyons. We moved down there at the end of December 1951, and within a few days it was obvious that he and I were not going to get along. It would be easy to run him down, but I suppose the truth of the matter is that he had considerably different ideals or philosophies of life than did I, and many of them were simply unacceptable. There were a host of minor irritations; for example, I was told not to instruct the third-year students that there were several theories about the cause of pancreatitis, but to give them one line—that the cause was gallstone with regurgitation; it was said that the students were not old enough or knowledgeable enough to understand that there may be multiple causes. As a result of those experiences and several others, I submitted my resignation after I had been there about a month. I agreed to stay on in the job as assistant professor until Sterling Edwards arrived from Boston, where he was completing his training. During that time I was looking, as John Kennedy says, into the "dark and final abyss," because I assumed that Champ would go after me tooth and nail after that (and he did). So, without other prospects I returned to Rochester at the behest of my many friends there and worked there for eight years before I moved to Nashville.

Johnson: Were you a general surgeon at Rochester? Was Jim DeWeese on the attending staff?

Dale: Jim was about four or five years behind me, but he and I were always friends. I had been working up in the physiology lab with Hermann Rahn on atelectasis and one day I got to thinking about the problem of putting in a crossover graft for misplaced great vessels. So I did one of those on a dead animal, and that sort of interested me in vascular and I saw that you would need a graft to do this. By that time I'd been working in the lab for three years, I was assistant professor of physiology, and I was assistant professor of anatomy because I was teaching surgical anatomy, so I had three appointments. Merle Scott was chairman of surgery, and he called me down one day and said, "I would like for you to come back down to surgery on the second floor (physiology was on the fourth floor) and take over the surgery lab and try to get it going, because it's never amounted to anything." I talked to him about it and asked what kind of money was in it, and it turned out there wasn't any money, there wasn't anything except a space, but one way or another he persuaded me to come down. Our first money came from everybody there donating 10 percent of their gross to the department. At any rate, I came back down and was director of the surgical experimental laboratory. I held that position until the time I left.

Jim came along, and he was interested in working in the dog lab, primarily on heart and lung, but also some grafts. We had picked up a fellow from Scotland named George Mavor, who was doing some grafts also, so there were three of us trying to do grafts. I was using the saphenous vein, and those fellows were using homologous artery and probably an early version of a synthetic tube. With three of us operating, it didn't take us very long to accumulate some material, and it looked more and more to me as though the saphenous vein was the better of the three. Interestingly enough, the first seven saphenous veins that I did all failed. Fortunately, we did an eighth one, which stayed open. It looked at that time as if the saphenous vein was such a fragile and difficult thing to deal with that maybe it wasn't going to prove to be useful. That's what I thought the first time I did a renal artery repair. But of course, as you go along you learn how to do it. After a year or so of working along that way, my secretary told me that her grandfather had a bad toe that looked terrible and that he would like to come over and be the first clinical patient to have a vein graft. I explained to her what she already knew, which was that we had never done one of these before, but she said her grandfather understood it. He came over and proved to be a delightful gentleman. I put my first vein graft into him. He lived for another fifteen or so years, and after I left Rochester Jim used to do arteriograms on him about every five years. The graft stayed open.

At any rate, that encouraged us, so I put an abstract of a paper in to the vascular meeting. The authors included Jim DeWeese and Merle Scott. We had something over a hundred experiments, and I think we had seven patients at that time. After I gave the presentation in San Francisco, Denton Cooley got up and remarked that in Houston "we operate on patients, not dogs." I don't remember how it's recorded, but my response to that was that the dogs were apt to give you a truer answer because you could do more of them under more controlled conditions. At any rate, it wasn't any big problem and was sort of funny. About 1957 we got a new dean, and the new dean wanted us to have a full-time financial program or compensation program. After the details of his plan came out, I told him and our department chairman that I just couldn't go along with that. I thought it was "un-American," denying my freedom of getting ahead. I told the dean that if he was dissatisfied with my teaching, all right, I'm out; with my research, I'm out; with my personality, I'm out—but don't limit the number of patients that I can operate on, because I intend to build this vascular surgery section. We hassled around for a few days, and Merle Scott suggested that I stay on for the time being with an agreement to leave on short notice whenever I wanted. I said that would be fine and stayed from that February to the next November. In November the dean sent me his little piece of paper requesting a report on income received to date. I went to see Merle Scott and said, "Dr. Scott, this is what I object to and I'm not going to be able to fill this out, which means that I am going to have to leave." He was very nice and suggested I stay as an associate professor with greater leeway on money. I said that would be really selling out to do it that way. He asked me to reconsider, but by that time I'd been considering it about three years. I said "No, sir." He called me back in a couple of days and said the dean was furious and had told him to fire me at once and get me out of the hospital. Merle Scott told the dean that if he had to fire me, then he went, too. I said, "Well, I appreciate your loyalty, but we have to be practical. How long would you allow me to stay until I can find a place?" He said he would tell the dean that I could stay as long as I wanted, within reason, so I said okay. That was in the winter of 1956.

I started looking around, and in April I came down to Nashville and when the plane banked on that final approach into those green hills, I said, "I gotta go back."

Johnson: Homesick, weren't you? How far is Columbia from Nashville?

Dale: Forty miles. So we landed and I went over to see Bill Scott and we started talking after lunch, maybe about one or two o'clock in the afternoon and talked until about five o'clock. The first thing he said was, "Come on, I welcome you." Then he asked what I wanted to do. I said I wanted to develop vascular surgery, and I showed him a notebook that I had been keeping on patients, with the preop arteriogram, and the postops, and some evidence that something had been done. I showed him the other paper I had presented and he said, "Well, that's fine. I will do anything for you I can." So I said I would like to work in the lab. Of course, you know he loved that, because he didn't have anybody working in the lab. I said I would bring three grants with me, and he loved that too. So we got started off on a good footing. Bill was always the most sup-

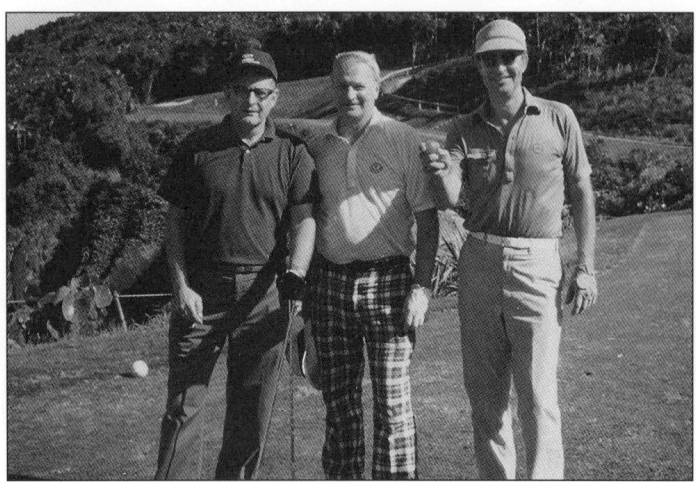

George, Jim, and Andy, at Mahogany Run, St. Thomas, Virgin Islands, 1984.

portive guy imaginable. He did more things to help me. He was a great friend.

Johnson: Were you at Vanderbilt when you first came down?

Dale: No, I had an office out in town. The guys at the medical center asked me to have an office over there by Vanderbilt and I said, no, that will tie me too closely to Vanderbilt. I said I wanted to have a private practice and didn't want to be known just as a Vanderbilt doctor or Baptist doctor. So I rented some upstairs space in the building and started out there. I turned down the Vanderbilt office. But I went over there every Wednesday morning to work in the out-patient department and I put my name on it.

Johnson: And your lab was at Vanderbilt?

Dale: Yes. We kept the lab going for I guess about ten years, until my volume of practice became so heavy that I was putting a half-day in the lab every week, usually Tuesday morning. I was fortunate to develop enough practice so that I finally didn't have any time to put in and we closed down the lab work after about ten years. Meanwhile, Malcolm Lewis had come along and started renting space from me, then we started sharing expenses. I got him interested in the lab program, so he would do some of the dogs too. That's kind of the story.

Johnson: How did you get to St. Thomas'?

Dale: Well, I got trapped there, in a sense, because in the early 1970s I realized that vascular surgery was going to be something more than just an occasional case and I thought that there was a need to have a more organized service, a vascular service. And I got the Tennessee State Medical Association to fund a fellowship at St. Thomas' for two years, which they did with the understanding that at the end of the two years, if the hospital wouldn't pick it up, goodbye. But it did. Bill Edwards had come back by then, and, of course, he immediately developed a large volume practice because it had been left to him by his father. I knew I would never develop a volume like that for a lot of reasons, one being that I didn't want to work in the emergency room all night like he was doing. We had a fight with the cardiac guys about their doing vascular operations. We won, so it was just Bill and me. Joe Mulherin came along as a fellow in 1975 and joined Bill at the end of his fellowship. It ended up that the fellow would scrub with me on even days of the month and with Bill on odd days of the month, regardless of what it was, and there was no saying "I've got a good case and I wish you'd scrub with me." Then we had a problem with Joe because it wasn't fair that he didn't have anybody to scrub with him. At first, he operated after Bill finished, but when he started operating earlier it made him a real problem. Somehow we scrambled it out.

Johnson: In conclusion, when did you meet Corinne?

Dale: I first met Corinne when she was at Sweet Briar, just a very casual meeting, and then I didn't see her again until I was in medical school, about my fourth year. Corinne had finished school, and she came over to work at the hospital on pediatrics, so I ran into her again. One of my best friends, Fred Gray, started having dates with her, and we would double-date because he didn't have a car and I did. I really got to know her on those double dates. It seems strange, but when Fred finished and left to go to Barnes Hospital, I told him, "Fred, if you leave here, and leave that girl, I'm going to marry her and you'll never see her again." He said, "What do you mean?" And I said that she was the best girl I'd ever seen. I picked her out before I ever had a real, formal date with her, so that as soon as he left I was hot on the trail. She laughs because she was bridesmaid in a wedding in a small town in West Tennessee and she says that I wasn't even invited but I showed up there on a Friday afternoon, and the father of the bride didn't know what to do with me. They didn't know who I was or anything. Of course, I told him my name, so they took me into their home, the guest bedroom, and Corinne was amazed that I stayed with the bride's family. The next day the bride's family took Corinne and me to lunch and then put us on the train back to Nashville. I could see at the time that she was the best girl I'd ever seen.

Herbert Dardik

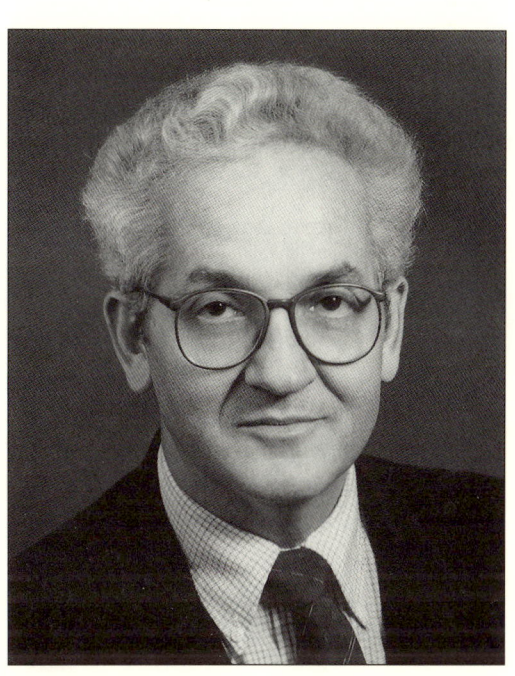

H ERB DARDIK grew up in a deeply devout Jewish family in northeast New Jersey. In spite of numerous setbacks, including a recent bout with cancer, he has remained on top. His persistence and belief in following through on an idea while still being involved in a busy private practice is an example for others. He was interviewed May 24, 1988.

Dale: Herb, let's start out with your background. Who were your parents and where were you born?

Dardik: I was born in Long Branch, New Jersey, on May 17, 1935. Long Branch is known as the nation's first seashore resort. I was the fifth of six children. It is my younger brother, whom everyone knows, who was involved with me in vascular surgery.

Dale: Irving?

Dardik: Yes. He made his mark in the sports world as a well-known sprinter and established the Olympics Sports Medicine Program.

Dale: What was your father's occupation?

Dardik: My parents were emigrants from Russia, born in little towns and married in Russia when my father was twenty and my mother was fifteen. My father escaped the Red Army to come chasing after my mother who, although they were married, had come to America with her family in the early 1900s. They had no papers and had to remarry in the States. My father told me he arrived with a nickel in his pocket. When my father came here, his interest was in scholarship and, having a very strong background in the Braag studies, he became a Hebrew teacher. In the early 1930s, before I was born, he developed spondylitis and later became kyphoscoliotic. As he got older, he became virtually wheelchair-bound. He didn't accept it very well, but he did his work as best as he could and took care of us at home. My mother and father had reversed roles because of his illness. He taught, and he was also what we call a *shochet,* the person who does the ritual slaughtering of animals in order to make certain that they are kosher. He was called a reverend and he was one step removed from being considered a rabbi.

Dale: What about your mother? Did she work outside the home?

Dardik: Yes, my mother had to become the working person and support the family, so she joined the labor force as a seamstress in a factory in our town. I remember as a child occasionally going by to deliver something, and she was in a line of women turning out bundles, like the picture of the immigrants on the Lower East Side of New York. She was the person who was out every day. My father did the cooking, sent us off to school, and did the laundry. On Fridays Irving and I would quickly do the kitchen floor so my mother wouldn't have to do it when she came home for the Sabbath. My father was a real romantic, and despite his infirmities tried very much to have this type of relationship with my mother. He was also volatile. My mother was much more of a cool person who took things under advisement and remembered things for a longer time, and I think that is where I come from.

Dale: What about your early schooling?

Dardik: My parents were very oriented towards education. I did quite well. We all went to the public school system in Long Branch and graduated from high school there. I would consider myself at that point in life a good student.

I knew that for me to go to college it was absolutely necessary for me to get a scholarship. I had my heart set on the University of Pennsylvania, but got only a half-scholarship there. I did get a full scholarship to Rutgers and to NYU at the Heights. I went to the Heights and really fell in love with the place. It was a beautiful little oasis in the Bronx, and the Hall of Fame was there. I remember walking down the hallway for my interview, seeing some beautiful young ladies, and thinking, "Gee, this is wonderful!" Then I got up there and discovered to my chagrin that it was an all men's school. This shows you how naive I was; the beautiful young ladies I had seen were secretaries.

I found myself in a very interesting situation. Here I was from a small town in New Jersey, in competition with a predominantly Jewish bunch of kids who were highly competitive and all oriented to go into medicine. I had told my parents before I left for college that I didn't know what I wanted to be, but I knew one thing for sure, that I was not going to be a doctor. And there I was in college taking courses—and I remember, during a chemistry laboratory, that I was lost a little bit while doing a qualitative analysis. So I asked those on my left and those on my right, "What do you think? How do you do this?" Immediately everybody hid their work. So I made up my mind and said to myself, "Dardik, you are going to show these people something." What happened was that I got almost all A's and won all the biological prizes. I really zoomed forward and the next thing I knew I was at Bellevue Medical Center.

Dale: What else did you do in college?

Dardik: I had a very sad experience in junior high school. I went out for the track team as a freshman in high school and Dr. Strayer—I still remember his name—examined me and listened to my chest and said, "Oh no, you better go see your own doctor. I am not clearing you at all." I was frightened, so my parents took me to Dr. Bender, and Dr. Josephine examined me, listened, and said, "Oh, my goodness." He told my parents, "Don't even let him take the garbage out. This is a very sick boy here. He's got a murmur." So during high school I was an invalid kid.

Later in medical school I had my physical examination and the doctor said, "You're fine." I said, "I am not fine. I have had this murmur all my life." He said, "No, it's just a little functional murmur." I was grateful to be well, but to have learned after all these years that I could have truly been active was hurtful. I thought it was awful that a doctor through his own ignorance could really destroy a youngster going through high school and college.

During college my major interest was music, because as a high school student I wanted to be a pianist.

Dale: Do you still play?

Dardik: Yes, I do. In fact, it was required of us in the family to take piano lessons, and I did enjoy it. I remember seeing a movie about Chopin, *A Song to Remember* I think, and I walked out of that theater and said, "I am going to become a pianist." I really started to work hard at it and I thought I did very well. In my senior year of high school, before deciding on science, I had applications all ready for Julliard, Oberlin, and Rochester. But one day my piano teacher, Mrs. Resznikoff, said to me, "Herbert, you're a hard worker, but your brother Irving has talent." That was so deflating. It was awful, but I have to say in retrospect that she really did me a favor, because had I pursued a musical career I would probably be playing in a bar or maybe for Radio City.

But the first purchase Janet and I made after we were married was a Knabe piano, which we still own. I was an intern at the time, and she had just started teaching. As my finances improved, we got a second piano in our house, a grand, and we love it.

Dale: Where did you meet Janet? When were you married?

Dardik: That's also interesting. In order to make my way through college, I used to work in the summertime down at the Jersey shore at the fun house, running the merry-go-round or the Ferris wheel without stripping the gears. In addition, my father taught me how to perform services on the High Holidays, Rosh Hashanah and Yom Kippur. There were a number of hotels that were always looking for someone to perform services for the older people who couldn't get to temple or synagogue. So for a few hours on Rosh Hashanah I would do these services, for which I earned $125. My brothers, who had better voices, earned a little bit more, but I never had a good voice, so I got the low price. At that time $125 bought me several months of room and board in college. In September 1956 I had just graduated from college and was getting ready to start my first year of medical school at Bellevue. After the services, the grandmas would come by and try to fix me up with some granddaughter. But that year I remember seeing a young lady in the back, wearing a black dress with a white frilly collar. I figured to myself, let me hang around and maybe a grandma will come by, and, sure enough, it worked. Grandma came by and introduced me to this young lady, who happened to be Janet. We talked for a while, exchanged numbers, and I said I would call her, but I never did. The following summer I had the same job in Asbury Park. In the mornings my father would wake us up to go down to the shore and grab a swim. I used to go down to a place in Deal, New Jersey. It was really for higher income and well-to-do people. I knew someone who ran a club next door and I used to sneak in. One day I saw Janet, walked over to her, and said, "Do you remember me?" She looked at me and said, "Oh sure, the rabbi." That was her view of me. Well, needless to say, that summer we had inexpensive dates by the beach in the morning. I couldn't afford anything else. By the end of the summer I gave her my Phi Beta Kappa key. I was already starting my second year of medical school and she was starting college at Douglas, which was the women's division at Rutgers. By Christmastime we were engaged. That is how we met.

Dale: How did you become interested in surgery?

Dardik: I always had been interested in anatomic structure; I loved anatomy, I loved pathology, and I had always loved to do things with my hands as a child. A lot of it dates back to that. I used to construct little model airplanes with balsa wood strips; now they come all prepackaged and you clip it. We used to have to pin it into shape, glue it, and put tissue paper on it. I used to build many, many models, so my orientation was obviously toward surgery. I enjoyed it.

I find that my son, who is now in medical school, tells me practically the same things that I felt. In medicine, I can remember, I listened to the heart, but I couldn't hear the murmurs that everybody was talking about. Gradually I knew that surgery was where I was heading. I also like to be able to do something. I found that although I did enjoy medicine, it was very philosophical, with thinking about the case and then saying, "Let's give this medication and then we'll see how it works out." I like to see results and I like to do something. I also felt that as a doctor I wanted to do everything that was possible, as opposed to diagnosing and giving it to someone else to treat. The only time in medical school when I was not going to become a surgeon was in my third year, when I rotated through surgery at Bellevue. Doctors Mulholland and Doubilet were there, and I remember being a student holding retractors and thinking it was an awful bloody mess. I didn't really like the environment at that time in surgery.

Dale: Were they not good operators?

Dardik: It was rough. In retrospect, it was a lot of rough surgery and, I thought, an environment that lacked culture and dignity in the operating room. It was more like a butcher shop and I thought this was really not for me. In my fourth year I rotated through St. Vincent's, and Dr. Louis Rousselot was chairman there.

I knew that this was a man who was world-class with shunting procedures, but what impressed me and brought me back to surgery was an event one morning when he was doing a breast biopsy in a young girl. He came into the operating room and held her hand as she was being induced, was very calming to her, and told her to relax. I thought, oh my gosh, this is a real human being; he is treating somebody very nicely and it is a nothing case, so to speak. I thought to myself, if he can do it, I can do it, and that was what reconvinced me. From medical school I went on into my internship and subsequent residency at Montefiore Hospital in New York.

Dale: Who was the chief there?

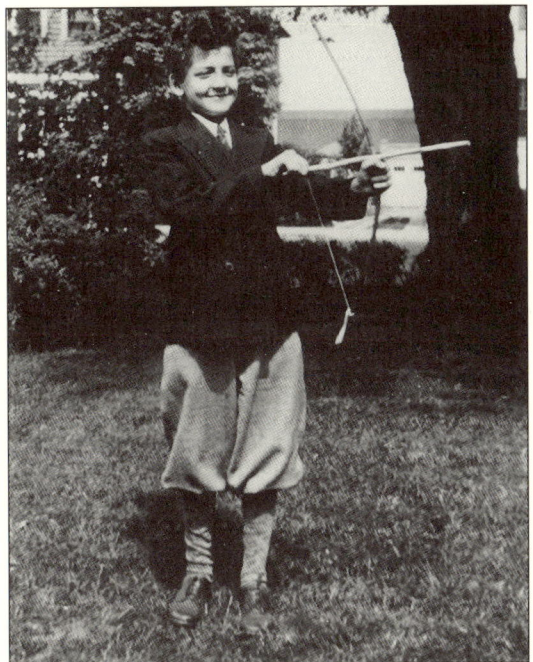

Herb as a youngster

Dardik: Elliott Hurwitt. In those days we took a mixed internship, and most people took a rotating, so we didn't have obstetrics. My big brother was a surgical resident in his first year, and one day he said to me, "Herb, I have had it with surgery; I'm going into psychiatry. I just turned in my resignation. You're not the kind of person who should go into surgery either. Go into something else. These are animals." I remember again what I said to him, "You know, I think surgery maybe needs somebody like you or me. If you can't make it, I am going to do it, and that's what surgery needs—a different kind of personality from what we're seeing around here."

I was very much impressed by Dr. Hurwitt and Dr. Rousselot, and I remember that as a child my role model was a Dr. Kazmann. He was the chief of surgery in Long Branch and I remember, not dreaming I would ever go into surgery, that this was a real role model. Everyone knew old Dr. Kazmann. Along the way I met others who were fine people in addition to being excellent surgeons, and they were the kind of role models that drew me. When Dr. Arthur Aufses, Jr., gave his presidential address to the American College of Gastroenterology, one of the things he pointed out was how important it is for senior surgeons to be proper role models, aside from just being excellent surgeons, because the impact is there. His father was "the" Arthur Aufses of New York, father of thoracic surgery, whom I also knew and who was a very, very nice man.

Dale: Did you finish your residency there?

Dardik: I finished all my training at Montefiore in 1965. I had joined the Berry program because this was during Vietnam War, so at that point I joined the air force and was very fortunate in being assigned to Andrews Air Force Base in Washington, D.C. I spent the next two years there, which was wonderful. I was the only two-year man with two senior career people over me. I had the opportunity to do a lot of surgery and was on my own.

During my training as a resident, I was convinced that I was going into surgery, but not vascular surgery. Dr. Haimovici was the chief of vascular surgery at Montefiore. I liked him and he liked me, but I just couldn't take the idea of doing a fempop in the morning, arguing with him at night that I thought it was closed while he thought it was open, then finding two days later that it would be closed and begin the series of amputations. I just didn't like it. While I was in the air force I had already picked out my office and the colors of the office at the Monmouth Medical Center in Long Branch. But during my air force time, when I was really on my own, I was doing fempops with saphenous vein and getting pretty good results. I had the time to sit there and work out those little fine anastomoses, so I thought, "Gee, maybe it is fun and I'll do some in practice."

Elliott Hurwitt died in 1966, and his successor was Dr. Marvin Gliedman. My brother, Irving, was chief resident, first with Hurwitt, then with Gliedman, and Marv Gliedman offered Irving a job. Irving wouldn't take a job unless I would join him at Montefiore, because he had been going to join me in Long Branch. So I flew up and met Marv Gliedman. I was seduced into giving up going into private practice in Long Branch to come up to Montefiore. I figured I could try this academic environment, and if it worked out, fine; if it didn't, I could always go into practice, but I thought the reverse might be more difficult. So in 1967 I came back and joined the full-time staff at Montefiore Hospital. My immediate assignment was to run the surgical program at the Morrisania Hospital, which was a municipal hospital in the New York City system, under the control of Montefiore. At the same time, I got involved doing a lot of dog work at Montefiore.

You might be interested to know how Montefiore's name actually came about. It comes from a banking family that lived in Italy. Their original name was Blumberg, but Blumberg was not a very prestigious name. Since Blumberg meant "flower mountain" in German, they translated it into the Italian "Monte-fiorre." The anglicized version is Montefiore.

My brother and I spent all our time running it. It was a glorious two years for Irving and for me, doing between the two of us thirty to thirty-five cases a week with the resident, and at the same doing a lot of fun research. When the full-time staff started coming into the clinical side, our work volume dropped and Irving became disheartened and went into private practice. I hung in a few more years, but then I became unhappy because of the number of cases I had to share with everybody. My volume per week was five, six, or seven cases and I wasn't prepared to go into retirement. Unfortunately, Dr. Gliedman didn't listen to my complaints, and Irving convinced me to go into practice with him. He was doing very well economically, of course, but the volume of work he was doing in general and vascular was stupendous. I thought, "I am not going to get rusty," so I joined him and another older person.

We all worked at Montefiore, but in addition, because of his big volume, we spread out to other hospitals in New York. I didn't stay with that situation too long, because I again became unhappy. Because I was so busy running around, that was the one year that I did not write a paper. When I started my residency, it was my goal to write at least a paper every year, and I did that from 1962 onwards, but in 1971–1972 I did not write a paper. I felt I was not delivering optimal care, because I was rushing from hospital to hospital. After about eight months of this, I told Irving I was getting out to do my own thing, concentrating more on vascular. I told the other person I was leaving, and within five minutes Irving told him he was leaving, too. The two of us joined forces and it was phenomenal. We really started to concentrate at Montefiore and I would say we truly had the largest practice in general and vascular.

He and I had an interesting arrangement—he would take more of the night call so that he could be very much freer during the day, because he was very anxious to run and jog. I gave him time during the day to work out and he gave me the time at night to do the papers. A year after we went into private practice, Irving was doing a thrombectomy with a bovine heterograft in the axillofemoral position. He called me up at 4:00 a.m. and said to me, "Does the umbilical cord have blood vessels in it?" I said, "Irving, it's four in the morning; why are you bugging me now? Let's talk about it in the morning." The following morning I asked him what he was talking about. He said, "As I was cleaning out that thrombus, it looked like jelly, and I thought about Wharton's jelly. I thought, instead of this bovine, maybe there is something in there we can use." I said, "Well, let's look into it," but he said, "No, forget it." That's Irving, basically: he has bright ideas, and then he drops them. I followed through with it and saved some umbilical cords. I brought them home in a huge jar with formalin and put them in the basement. They were there all summer and in the fall my wife said, "I need to do the laundry down there. Get rid of that—that is absolutely disgusting." So I threw it out. But afterwards I thought to myself, that's silly, so I went out there, took my little son's dissecting kit, and dissected this material on the redwood table. It was all formalized and looked just awful, but I thought maybe it would be good for a patch or something, so I drove over to Irving's house and we both agreed to get fresh stuff. We went down to Englewood, the neighboring hospital around the corner, and asked them to save us some umbilical cords, which they did. They thought we were crazy, two strange brothers, but we collected cords. It took us about six months to learn the technique of how to dissect the vessels out. We did a lot of bench work. One day we carried home from Montefiore one of those little extracorporeal animal pumps, and hooked it into a circuit and let it pump all weekend. It looked great, so we decided we really needed to get some animal work done.

This is the sad part of the whole story. We approached Frank Veith and Gliedman. At that time, Gliedman was angry at me, because I had been his bright young kid and I had gone into private practice. I remember to this day that he said, "No, you're in private practice and we won't support you with this and not only that, it's not that great of an idea." So Irving and I walked out, and, having been raised in a very religious environment, we both agreed—you know the Bible says you are supposed to give a tenth of everything back to charity—to take all the money and put it back into the project.

We scouted around and found Sterling Forest in New York State, about an hour and a half's drive from New York City. It's a conservation area of many, many acres. They have industrial areas, one of which was owned by New York University and was the site of the Laboratory for Experimental Medicine and Surgery in Primates. It was run by Dr. Moor-Jamkowski, an immunologist. We thought to ourselves, if we are going to implant human tissue into an animal, let's get it into the closest animal we can, a primate. So we called Dr. Moor-Jamkowski, who said it would take six months, but I got on the line and said, "But Dr. Moor-Jamkowski, this is fascinating. We are taking xenograft tissue, we've got human tissue, now let's see what happens with the rejection." The next day we had a baboon. It was so amazing! We began a series of events where we went up to this place once or twice a week. It cost a fair amount of money. We suddenly found ourselves with $50,000 to $70,000 invested in baboons; every time we had to x-ray them, it was $17; $2.50 for food; shots. I knew they were getting a good deal; some of these animals were re-do animals, because I saw evidence of other experimenters. Basically, we put xenograft tissue into the aortic position, and we got pictures that were gorgeous—very, very nice. We used the entire cord at that point. After six weeks, we started to reoperate, and, to our chagrin and horror, we discovered that in every one of the animals, the graft had turned into an aneurysm. We realized two things. Number one, it may be too weak, and number two, it was probably getting rejected after all.

So we did a few more experiments. In one of them, we wrapped it with mesh, and then we began treating it with formalin, glutaraldehyde; we learned all the chemistry. I had some thoughts about using peroxide, which would oxidize the aldehyde group to a carboxyl, making it more of a negative charge—we played around with all these things. It was a lot of fun.

In the meantime, we were going crazy because we had our private practice and ran into a very bad political situation when I wrote the first paper on the experimental use of this procedure in baboons. I was going to send it off to *Surgery, Gynecology and Obstetrics,* and I thought to myself, I ought to put Montefiore on this also, because that's my home base. Before this, when I had been doing intramural work at Montefiore, I described the lateral approach to the peroneal artery. Frank Veith had just come on board at that time into vascular, and we were very friendly, so I put his name on it. In fact, one of the reasons I dropped out was that I was supposed to become chief of vascular after Haimovici retired, but Gliedman pulled the rug out from under me. When Frank became chief, I was very disheartened, so between that and my not doing a lot of cases, I dropped out. Now I wanted to have this paper published, and I thought I should have Montefiore on it, too. So I put it through the research committee, and it came back to me—I still have it—all penciled in green: "You can't publish this without our names on it," from Marv Gliedman and Frank Veith. I became very upset and very obstinate at that point. I was willing to share authorship—in fact I have written an editorial that was published in *SG&O* on the problems of dealing with multiple authorship. I felt very strongly that when I worked intramurally, with the support, advice, guidance, or in the milieu of somebody—yes, okay, fine, I can understand that. But here I had been rejected, I had been told it wouldn't work, I went out of the institution, and we did it all with our own funds. I didn't feel that deserved coauthorship. Gliedman pulled back, but Frank really started open warfare. It was awful. I went to a lot of people who said, "Oh, Herb, we know you are right," but when I asked them to speak to Gliedman or Veith, everybody backed away. There was only one person who was wonderful, Harold Laufman, whom you must know. He was a principled man; I had done some other work with him, and he had helped me learn how to write. We did the Dextran project, a clinical project in the state, and Harold made me rewrite it ten times, fifteen times, but it was great. I went to Harold with this problem and he understood. He got on the phone with Loyal Davis, and the paper was published. I think it did have Montefiore on it, but along the way there were a lot of difficulties.

The paper was published in 1974. We had a previous publication in 1972 with the baboons, in the *Journal of Primatology*. Dr. Moor-Jamkowski suggested that, because he said you should have primacy; just put it someplace and you can always show that you had it. We said fine.

But the first real surgical one was in *SG&O,* and the first human was done in 1974 at Union Hospital. Again, because of our political problems at Montefiore, we couldn't put patients there. We had a lady, Mrs. Barnett, who had had multiple failures before, and there was a question of doing an amputation. She had an inch or two of artery and in the previous years, knowing of your original work with small vessel bypass and some others, I had become interested in that and started to do them. I went to her and explained what we were dealing with and she said to me, "If it is spaghetti you are putting in there and it will work, I will agree." It was in October—I think it was Halloween—that we did her and another patient, and it worked. We did a series of about seven or eight patients, and the problem we ran into was that within forty-eight to seventy-two hours most of them thrombosed. We went back and cleaned them out, and then they worked, but we stopped putting them in clinically because we knew there was something going on. We thought it was the glutaraldehyde, and it turned out that was it, because we were taking our lead from the heart valves, where they were treating with glutaraldehyde and storing in glutaraldehyde. We did the same. But there was probably too much aldehyde in a long graft, compared with a little heart valve tissue, so we went back again and treated with glutaraldehyde and alcohol. That did the trick, so at end of 1975 we began our second series, which continued, and that was the series of ten years that I reported last year at the Society for Vascular Surgery in Toronto.

Now, that is a potpourri of a lot of different experiences, because in 1975, 1976, and 1977, I think, we were not as good as we were in 1983, 1984, and 1985. But we learned a lot, and, of course, during these years different things happened in vascular surgery; PTFE was on the scene, and in situ came on the scene. As I described in one of my papers, we went through phases. Whereas in the mid-1970s we used the umbilical vein almost routinely, we now use it once or twice a month.

Dale: How many umbilical vein grafts do you think you have placed?

Dardik: I have placed now over a thousand. We used to do a hundred a year, now we do maybe twenty, maybe even less than that, and we really try to use the veins.

Dale: What would you advise a child or a young person who is showing interest in going into medicine today? It has changed so much, don't you think?

Dardik: To me, you should become a doctor not because of the economics, but just as if you wanted to become a priest or a rabbi; that is the kind of commitment you should have. Also, you should be paid very well. It's bad to be corrupted by money, but it is bad to have no incentive. I recognize all those things, and I don't presume to have the answer, but number one should be that the person has a commitment to medicine. If you are not inclined to academia, then treat people, and that's where I think I have done something. I take care of people, I try to do some clinical research, I try to contribute, I write, and so I have encompassed just a little bit of everything. That is what I would tell a younger person.

Michael DeBakey

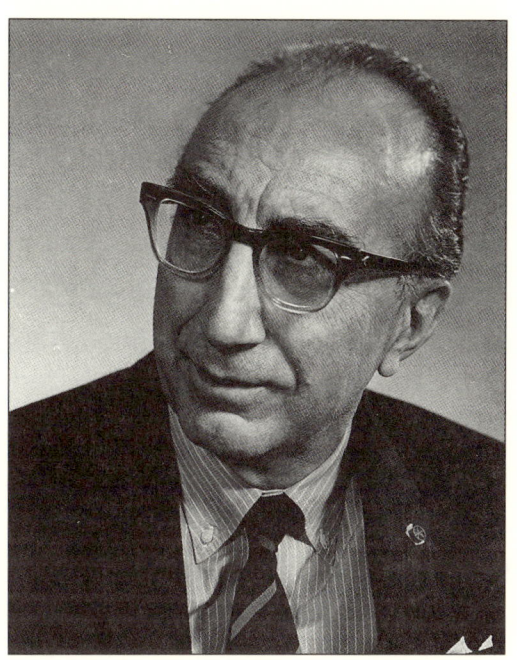

M IKE DEBAKEY is the most internationally famous surgeon of the century, a distinction based on achievement,
service, and vigorous longevity. A longtime academician,
DeBakey has long since demonstrated superior skills, even virtuos-
ity, operating upon scores of patients daily as well as teaching and
successfully administering Baylor's Department of Surgery as chairman. He has also served the Baylor College of Medicine as its president and its chancellor. His biographic details in *Who's Who in*

America require a ten-inch column of fine print; a list of his writings would fill many pages. Mike DeBakey is also an articulate speaker and a warm person. He was interviewed June 6, 1985.

Dale: Mike, who were your parents, and where did you grow up? How did you become interested in medicine?

DeBakey: I was born on September 7, 1908, in Lake Charles in southwestern Louisiana. My parents were exceptional people—industrious, compassionate, scrupulously honest, and deeply patriotic. They instilled in their children high ideals and values and the desire to make some contribution to society. There were doctors in my family, and among my father's businesses were several drugstores, so I came in contact with a lot of doctors—it was a small town and his drugstores were a hangout for all the doctors. Those factors influenced my desire to be a doctor.

I went to Tulane for my bachelor's degree and later my M.D. While I was in college getting my bachelor's degree, there were some influences that made me think of other careers. I was interested, for example, in biology—I had an excellent teacher—and my professor wanted me to continue my studies in biology rather than go into medicine. Somehow I overcame that.

I had a similar experience in physics. My professor encouraged me to pursue a career in physics. I had very good relations with my professors in college—in fact, they recommended to the dean that I be admitted to medical school at the end of my sophomore year in college and get my bachelor's degree when I finished my second year in medicine. During my first two years, I took the medical curriculum along with other credits that I needed to get my bachelor's degree at Tulane. So I did get my bachelor's degree with my classmates from college.

Dale: You did both in six years. That was unusual in those days.

DeBakey: My professors were very nice to me and supported me in every way. I did have a good scholastic record.

Dale: Then you went on to intern?

DeBakey: As a medical student at Tulane, I had come under the influence of Dr. Alton Ochsner, the professor of surgery, who was very energetic and had a deep interest in students. He had a great influence on me. He invited me to work in his research laboratory when I was a junior medical student. That's why I developed such a serious interest in surgery. At that time there was no specialty of cardiovascular surgery. I was also influenced by Dr. Rudolph Matas, Dr. Ochsner's predecessor as chairman of surgery at Tulane.

You will recall that in 1938 Bob Gross had successfully ligated a patent ductus, and that created quite a bit of excitement and interest. Shortly after that, I assisted Dr. Ochsner in performing a similar ligation of a patent ductus. It was during the 1939 meeting of the American College of Surgeons in New Orleans, so there were a number of visitors in the surgical amphitheater.

I was assisting, standing on the other side of the table, of course, and Dr. Ochsner said, "Now see if you can get your finger around the aorta from your side." Remember that the only reason we would operate at that time was if an infection set in; the risk was great. And, of course, the infection made the tissue friable and easy to tear. Soon I got my finger *into*, not around, the aorta. I knew my finger had torn the artery and gone inside it because I felt it happen. I was terrified. I leaned over the operating table and whispered to him that I thought my finger was inside the aorta—that I had torn into it.

Here we both were with all those prominent surgeons looking down from the amphitheater. I could see a tragedy developing. But Ochsner said, "Just keep your finger right there, and let me put some sutures around the side of it," which he did. I was also afraid that he might drive that needle through my finger and give me an infection, but I couldn't pull out my finger; that was the only thing that kept the patient from bleeding to death. Even so, there was a little pulsation of blood coming out and around my finger. Believe it or not, Dr. Ochsner finally got the sutures in, and we got that patient off the table with a cure.

Dale: What was your position at Tulane?

DeBakey: I had just returned from a year at Leriche's clinic in Strasbourg, France, as what they called *assistant d'etranger*, meaning that I was a foreign fellow. From there, I had gone to Heidelberg in

Germany, where I spent a year with Kirschner, who was professor of surgery there.

Dale: So you spent a year each with two legendary surgeons, Leriche in France and Kirschner in Germany. How did you choose them?

DeBakey: Dr. Ochsner encouraged me to study abroad with them, and my parents wanted me to have the best possible education. In those pre–World War II days, European surgeons were recognized as world leaders in the field. I went to Leriche, who was a pioneer in vascular surgery, because I was interested in vascular work. In his clinic I met Jean Kunlin, a younger surgeon, who in 1948 did the first femoropopliteal arterial bypass. And the other young man who was there—a foreign fellow like me—was João Cid dos Santos from Lisbon. He was the son of the older dos Santos who developed aortography. The son later developed thromboendarterectomy in the late 1940s.

Dale: Tell me something about the personality of the famous vascular surgeon, René Leriche.

DeBakey: He was an intellectual, a great scholar, with more of a philosophical inclination than you would consider the usual surgeon to have. He had a great fund of knowledge in art and literature as well as in science. His lectures were wonderful, because he could call upon this background of knowledge to intersperse anecdotes that were most interesting.

One that I remember shows what an impressive speaker he was: Fifty years later I recall it in connection with a lecture he was giving on renal failure. He told us that the fellow who originally described it was the man in the famous Flemish painting called *The Anatomy Lesson.* This anatomist lived about the same time as Napoleon, so he told a story about Napoleon.

Dale: What was the story?

DeBakey: Napoleon was driving along a road beside a canal when suddenly he came to a barricade, where a guard stopped his carriage. The driver said to the guard, "I have to get through; I am carrying an important person." The guard replied, "I don't care how important he is, or who he is. It is the rule here that the head of sanitation has made. When we wash these roads, they are blocked off. I don't care if you've got Napoleon in your carriage." The driver told Napoleon what the guard had said. The emperor congratulated the guard and told him that he was absolutely correct: "I want to tell your boss—that's the head of the Sanitation Department—what a good job you are doing. I'm going to send him a note to that effect." That's the kind of anecdote that Leriche frequently used.

Dale: Was Leriche a good surgical operator?

DeBakey: He would do good work if he was interested in the procedure. For example, he had a special interest in sympathectomy. And he was very meticulous about doing that operation. In fact, he was so meticulous it became boring. It was like Halsted, tying every little capillary. But he'd take two hours to do a lumbar sympathectomy; you and I do them in twenty minutes. Yet it was nicely done. I had a feeling, however, that he was not greatly interested in the technical aspects of surgery and that he preferred to write philosophically. Remember Leriche's book on pain? It is a philosophic treatise that is both provocative and interesting.

He would ask questions, provocative ones like "Why does calcification take place?" Some of his concepts were not very scientific, but he was an interesting man, certainly a stimulating person to be around.

Dale: I believe that he visited our country many times.

DeBakey: Yes, he did visit, and he did stimulate me; there's no question about that. He kept on asking provocative questions to his own people, and I think that added to their great contributions. I worked with them in his laboratory and wrote papers with them.

Dale: What was your overall impression of the French school? I have had the impression that often they jumped into a clinical problem without having any experimental background.

DeBakey: In general, I had the impression that they were very rigid; the structure was quite inflexible. But they are not very scientific, despite the fact that certain types of biologic science did start in France—remember Pasteur. But the scientific process was not highly developed in France.

The French are interesting in many ways. For example, in contrast to the British or the Germans, who are very precise, the French are imaginative and creative. The attitude of the French was different. Sterilization began there, but the French received it rather casually, and eventually the English did a better job. When I went to Kirschner's clinic in Heidelberg, Germany, I was completely astounded by the differences.

Dale: What were they?

DeBakey: In France, we would hang around waiting for Leriche to arrive before we made rounds in the morning. He might get there at eight o'clock and he might not get there until ten o'clock. We never knew what to expect, so we stood around and waited. But in Heidelberg, Kirschner started his rounds at seven o'clock, and anybody who arrived one minute after seven got a tongue-lashing. He was very strict that way.

Dale: Was that what began your habit of working early?

DeBakey: No. My father and Dr. Ochsner did that. I was always an early riser because I grew up that way. My father got up at four-thirty or five every morning. He thought it was essential to be out of bed by then. You must remember that in those days, the children had chores to do before we went to school. So we all rose early—the entire household. Of course, we had breakfast together. Then we had to prepare things and make sure our homework was all in order before we went to school. So we were up early, and I was accustomed to it.

Dale: So you returned to Ochsner and stayed in New Orleans until the war?

DeBakey: Yes. I wrote my thesis for my master's degree on peptic ulcer. At Tulane, I was working with George Burch and some of the other people in the Department of Medicine on the circulation. One of the things that we needed was to develop a pulsatile wave pump, so I made a search of the available pumps and went to the engineering school to talk to the people there. Because there wasn't much money available for research, we did everything ourselves. I used to smoke the old kymograph drums myself. It was out of that research that I developed the roller pump. Now if you take a tube, for example, and put a roller around it, you can force blood through that tube. And if you interrupt it in certain cycles, you can create a pulse. That's how simple it is.

The way John Gibbon got the pump from me was that we were at a meeting in St. Louis where I had an exhibit on it, and he had an exhibit on the heart-lung machine. John showed me what he was doing and said that he was having trouble with his pump. I said, "Come over here and look at this pump and see whether you can adapt it." After I showed it to him, he said, "You know, I may be able to use that." And I replied, "I'll send you a sample." So I sent him one, he adapted it, and later acknowledged it in one of his papers, and that's how it became a part of the heart-lung machine.

Dale: How did you enter the military service during World War II?

DeBakey: I went to war in 1942. Dr. Fred Rankin called Ochsner and said, "Look, I want DeBakey sent here," and that is how I began. There were three of us who were surgical consultants for the army. It was a great experience. As a matter of fact, it was truly wonderful because I came in contact with so many fine doctors.

Dale: You worked out of Washington?

DeBakey: Yes. I would be assigned on temporary duty and then come back. I was a captain, later major.

Dale: How long would a trip last?

DeBakey: Sometimes I would serve on temporary duty as a consultant for six weeks. When I went to Europe, I stayed some four or five months with duty in several armies. That's how I came to collect the material with Simeone on vascular injuries. I had a protocol, and I would get somebody to retrieve the data during each of my visits. Simmie had the complete data on the Fifth Army. He was in the Massachusetts General Hospital unit, first in North Africa and later in Italy.

Dale: Did you have any unusual experiences?

DeBakey: Once I was almost court-martialed. While assigned to the Seventh Army, I wrote a report for the Surgeon General, with a copy to the general who was in charge of the medical people on the scene. My report questioned the Seventh Army policy of having only 50 percent of the surgeons working at any one time. They'd receive a large number of casualties who would be waiting to be treated. Some would die before they received treatment because there were too many of them for the doctors who were on duty. Other surgeons were being held in reserve, waiting to be assigned because they might be needed elsewhere. So we were short of personnel, the doctors didn't like it, and the surgical consultant didn't like it but couldn't do anything about it because the surgeon in command insisted upon doing it that way. My report was critical, but I gave him a copy of it and then left and went over to General George Patton's Third Army.

I had a wonderful experience with the Third Army because I stayed with Patton. His physician, Charley Odom, had been one of my classmates at Tulane. After three or four days with Patton, I received a message from Paris to come there urgently, as I was going to be court-martialed! I was amazed. What had I done to be court-martialed? But Patton sent me back to Paris in his little observation plane.

When I arrived in Paris, Elliott Cutler told me that the commanding surgeon was furious and had accused me of all kinds of things. Cutler said, "The general wants to see you at his headquarters." I replied, "I've got a lot more material. I didn't put it all in my report; I can give you a lot more data showing that this commanding surgeon is incompetent." I was angry. I told them, "You see what's happened—you see that the casualties are about the same, but the incidence of death in the front-line hospitals is much greater here than in the Fifth Army. The reason is they just can't handle the load of wounded men, especially those in shock, because the number of available personnel is inadequate. Yet there's a hospital just ten miles away doing nothing—sitting around doing absolutely nothing!" Then I left. That general was relieved, and the policy was changed.

Dale: Then you returned to General Patton?

DeBakey: I had a great experience with Patton. There were only five or six of us in the "Patton family" at his headquarters. Every night we would have a formal dinner, using his own linen, his own crystal, his own china—he carried all of these with him. He was a military scholar—an amazing fellow and quite an attractive man in that setting. Every night after dinner, he'd serve drinks and we would sit around the fireplace in the castle he had commandeered—it was wintertime—and he'd tell us the background of military engagements that were historically important. Patton believed that the geographic conditions for a battle determined the outcome.

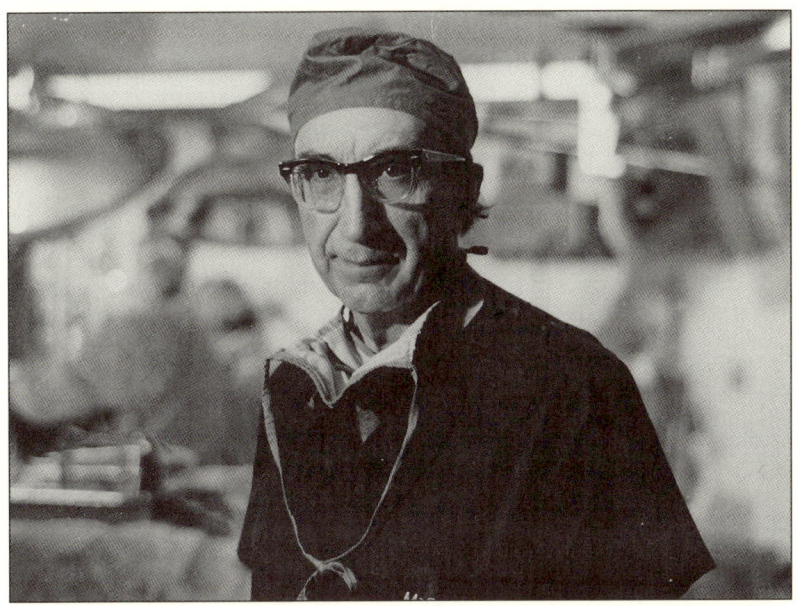

Mike in the OR

And he knew all of those. It was an unusual opportunity to get to know him.

Later on, I was in the Surgeon General's office when the word came that he had suffered a broken neck in a jeep accident. He was quadriplegic and survived only a short while.

Dale: What did you do when the war ended?

DeBakey: After the end of the war, I stayed on. We had already set up specialty centers, such as plastic, orthopedic, hand, and others. The fighting had ended, but the wounded men lingered on in those centers, needing treatment. Naturally, everyone wanted to go home. I called about a hundred surgeons and asked them to stay in service—to remain to care for our wounded men. I was able to get them all to stay. Not a single one refused. It was amazing. I explained the situation to them: "You can go home if you want to, but we have an obligation to these wounded men. We don't have enough people to care for them properly. So we need you." They all stayed on!

Dale: That's unknown to the general public.

DeBakey: No, it was not known, not recognized at all. It was extremely gratifying for our doctors to do this. I thought it was a wonderful gesture on the part of the surgeons.

In addition, I thought that having all the records furnished was a wonderful opportunity for follow-up studies that would allow us to learn about the natural history of diseases such as hepatitis. I proposed this to the National Research Council. They became interested, so I spent some time with them.

Then I organized the Committee on Veterans' Medical Problems. That led to the establishment of the Research Section of the Veterans Administration, and led me to participation with the Hoover Commission, which later supported the National Library of Medicine. I used to go to the library to study research material. Here was the greatest collection of medical books in the world, housed in an old firetrap building. The army simply couldn't take care of it, because they always had a low priority for library funds.

The Hoover Commission formed a medical task force whose most important recommendation concerned the National Library of Medicine. Mr. Hoover himself became interested. In the final analysis, it became established as the National Library of Medicine, which is what it is now.

Dale: Did you return to New Orleans?

DeBakey: Yes, although I still had work to do in Washington. I traveled back and forth, but in 1948 I moved to Baylor in Houston. I had turned them down twice before.

Dale: Why did you turn down their first offers?

DeBakey: At the time, the school did not have a service and they did not have a hospital. It was a third-rate place, and I did not want to be associated with it under those circumstances.

When I did go to Houston, I had considerable difficulty in the beginning because I was a little radical for them. The local doctors were reactionary—ultraconservative—and were dominated by general practitioners. There was a dearth of real surgeons there.

Dale: Who went with you? Who were your first staff men?

DeBakey: Nobody went with me initially. Later I recruited two young surgeons whom I had known. One was George Jordan and the other was Oscar Creech. George had worked with me in the research laboratory before he went to the Mayo Clinic to get his advanced training in surgery. When he finished there, I brought him to Houston. Oscar had been the senior resident at Charity Hospital in New Orleans while I was on the Tulane faculty. Later Denton Cooley finished at Hopkins, and Al Blalock recommended him to me. Houston was Cooley's home.

Dale: Were your younger associates received well?

DeBakey: There was no real problem. I recall one curious incident. One morning one of the younger surgeons had been assisting a general practitioner–surgeon do a difficult intra-abdominal tumor case. About eleven o'clock, he came to my office, quite agitated: "Dr. DeBakey, I can't continue to work with this doctor. He just let that patient die on the table, and I can't live with that kind of incompetence!"

I called the surgeon to my office and told him that his surgical privileges were suspended—that if he had a case to do, I would do it myself in order to protect the patients. He became angry and stormed out of my office. About an hour later, I had a call from one of his friends, saying, "Dr. DeBakey, Dr. ———— is very angry. I must warn you that he carries a gun and in the past has acted violently."

Well, I sent the erring man a message to come back to my office; he appeared about four o'clock. I asked him to be seated. "Look here," I said, "our conversation this morning was private. You have now spread it about to your own detriment. You have performed badly, and you know it! Now I'm not going around the rest of my life looking over my shoulder for you. If you are going to shoot me, pull out your gun and do it now!"

The man was momentarily stunned, and then broke down in tears, saying, "Dr. DeBakey, I respect you and admire you, and I wouldn't harm a hair on your head." So I jumped up from my desk and went to him, put my arm around him, and tried to quiet him. It was a rather fantastic scene, the two of us. Finally, I told him that I would help him get a job as a resident if he really wanted to study surgery. But he never again operated.

Dale: When did you first operate on an aortic aneurysm? Was the first one ruptured or elective?

DeBakey: The first one was urgent. It was a thoracic aneurysm which was beginning to erode the sternum. I did the same thing that a French surgeon had done some thirty to forty years before—although I did not learn about it until later—and that was to tie a ligature around the neck of it. Unfortunately, I made the same mistake that he did.

Dale: What is the correct method?

DeBakey: If you place a ligature around, it will cut through in time. You must sew it with interrupted sutures and bring the edges together. I just placed a ligature around the thing, so it ruptured later and the patient bled to death.

Dale: When did you perform your first abdominal aortic aneurysmectomy?

DeBakey: In the late 1940s there was great interest in aortic arterial homografts. The greatest stimulus was the work of Gross on coarctation. He replaced the narrowed segment of a thoracic aorta with an aortic homograft. Those findings were presented at a meeting, and the presentation inspired me, so I started working with homografts in our research laboratory. At the time, we had the good fortune to be affiliated with the City-County Hospital. The coroner was a nice fellow—a nice man, but somewhat lazy—and I was able to persuade him to let our team do all of the autopsies for him. That gave our residents a tremendous experience. It also gave us the opportunity to collect a lot of homografts.

Early in 1952, after working in the laboratory, I said, "It's time to do it." In those days there were no forms of consent, or institutional review boards, so we just did the operation. We thought the size of the homograft was right, but we failed to realize that when the blood flowed into that replacement vessel under pressure it would enlarge the diameter of the graft and cause the graft to elongate. We had to take out a piece, but it worked.

Dale: Who helped you with that operation?

DeBakey: Several members of my team. We were exhilarated. We didn't know that Dubost had done the same thing some months before. It hadn't been reported. We found out about it later.

Dale: What about plastic arterial grafts? How did you get into that?

DeBakey: We realized, as did others, that homologous arteries just weren't the answer. There were too many patients, we didn't always have the right sizes, and they weren't easily available.

Arthur Voorhees of New York had reported the successful use of Vinyon-N to replace dogs' aortas. That caught our attention, and so we started working on that. I went to a department store in Houston and bought sheets of various plastic materials, such as nylon, Dacron, and Orlon. I cut these into different sizes, even Y-forms. I would sew the edges on my wife's sewing machine. You might find that strange, but my mother had taught me to sew on a machine.

Dale: That was serendipitous.

DeBakey: I would produce these plastic grafts at home and take them to the laboratory, where we'd put them in dogs. They worked fine. Finally, we reached the stage where I said, "It's time to go to the patient." Again, we didn't have any consent form. But we did have a patient at the Veterans' Hospital with an aneurysm of the abdominal aorta. We made up some extra-large replacement grafts out of Dacron. Later we tested the other materials, but none of them proved as satisfactory as Dacron, and it is still the best material. In 1953 or 1954, when we put the graft in that patient, it worked fine. He lived thirteen years before he died of a heart attack.

Dale: Tell me about the further development of Dacron grafts. They are certainly commonplace today.

DeBakey: We put more in, but we realized that we needed expert technical help. I had a patient who owned half an interest in a sock factory in Reading, Pennsylvania, so I went there to learn if there was a machine that would knit Dacron grafts. He gave us some support funds and referred me to the Philadelphia Technical Institute, which later developed a machine to make the grafts.

Dale: Did any other commercial enterprises help?

DeBakey: I went to the research people at DuPont to inquire about artificial fibers. They had a policy at that point which made them reluctant to work with us because of the possibility of lawsuits. Their refusal was amazing. So we had to work undercover. A couple of their men did help us to develop the grafts we needed.

Dale: What about the aneurysm operation on the Duke of Windsor?

DeBakey: A doctor in New York called me about him and said he had a large aneurysm that he thought would soon rupture. I said, "Well, why don't you fly him down here, and we'll fix it." His doctor replied, "He won't fly." When I asked why, the doctor said, "Because his wife, the duchess, is afraid to fly." So I said, "Well, send them on a train." And they did come on a train. He was a good patient, and I had no trouble at all. He was very cooperative.

Dale: Did you put a tube graft in him?

DeBakey: I think we used a Dacron tube. He did well. Every day I had to send a medical report to the queen. She was very fond of him.

Dale: Was there anything to the rumor that he jumped his hotel bill and that the queen paid it?

DeBakey: I never was able to pin that down. It was suspected. Neither he nor anyone else paid me anything.

Dale: Really?

DeBakey: I did not send him a bill. I was hopeful that he might make a contribution for our research program at Baylor.

Dale: It has been said that he never paid off a golf bet when he lost because it was such a privilege to play with him. So he gave you the privilege of operating on him.

DeBakey: That's what I've been told also. That kind of thing never bothered me much. Many times I've operated on well-to-do people and not sent them a bill, hoping that they would make a donation for our department. Sometimes I was disappointed, but there have been other patients who made contributions, and that was gratifying.

Dale: Before we go, will you comment on your relation with Denton Cooley? You worked together for a long time.

DeBakey: I have no objection to telling that story; he played a part in the development of our department. Of course, he was ambitious, but I encouraged all my people to have high aspirations. He had an opportunity to develop a separate service at St. Luke's Hospital, which I encouraged because that increased the scope of our surgical department.

What led to Cooley's separation from our department was his unfortunate implantation of our artificial heart in a patient before it was ready for clinical use. The premature human implantation was a deep disappointment to all of us working in the artificial heart program. Later, a formal investigation was necessary, because as principal investigator for the Artificial Heart Research Program, I had to justify the use of this new device for a human being. Anything new had to be approved prior to human use. The Institutional Review Board had never received any such request for human use, because at that point I had no scientific basis for requesting that it be done on humans. At the time, the longest animal survival was twelve hours. Among seven calves in which we placed that particular unit, only two survived eight to twelve hours. Most of them died on the operating table. So we were nowhere near the stage where we could recommend it for human use.

Meanwhile, a fellow by the name of Liotta who was working with us had been talking to Cooley about using our device in a human being. During the inquiry, when he was asked why he did this, he said, "Dr. DeBakey wouldn't let it be done on a human being." But Cooley told the inquiring committee that one of the animals had lived forty-four hours. We did machine-pump that calf for forty-four hours, but it was dead from the time of implantation. We had the calf on anticoagulants, and we were interested in what happened to its blood, so we pumped it for forty-four hours. Cooley had never asked me about putting the artificial heart in a human. Four or five other members of the department were working in the laboratory with the artificial heart, but Cooley had never shown any interest in the laboratory work. He never did any work in the laboratory that I know of. Because there had been tremendous publicity, the National Institutes of Health, which was funding our artificial heart program, demanded an investigation. The Baylor investigating committee, which included members of the Board of Trustees as well as the faculty, recommended that Cooley be separated from the faculty.

Dale: So that's the way it was resolved?

DeBakey: That's the way it ended. He left the school and, as far as I am concerned, that ended the whole thing. The unfortunate thing is that a reporter came in with the specific purpose to create a sensational thing about a feud between us. As far as I am concerned, there was never any feud. I have always been too busy for such negative activity.

Later, when Cooley was sued by the patient's family, they subpoenaed me to testify. I told the judge, "I was out of town when all this happened. I had nothing to do with it." It is true that they used a heart device that had been developed in my laboratory—but that's all I knew. I couldn't add anything.

Dale: What was the verdict?

DeBakey: They threw the case out.

Geza de Takats

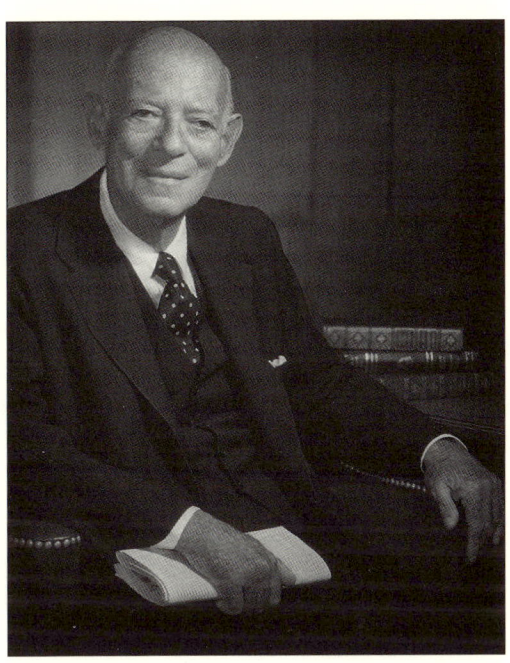

W HEN GEZA DE TAKATS died in 1985 at age ninety-three, he was the oldest surviving founding member of the Society for Vascular Surgery, of which he was president from 1952 to 1953. Born in Budapest, Hungary, and a hero of World War I, he was a duelist while a youth and a sage in old age. He might be called the midwife of vascular surgery as it emerged from general surgery in the 1950s.

De Takats went to the University of Rochester as a visiting professor in the early 1950s, discussing cases at the bedside and predicting the virtues of low-dose heparin prophylaxis twenty years ahead of its time. In an era when rush and bustle were the order of the day for surgeons, he invariably exhibited charm, thoughtfulness, and friendship for his colleagues, whether young and aspiring or nearer his own age. He was a gentleman of the old school—courtly and courageous. His interest in his friends and their activities continued to the end of his fruitful life. He died on October 3, 1985. Geza de Takats truly became a legend in his own time. He was interviewed March 3, 1978.

Dale: What led you to enter the medical field?

de Takats: My father, grandfather, and great-grandfather were all ophthalmologists, so it was natural for me to enter the Medical School of the University of Budapest in 1910 when I was eighteen. I was born in 1892.

Dale: From the story "The Maltese Knights" in your book *Breach of Etiquette,* I learned that you served as a surgeon in a Hungarian fighting unit in World War I. To me, that seems a long time ago. What happened?

de Takats: The assassination of Archduke Ferdinand in Sarajevo in August 1914 triggered the First World War. I already had completed four years of the prescribed five-year course in medicine in Budapest. At the outset, the Austro-Hungarian Army lost so many doctors, not to mention soldiers, from typhus and typhoid fever that medical students about to graduate were called to immediate duty. They shortened our course. I never received any instruction in obstetrics, which is why I still think that storks bring babies. I became a medical lieutenant. I was destined to become an ophthalmologist, following my father, but the combat injuries interested me, so that thereafter I wanted to become a surgeon.

Dale: How did you become a hero, or "goat," in 1916?

de Takats: When the city of Jaroslavl was evacuated after its defeat, I was left to care for three hundred wounded soldiers. The thought of a Russian prison was highly abhorrent, especially when the railroad line remained open and a telephone line was at hand. I found that a train staffed by Maltese Knights dressed in fancy costumes could be obtained. A few hours later all the men had been loaded aboard; we ran a gauntlet of fire but escaped. I thought that I probably was a hero and would get a medal.

The next day, however, the commanding general discussed with me my breach of discipline in bringing out the men when my orders were to stay with them in Jaroslavl. He further noted that, while I was due for the Order of the Golden Fleece, my disobedience would cancel it out. However, the attendant Knights did receive decorations!

Dale: How did you come to the United States?

de Takats: After demobilization, I studied surgery in Copenhagen with Professor Rousing. My father had become dean of the medical school. With his help, I received the traveling fellowship of the Rockefeller Foundation in 1923. I visited the surgical departments of Harvey Cushing, the great neurosurgeon; Allen O. Whipple in New York; and the Mayo brothers in Minnesota.

After a year, I returned to Budapest—I was thirty-two years old—and found that another person had become the chief of surgery there. The Rockefeller people allowed me to return to the States for a second year. Then I met Carol Beeler. We were married six weeks later and remained so for sixty years.

She was a biochemist, a graduate of the University of Chicago, and was in her first year of medical school in Cincinnati when I met her while she was visiting her sister and brother-in-law, who lived in Rochester. They often played bridge from nine to two in the morning. Carol and I sat there, since we didn't play cards, and became engaged. Carol returned to Europe with me, and we lived there a year.

Dale: Did you have any experience with any of the early French vascular surgeons, such as René Leriche?

de Takats: I didn't know him then. There wasn't any vascular surgery that long ago. My first case was a periarterial sympathectomy on the subclavian and brachial arteries in 1920. The indication was wrong—he had scleroderma—but I had heard about the technique from an article by Leriche, so I did it.

Dale: Was that in Budapest, and did it help the patient?

de Takats: Yes to the first, and no to the second. I was stumbling in the dark. But later, with Dr. Allen Kanavel in Chicago, I became involved with many sympathectomies.

Dale: Did you work with Kanavel, the pioneer hand surgeon?

de Takats: Yes. He was a marvelous general surgeon who did many sympathectomies. He also did much brain surgery, but was known chiefly for his hand surgery. He gave me a surgical fellowship at Northwestern in Chicago, and I really came to stay there permanently at the end of 1925. My three-year surgical fellowship allowed me to do some teaching, more research, and to build up my private practice the rest of the time. Kanavel said to me, "There are too many surgeons doing gastric resections, cholecystectomies, and thyroids. Why don't you select a specialty that we don't have here?"

About that time, I read a description in a Scandinavian journal of injecting hypertonic glucose to produce a clot. There was a rather large group of people with vein problems, so I said to Kanavel, "Why don't we start a vein clinic?" He was delighted because no one had been interested in that. Also I was asked to give a course in local anesthesia, because at that time no one in the United States was doing any major surgery under local, and I had been trained to do a lot of it. You may remember that Finsterer, a surgeon in Vienna, did many gastric resections that way.

Dale: In fact, he visited Rochester at age ninety-two and performed one, to our amazement. John B. Murphy was a pioneer vascular surgeon in Chicago. He did the first end-to-end anastomosis of a human artery just before the turn of the century. Did you know him?

de Takats: John B. Murphy had a large clinic at Mercy Hospital. Doctors came from all over the Midwest to hear and see him. He was quite controversial and was disliked by many doctors. Chicago was full of doctors, so there was great rivalry. They fought each other day and night.

Dale: Why did they dislike Murphy?

de Takats: He was quite aggressive and often abrasive. For example, after President Theodore Roosevelt was shot by an assassin in Milwaukee, he was placed on a train to be treated in Chicago by Dr.

Arthur Bevan. Murphy met the train at a suburban station and took the president into his care—he more or less abducted him. That did not help his image.

Dale: When did you first perform a lumbar sympathectomy in Chicago?

de Takats: There were a number of patients in the clinic at the University of Illinois who had Buerger's disease—at least we thought so at the time. Today they would probably be classified as arteriosclerotic problems. In any event, I talked to René Leriche and René Fontaine when they visited Chicago and did it after that. It was in the early thirties.

Dale: John Homans was a pioneer vascular surgeon in Boston. Did you know him?

de Takats: I had a traveling fellowship and went to Boston. He took me on rounds with him. He was famous for his hard treatment of the residents; he thought it stimulated them.

Dale: That was the common wisdom of surgical teachers at that time. Dr. Barney Brooks certainly followed that policy in Nashville.

de Takats: Homans asked one of the residents, "Where are the oscillometer records of this patient?" The resident replied, "Dr. Homans, we have none." Homans cried, "Jesus Christ, even de Takats has an oscillometer!" But Homans treated me well—his manner hid a fine, friendly man. He took me to a football game, put me up at the Harvard Club, and supported me generally. He, Dan Elkin of Atlanta, and Norman Freeman were on the vascular subcommittee of the National Research Council. They put me on it also.

Dale: The French school surgeons led the way clinically then. What is your idea of their work?

de Takats: I had great admiration for René Leriche. He was a genius with magnificent ideas, of which he could prove none—they were all intuitive. Many of those ideas were correct, but a lot of them were wrong. On balance, though, adding up the plusses and minuses, he came out ahead. Let me give you an example: He inspired Jean Kunlin to inject the stellate ganglion of a German prisoner of war with Novocain, which at the time everyone thought was a crazy way to treat an injured arm, but it turned out to be a useful therapy.

Dale: When did Ormond Julian come onto the scene in Chicago?

de Takats: Ormond came out of service to the hospital at the University of Illinois, where Warren Cole was chief of surgery. At the time, I was running a vascular service at Hines Veterans' Hospital, where the chief of medicine allotted us thirty beds because the surgical service had no place for vascular patients. They would do the diagnostic studies, we would operate on those who needed it, and they would perform the postoperative care. It wasn't a good arrangement, but it did last a while. When Charles Puestow became chief of surgery, he took us back on his service where we belonged. We started with thirty beds and ended with ninety.

When Ormond Julian arrived, we needed help badly. I was only a consultant—over there twice a week. Ormond got into it and started real vascular surgery in Chicago.

Dale: When did vascular reconstruction with grafts begin in Chicago?

de Takats: There were a few people involved; Ormond Julian was one. He admitted a man from Peoria who had a large aneurysm which had been embolizing, with clots passing down into the legs. We had previously explored it surgically and wrapped the external part in cellophane. That was done at the time in an attempt to cause scarring, so the aortic aneurysm wouldn't rupture. When Ormond explored him, the adhesions and scarring were so severe that he stopped and did not remove the aneurysm. Soon thereafter Charles Dubost did the first reconstruction of aortic aneurysm in Paris, so Julian missed the first, and Dubost thereby established priority.

Dale: I am not strong on "firsts," because developments usually lead several people to do the "first" at about the same time. The quickest writer may get credit.

de Takats: You are correct. Sometimes it seems as if the paper was prepared before the patient leaves the hospital in good shape.

Dale: Was there an artery bank, as we had in Rochester?

de Takats: Yes. Julian used it, as did Harold Laufman at Northwestern University. They were trying to start individual artery banks. I brought Oscar Creech here from New Orleans to advise us how to develop a cooperative municipal artery bank that could be used by all. I am proud that I persuaded all the Chicago hospitals to

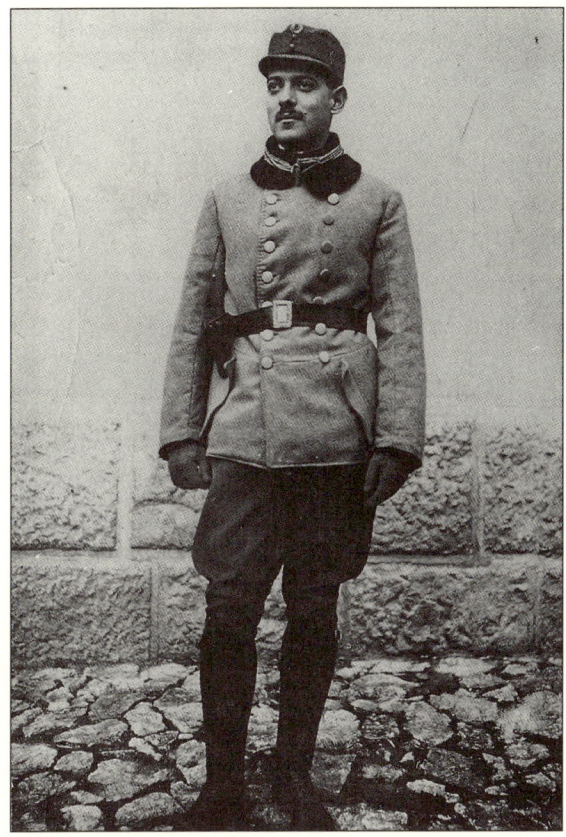

Geza de Takats, December 1915.

cooperate in establishing a bank at the Cook County Hospital, where a pathology resident received the arteries and prepared them.

Dale: What method was used then?

de Takats: They were removed sterilely, frozen, sterilized with ethylene, and stored. About three hundred of those banked arteries were used. The Red Cross distributed them.

Dale: Were they available to any surgeon who asked?

de Takats: We knew which surgeons were capable, and allocated grafts to them. When synthetic grafts were developed, the artery bank became outmoded.

Dale: When Arthur Voorhees's paper on replacement of the dog aorta with Vinyon-N was presented in 1952, did you think it was important?

de Takats: I thought that if you could use an artificial material taken off a shelf, it would be a great improvement over the artery bank, which required a postmortem operation, preparation, and maintenance.

Dale: Wheelock Southgate placed the first synthetic graft in Rochester at the Genesee Hospital. Who did the first in Chicago?

de Takats: I don't know. Julian and Laufman were both going hard, so it must have been one of them. Everyone was elated that something might replace the troublesome arterial grafts.

Dale: Did you have any experience with the heterologous bovine graft that Norman Rosenberg and I tried in the late 1950s but later found to be useless?

de Takats: We tried them in the laboratory; we had obtained a grant from a large pharmaceutical company to work on it. Our results were poor, and there were some others who reported the same. Our financial helpers were quite anxious to suppress our report.

Dale: The same company gave me the same trouble, much as did another monster company that refused to tell us what caused the discoloration on their Teflon tubes. Did they stop your report?

de Takats: No.

Dale: Dos Santos first described this in 1927, but it was almost thirty years later before it became commonly used. Did you have experience with visualization of arteries by angiography in the early days?

de Takats: I had a long friendship with João Cid dos Santos of Portugal, who performed the first endarterectomy in 1947, and knew all about his father's work. Also, I knew that Barney Brooks had done the first human arteriogram in Nashville in 1922, using sodium iodide. We began to do it in the fifties. The radiologists had no interest and in fact did none of them, nor did they develop the field in those years. They came later.

We wanted to obtain carotid arteriograms, of which the old European literature had good reports. One was done, and it incurred the wrath of Loyal Davis, the chief of neurosurgery and stepfather of Nancy Reagan. He hit the ceiling because he thought we were invading his territory. In other words, he thought it was a neurosurgical problem and said that no member of his service should perform such a dangerous procedure.

Dale: It's the old story of the wisdom of the establishment versus the risks of progress. When I reported the first femoral arteriogram at grand rounds in Rochester in 1952, one of my respected teachers objected, "You young fellows are going to kill a lot of people with this." For those early ones, we exposed the femoral artery in the operating room, covered the wound with a towel, transported the patient down the corridor to the elevator, and went down two floors to the radiology department. There a needle was placed in the artery, the injection done, films developed, and the patient returned to the operating room for closure of the wound. It was cumbersome, to say the least, but we forced the issue. The radiologists had no interest in that development; they later changed their minds.

Back to Hines Veterans' Hospital in Chicago. What kind of patients occupied your ninety beds?

de Takats: They were mostly old war injuries, with some cases of lymphedema mixed in, because we admitted dependent females. We also performed many thoracolumbar sympathectomies and the amputations that were necessary. At that time, the orthopedic surgeons restricted their practice more. They had no interest in amputations. The ones they performed were criticized by the artificial limb makers as being difficult to fit. We did the Gritti-Stokes procedure, which they liked better.

Dale: Has that now been generally abandoned as a difficult stump to fit?

de Takats: Perhaps so. Maybe we were wrong.

Dale: There are several approaches for thoracic sympathectomy. Which did you use?

de Takats: Originally we performed this procedure through the neck, but changed later to the transaxillary thoracic route, which Atkins had reported and which was pushed by Robert Goetz. We also used Reginald Smithwick's posterior approach. He believed that the resection of ganglia should be done in a preganglionic manner. We finally thought that there wasn't much difference between the pre- and postganglionic methods.

When we changed to the transaxillary procedure, it became easier. I recall a woman with excessive sweating—hyperhidrosis. I said, "Let me fix one arm and then you decide whether you wish the other one done." The only available room was a small one usually used for eye surgery; there was only a student available to help. The procedure by that method was so easy that the accommodations and help didn't matter. That lady from Kalamazoo, Michigan, had an excellent result. It was simple.

Dale: You discussed the possible use of heparin as a prophylactic agent against deep venous thrombosis far before Kakkar of London and others popularized this. It must have been about 1954 when you were visiting professor at the University of Rochester.

de Takats: We had a good time, didn't we? Merle Scott, your chief, invited me to lunch at a restaurant near the hospital where we had so many martinis that we almost missed giving the lecture. But they said I did better than if I'd had none.

Seriously though, you recall that after McLeod's discovery of heparin in 1916, it did not become clinically available until 1936 in Scandinavia and Canada. One of the things that impressed me quite early was that Crafoord found he had to give different amounts of heparin to different people, and that it was not related to their weight. I tried to develop a heparin tolerance test. It was thought that heparin was of uniform strength. We didn't know any better, so we gave them all the same dose. A clotting test was then done. It showed that people's tolerance varied—even the same patient's tolerance would vary from day to day and postoperatively—so some people got too much and some people got too little. I tried to learn how to set the dosage. We were looking for a bedside test so that an intern or nurse could run simple clotting times at the bedside to see what the next dose would be.

Dale: That's what kept me up all night many times when I was an intern. What about caval ligations to prevent clots embolizing to the lungs? Did you do those?

de Takats: Yes, we did a few caval ligations, but not many because we thought that most of our patients did well on heparin. Let me tell you of a curious experience that I had with a caval ligation. She had thrown several emboli. I made a lateral extraperitoneal incision and found that she had a tremendous number of lymph glands around the vena cava, and I, being naturally of a rather cautious nature, backed out; she never threw any more clots.

Dale: It amounted to a sham operation—and the clots ceased spontaneously.

de Takats: She stayed well and lived many years. She sent me a Christmas card every year and died about thirty or forty years later without further trouble.

Dale: What drugs were you using then for pulmonary embolism?

de Takats: We had a triple drug treatment in use on our wards whereby the patient received intravenous atropine, papaverine, and lidocaine, because I had become convinced that many of the immediate deaths were due to arterial spasm.

Dale: How did you happen to use papaverine?

de Takats: Papaverine was originally used by the Viennese surgeons, who suggested it for acute arterial occlusion with spasm of the artery. We used it for acute arterial occlusion, and it seemed to produce some vasodilation. When we began to perform angiograms, particularly of the upper extremity, we always injected papaverine before the dye, because I was convinced it was a very potent smooth muscle relaxant. Now we use priscoline.

Dale: Did you know Rudolph Matas, the great New Orleans surgeon who did so much work on peripheral arterial aneurysms?

de Takats: I have some very pleasant memories of him. We had white, plastic-covered chairs. He sat down in one and spilled coffee on it. We decided that we'd never have it washed or cleaned up, and we had a sign on it saying that Matas sat here. By the time I knew him, he had retired and he didn't see well.

Dale: What about Barney Brooks of Nashville? Did you know him?

de Takats: No, I never knew Barney Brooks personally. He did reject one of my first papers on causalgia because he said there was absolutely no evidence that hyperemia would produce osteoporosis. I was very grateful to him in the long run. My philosophy in life has been that every time you have a mishap, every time you feel "sat upon," it really works out for the best. I left Northwestern because of some difficulty I had there, and I couldn't have done what I accomplished without going over to Illinois.

Dale: Let me say, as we conclude our talk, that the series of short stories that you published were great. I particularly liked the one about the pistol.

de Takats: You mean about the duel? That was a personal affair that takes me way back. I must have been in my twenties. In that part of the world, in Austria and Hungary, but not so much in Germany, they had real duels. In Germany they had a lot of fights in fraternities, but this was different. If you insulted someone in any of a variety of ways, he sent two representatives and then you had to meet him either with a pistol or sword. Mostly it was a token thing, because you wouldn't want to kill or shoot someone—you shot above his head—but some people were injured and finally it became illegal. It was a customary thing, and if you did not provoke him to a duel, or if you refused to have a duel with him, you were not a gentleman.

Dale: Was yours a token duel?

de Takats: It occurred after I whispered sweet nothings into Lilly's ear in 1916. Her brother became unhappy and required satisfaction by three shots (each at the other) at sunup. Fortunately both parties fired into the air, so no one was injured. The only winner was the girl. She acquired inordinate prestige and status.

Dale: What kind of pistols were they?

de Takats: Most of these were army equipment made in the German part of Czechoslovakia. I brought one of them over to America and kept it in my bedside drawer. There were five terriers who made a dreadful racket every morning about five in the morning by barking. I was going to shoot one of them, but I found that I couldn't get any ammunition for my gun. There was nothing that would fit it. I tried; I went down to the local stores here, and there was absolutely nothing, so I turned it in to the Illinois police department. They were crazy about it because they had never seen anything like it.

Ralph Deterling

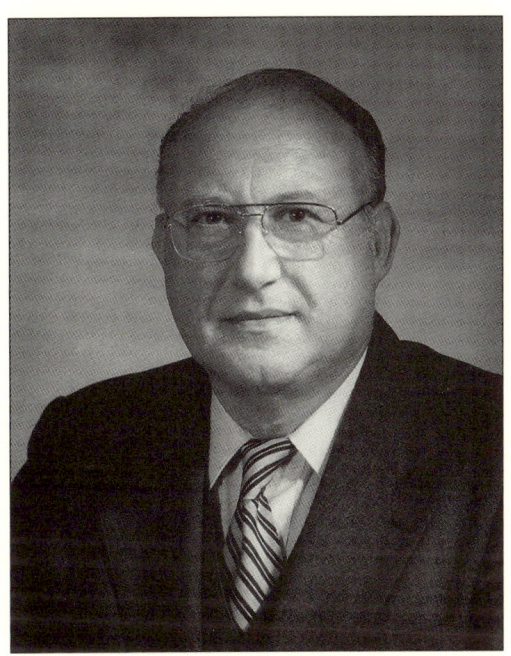

RALPH DETERLING typified the vascular surgeons of his time: He was aggressive, inventive, and courageous without consideration for personal effort and sacrifice. His early endeavors in homografts stimulated the development of prosthetic materials, and he had a permanent effect on Tufts Medical School. Deterling passed away in August 1992. He was interviewed December 8, 1986.

Dale: Ralph, let's talk about your early life.

Deterling: My father, of the same name, was in business and traveled a lot, so we didn't really have a firm family base. We spent most of my early years in Williamsport, Pennsylvania, where I was born in 1917, because my mother's family was there. They shared taking care of me when Mother was sick or away with Father. I went through most of the school system there, including high school. In 1933 Father's business shifted to San Francisco, and we visited Stanford. Although I had applied to the University of Pennsylvania and Penn State, I was taken with Stanford and was admitted, to my delight. I had a very fine time in college and applied to medical school.

Dale: When you say you had a fine time in college, what did you do besides study?

Deterling: I was very interested in sports, but had a sizable and sometimes painful hernia. We're talking about the late 1930s, when hernia was a big operation. So they allowed me on the fencing team and I became an alternate to the varsity. I did some swimming and some tennis, but it was strictly noncompetitive.

Dale: You didn't have your hernia fixed?

Deterling: I did. That was in 1935 and I was kept flat in bed for two weeks in the hospital, which gives you some idea of recovery in those days. It is still alright, so it was a good repair.

Dale: Tell me about the fencing.

Deterling: There was a lot of exciting hand-eye coordination and rapid, almost anticipatory, activity, which is what I liked. It was one-on-one, with no lapse time. That was really the thing that attracted me, rather than the activity itself.

Dale: Were you were interested in anything else, music or other hobbies, at Stanford?

Deterling: I was very much interested in music and was an avid reader and stamp collector. My grandmother started a German colonies collection. I wasn't too interested in it until I got into late high school. One of my father's hobbies was investing, and he said, "If you are seriously interested, what you should do is not collect the world but concentrate on something." I stayed with the U.S.

stamps and have done so since then. It is now quite a valuable collection.

Dale: You left Stanford and went to medical school?

Deterling: That was a story. I was fond of a gal who lived in Burlingame, near Palo Alto, but I had applied to both the University of Pennsylvania and Harvard. I was accepted at both and actually put down a deposit for Vanderbilt Hall at Harvard. Then things started to look more serious with the gal at Burlingame, so I decided to apply to Stanford, was accepted, and went through medical school there. Bev was very pleased that I did, and I have had no regrets.

Dale: Who was the surgical chief then?

Deterling: Emile Holman, who fired me up about vascular work because of his interest in arteriovenous fistulas. He was very demanding, not in the unreasonable sense, but a perfectionist. I was only a fourth-year student when I helped him on a big traumatic AV fistula of the neck from a hunting accident. He stayed up all night with the patient and boy, did that impress me! The head and neck were not exactly his main area of expertise, but it was so impressive that my eyes bugged out and I said, "This is it." I helped a little bit in the lab and from that time on felt that vascular work, which was just starting to yawn and wake up, would probably be the area of greatest satisfaction.

His friendship and support were paramount when I came back from the East Coast to practice. He did a lot to help me get very tough hospital appointments. Everybody from the army wanted to go back to California.

Dale: After Stanford, where did you have your residency?

Deterling: I wanted to go back to Pennsylvania, and the University of Pennsylvania took fourteen or fifteen interns. It was a two-year rotation, and they took all but four from the University of Pennsylvania. The dean at Stanford told me, "Well, you're going back there for the summer; why don't you drop in on Philadelphia? I don't think they'll take you, because they've already picked the four they want, but it wouldn't hurt to see the place and meet the dean." The dean at Penn was William Pepper. He granted me an interview, and we hit it off well. I thought I had nothing to lose; I was totally relaxed and had a very firm purpose in life. Some time after that, the dean back at Stanford said, "I don't know what you did with that guy, but you're one of his new interns." So we had quite a nice group. There was one from Hopkins, one from Cornell, one from I forget where, and me. While I was there, I wanted to get one of their two surgical residencies. There were two chiefs, the old father figure, Eliason, and the young upstart, Ravdin. They each had the right to appoint a resident every other year. I had to apply for the 1943 appointment, as 1942 was Ravdin's.

In the interim I had an opportunity to be an assistant orthopedic resident because Paul Colona was just starting a new program and wanted to steal fractures away from the general surgeons in Philadelphia. That's where I had my contact with fractures; Eliason had the contract with the 30th Street Station of the Pennsylvania Railroad, and we got all of the accidents from there. So I spent one year with orthopedics and enjoyed it very much. John Kirklin was one of my interns once, very dedicated and topflight, as you might expect. I have never regretted the experience of seeing Colona develop a department. I benefited greatly from seeing his organizational ability. It was good exposure.

Dale: Then the war came along.

Deterling: The war came along and I got my "greetings" and went out to the Schuylkill arsenal for my induction exam. I had rather severe asthma at that time, and they were excluding asthma, stomach ulcers, and things that could get worse without warning. I wasn't happy at all, first because all my friends were going and, second, because the Twentieth General was the University of Pennsylvania Hospital and all my friends were in that. I felt really disappointed, and then angry when I got word that the hospital was denying all appointments unless you were 4-F. My board in California kept me 2-A. I said, "Well that's fine, except I lost my residency at Penn." This was in July 1942; I called about eight or ten places and finally somebody said, "I think they're hurting at Mayo, because they skimmed off an awful lot of guys there. Why don't you try there?"

So I flew up and saw the director of the foundation, and we hit it off well. I think even if we hadn't, he would have said, "Okay, you're a body and I think you're breathing." So I started there in October

1943. I had some exciting experiences, although not in great depth, in vascular research. Vascular was under John Waugh, who was mostly a general surgeon, and general surgery was mostly cutting legs off or doing sympathectomies. The director said, "Why don't you talk with John? There may be a project or two he is interested in." I did that and he said, "You know, with your background and interest in AV fistula, why don't you do a physiological surgical evaluation of the systemic effects of AV fistula?" Then I enrolled in a Ph.D. program, and they laughed and said, "Some guys are optimists." I said, "What do I have to lose?" I finished the Ph.D. because I had a ski accident to my knee. I didn't do it intentionally! That is when I met my wife; she had to carry me around in her car with a full leg cast on.

Before then, the army called me up again to Fort something or other in Minneapolis. I spent a day and a half there and they made me 4-F, but the war was over. I then went into chest with Oscar Theron Claggett, known as Jim to everyone, and he took me under his wing. In those days you needed a year of tuberculosis experience, and then a year of lung work. We went up to the TB sanatoriums and did thoracoplasties and all sorts of stuff like that. When the Korean War came, Norm Rich and Sam Sealy, the general at Walter Reed, wanted me to send my thesis to them because they were receiving traumatic AV fistula cases, and there was controversy about the "collaterals." I think Dan Elkin had unintentionally started it. He felt that the big veins represented collaterals. It was really just the venous response to the shunting, and I had all kinds of experimental pictures of the development of collaterals and the effect of sympathectomy, so they seemingly benefited from my data. Now Leonel Villavicencio wants the thesis again, so history repeats itself.

Dale: You returned to New York at the end of 1947?

Deterling: Yes, in 1946 I had a paper at the forum on AV fistulas, and John Lockwood was in the audience. John had been at Yale, then went to Columbia, and was with George Humphreys, who became the chief when Whipple retired. John was impressed with the talk and chatted with me. I had met John when he and I were at the University of Pennsylvania. He was very interested in sympathectomy, so he asked me if I would like to come to Columbia. Well, I had already paid a deposit on an office on Post Street in San Francisco. My wife, Mary Ann, was just tickled pink, as her family was in southern California. I will never forget telling her that I was thinking about shifting gears and wanted her to be part of the decision. She said, "Whatever is best for you and what you enjoy most is good by me," so it was a complete turnaround and we ended up at Columbia Presbyterian just before a blizzard in December of 1947. It was a pip. About two or three days after we got there, friends called us from Minnesota and asked me if I wanted a dogsled dropped. There was one line of pedestrian traffic down the middle of Fifth Avenue. However, we weathered that.

I usually enjoy work of any kind, but I really dreaded that first six months. It wasn't a lack of friendliness or support, it was the challenge that I felt. Here was a guy from Mayo, which was sort of anathema to the Northeast. So smartass shows up in town and becomes assistant professor right after his training, while a lot of his peers, like Dave Havus and Ferdinand McAllister, were just getting out of the army. I don't say there was resentment, but there was "Let's see how this guy does." Everything I did was measured carefully. When you go through that every day, it gets a little thin. I did have a good chance to develop independence, judgment, and expertise. Later they took on the state hospital so I would have a resident service. We saw a huge volume of cases and had tremendous efficiency in handling them. All of this was a big plus.

I did manage to influence a lot of things, in terms of routine and methodologies. They had very slow operators. Hagenson would be eight hours on a breast, and Arthur Blakemore would be thirteen hours on a shunt, so it didn't take a hell of a lot to be a speed demon. I think a number of people, like Sam Harvey and Whipple, used the word "meticulous" so much that they actually teased the cells apart. To me, it was just being slow. You had McAllister, Havus, and some of the newer guys who were not that slow. They tended to be relaxed. Nobody gave a damn when you got through. I always had so damned much to do that I measured the day by the number of things I had to get done. I was not clock-driven, but I was very respectful of efficiency and I always told the residents, "You know, if you're not sure what you're doing, for God's sake don't bluster through watching the clock, because you'll get into terrible trouble and your patient won't thank you for it. But if you know what you're doing and you have good assistants, to take twice as long as you need to is irresponsible." That had been my way of teaching residents, and they moved along, too. Nobody was careless or irresponsible, and there were always graded responsibilities, so a guy didn't say, "I always wanted to do an aorta," and he was put on one. He had to earn it, so we had very good residents both at Columbia and up at Tufts.

Arthur Blakemore, whom I hated and loved, was the most aggravating guy to work with, because he was single-minded about himself and his things. He was my chief at Columbia. McAllister was still in the army, and I was the beating boy; whenever anything went wrong it was my fault. When Arthur was away, I had his whole service. After I started to get on my own, I would schedule a major case, and he would call me at home the night before and say, "Ralph, I've got some time tomorrow and I need you." I would say, "But Arthur . . ." "That's all right," he would reply, "we'll work it out somehow, but I'll see you at 7:30, okay?" and hang up. He was not a fast operator and my wife, who was used to the Mayo Clinic speed demons, saw me come home the first day I helped him with a splenorenal, and I was ashen. I had stood there for the whole damned day. We had the ultraviolet lights, the goggles, and drapes on the backs of our heads like the French Foreign Legion. She said, "Are you sick?" and I said, "I am, of the Columbia Presbyterian."

But Blakemore was pioneering things, no question. One of the things he was doing was using electrocoagulation for aortic aneurysm, combining the nineteenth-century technique and direct current. He had someone at Bell Telephone develop about a 31-gauge copper wire with seven coats of a flexible varnish that was very durable. He would pass it about four inches at a time into the aneurysm until it was packed solidly. We saw large aneurysms, so you would be there damned near all day pumping the wire in.

One day there was a particular lot of stamps being auctioned that I wanted very much. McAllister had just joined the staff, so this was a newborn freedom. I was helping Art wire a big aneurysm. I called

Mac and said, "I have to be out of the hospital. Will you cover me? Art is up in the OR pumping wire," and Mac said, "Sure, I have nothing much to do." So I got the subway, went down to Times Square, went to the auction, stayed and got my lot, was delighted, got on the subway, came back, changed and went back in the OR, and Art was still pumping wire, never knowing that I had had a wonderful afternoon while he was still operating. But those were the good old days!

Dale: How long did you stay in New York?

Deterling: From December 1947 until June 1959.

Dale: Who was the chief when you went to New York?

Deterling: Humphreys was chief the whole time I was there, and he was very supportive. He and I got into hollering matches, because he was very traditional and I was always impatient that things should have been done yesterday. In about 1948 he made me director of surgical research. We had already developed a fair effort in graft evaluation, and that leads me back to our friend Charlie Hufnagel. Charlie and I had met in 1946 at the forum. He was an aggressive, charging sort of guy and was working with Bob Gross in the lab. I had a very good friend from Stanford that I could stay with, who was at the General, so I asked Charlie if I could visit him. This was in 1946 and he said sure. So I went over and watched what he was doing at Children's and the Harvard Medical School laboratories. He was in bad graces with Bob because he didn't totally go along with this nutrient business. Bob felt that you had to have living cells in homografts you put in, although I am sure he was aware that the living cells didn't continue to live when they were put in somebody else. Nevertheless, he, and later Henry Swan, supported the same concept. But Charlie was a maverick and said, "Hooey, that doesn't make any sense," and he was freezing them.

One of the things I wanted to do at Columbia was to get an experimental program going on vessel grafts. I was helped a lot by the New York Heart Association, which was looking for something to put its money into; all I needed was a phone call to get $5,000. Of course, in those days, $5,000 was something. Nowadays it doesn't pay postage. I got Mary Parsley, who was a Ph.D. tissue culture expert with a lab that became our vascular tissue culture lab. We had a number of publications that came out of her work in that. A fellow named Bonsley had just come on the scene and was working with me, and we went into the frozen graft thing with enthusiasm. So the first bank in New York was our frozen tissue bank. Later Ed Keefer started one at Cornell with our help.

Dale: John Madden told me that Cornell had the first frozen tissue bank.

Deterling: Well, that is what John would say because John and Wes were good friends and Wes was in the group at Cornell. It was close, but they went with the nutrient thing. They stayed with frozen, but they did freeze-dry. They were having troubles, because they would get the split that you can get with a thick aortic wall that has multiple tissues with different freezing points. This would cause a disruption. I visited Luyet at St. Louis University; he was a big expert in freezing. That is where I met Rollie Hanlon for the first time.

I came back with a keener appreciation of some of the problems with straight freezing and with freeze-drying. So we stuck with relatively slow freezing, which is only a millisecond's difference. We were able to store them for months in deep freeze and used quite a few of them.

In April of 1950, in New York, I put the first graft in a young guy with coarctation. In those days, we were wrapping aneurysms below the diaphragm and putting rubber bands on. Art Blakemore was getting the pulse pressure and Fitzpatrick, one of the residents, was running the transducers and stuff to measure it. I said, "This is all foolishness. We ought to just replace the damned things." I still have Art's note in this trembly, scrawly hand, "Ralph, don't do it, the sutures won't hold." That was my brush with doing the first aneurysm resection.

Actually, in 1951 there was a fair amount going on with aneurysms by Dubost in France. It was exciting, because I had met Dubost and we exchanged ideas. I would visit him in Paris, have dinner at his home, and so forth. It got to be a rather collegial group.

Dale: What sort of guy was Charles Dubost?

Deterling: He was a charger. He was a very articulate person, with a very nice wife. He spoke good English and was a bon vivant. He had quite an apartment on Boulevard Paris and was very often in the United States at some meeting or other, as was Clarence Crafoord. So I saw those two often and consequently felt a kinship to them. They did a good deal to warrant respect.

Dale: Did you ever run into Kunlin?

Deterling: Oh yes. Jean was underappreciated.

Dale: What sort of fellow was he?

Deterling: Very retiring, I thought, as was Fontaine, who was his chief.

Dale: René Fontaine?

Deterling: René was a fire-eater. He was in the resistance and there were a number of people he didn't like, including a good friend of mine, Haimovici. He carried likes and dislikes to the limit. I remember visiting him in his home in Strasbourg and heard him tell my son John, who was with me, about his forays into the German areas, wrecking trains and things. My boy was about sixteen and God, he never forgot René Fontaine.

I think René Fontaine, and Leriche before him, had the same pyramid relationships. They were top dog and you didn't forget it. I rather suspect that Kunlin suffered a bit from that. Personally, I didn't think he was a Dubost. I met Kunlin at a meeting. We sat and chatted, and there was no question that he had contributed very significantly to the first vein bypass.

Dale: How did you happen to move to Boston?

Deterling: In about 1954 there was a big fight at Columbia Presbyterian between the head of the hospital and Dean Rapoley. They were two guys with big egos. The whole department was told to draw out of the full-time system and become part-time, and I was a little disillusioned by that. Once you became one of the part-timers, you got more referrals than you had ever thought of. My income tripled in one year and I got so damned busy I said, "You know, this is not for me." I couldn't do anything else. Finally I paid Bonsley to cover weekends just to try and get a breather. I had four sons I wanted to spend time with. My wife was increasingly unhappy, although she never said anything. But after we got to Boston, she opened up and said how much she had hated the latter New York period. It had become crazy, so I looked about for escape with honor and I went down to Duke to be looked at by Bill Anlyan. I met everybody, but decided that wouldn't be for me even if they wanted me, because there were too many full professors and a former president of the university who was a surgical professor.

In 1957 or 1958 Tufts, which was in a mess, said, "Would you like to visit here?" Well, all the people I knew in Boston were Harvard people, so I said, "It would be interesting at least to see what Tufts is." When I got there, I found that Gardner Child had gotten into a fight with the trustees at the New England Center Hospital for an unfortunate reason. The trustees told me later that they respected Gardner, but his goals were too far ahead to support fiscally. He wanted a ward service and all this sort of thing.

Their first full-time professor was Stewey Welch, who had come in about 1947. He had picked highly qualified people for the specialties: Bill Sweet for neurosurgery, who later went back to the General; Leadbetter, who went to the General later for urology; Swenson, from Children's, to do the children's stuff; and a number of other heavy hitters. After Welch left, there was a little bit of time until Gardner Child came into his authority. There were such strong people in each specialty that they said, "We're not going to be under any other surgeon or chief, and that's all there is to that." Gardner, who came from one of the Halstedian institutions, didn't see that at all. There was a constant polite battle between the specialty chiefs and Gardner, and then the trustees on top of that, so he said, "The hell with all these guys." He went down to the City Hospital and took the whole university budget with him, which caused more trouble.

Dean Hamon called me and said, "You have a reputation for being able to talk blisters onto track teams; why don't you come on up here and see what you can do?" I thought, I need this like a hole in the head. But I wanted to get out of New York. I don't think Callow was particularly happy to have me come, because he and I had the same field. There were only three full-time guys in the department, Rheinlander doing chests and general, Allan doing vascular and general, and Harry Miller doing tumor work and general. I finally got the nod and came up. I met right away with Allan and I said, "I know you are worried to death, but it can either be warfare or cooperation. I need your help; you have tremendous referrals and we need cases for the residents. I am supposed to be half-time here and half-time at the City, and I can't possibly compete with you as a new guy in town. I want you to be my chief of vascular surgery here and feel relaxed," and he said "Okay." It was just that simple. Hal became the head of the thoracic service and Harry became chief of the oncology service and we had a department. The two hospitals hated each other because of what Gardner had done with the funding, so I brought half the funding back to the center and tried to develop joint rounds. That was something. I said, "We're going to meet together because there is a different patient population down there and there is a different esprit. You guys won't hurt for mixing."

Dale: This was at Boston City?

Deterling: Yes. The first few of these combined rounds met twice a month. We would go down there or to the other place and everybody would sit there quietly, with no discussion or anything. I would say, "When I'm with you guys, you can't stop talking. Now why don't you just tell us what you think about this case? I don't think such and such should have been done, what about you?" Then one guy would say, "Well, I was going to say that." I would say, "Well, why the hell didn't you, because we're interested in what you have to say." Finally it got to be a very popular thing, but it was inconvenient. After a couple of years we had some rotations of residents between the hospitals. There were two independent residencies. We had almost no trauma at the medical center but we had it coming out of our ears at the City. They had problems with pediatric surgery at the City, which was a BU service. I had them come up, and it worked very well because we offered them the things they didn't have, and the things we needed they had down there. It may have been five or eight years before we had enough impetus to have emergency service at our place. There was a good relationship.

Then Egdahl and I decided we ought to have the Boston VA. The Brigham had the West Roxbury VA. So the Dean's Committee declared it BU and Tufts. There was quite a fuss by Bill Sweet. He didn't want to leave, so there was a certain amount of friction there, but it didn't last long and it became a very, very worthwhile facility for the students. Then Mannick came in, and that was good. We hit it off. We used to actually have one luncheon a month at the Harvard Club to talk about mutual problems. Then Mannick went to Brigham.

Dale: Where did he come first?

Deterling: He became chief of BU after Egdahl was bumped upwards. He went to the Brigham later, where he is now.

Dale: How did you begin your relationship with the green journal, in which you were active for so many years?

Deterling: That goes back into the myths of history. Henry Haimovici was very committed to the International Society of Cardiovascular Surgery. I think it began as an outgrowth of the European Society and Malan and Arnulf and so forth. When he was alive, João Cid dos Santos would give some strength to that argument. But it was really an international thing that Henry pushed, and everybody agreed it should be done. The success was nailed down when people such as Frank Gerbode and Harry Shumacker supported the international society, because they were international themselves and knew these other people very well. It was good old boys getting together every two years at our congresses. Henry became the secretary general and Holman was the first president, if I recall. We had our first actual congress in Lisbon in 1953. We had an organizational meeting in 1951 in Atlantic City. That is when the *Journal of Angiology* became the official organ. Well, Henry got into a fight with Saul Samuels, who was on the editorial board. Saul was troublesome and started this International College of Angiology. Henry was right on top of that and said that they could have the *Journal of Angiology* as their official organ, and we became the *Journal of Cardiovascular Surgery*. That was decided in Munich in 1949.

Dale: That was started then, the green journal?

Deterling: A group at the Four Seasons Hotel in Munich—Malan, Arnulf, Henry, dos Santos, and me—agreed that this was a good idea. A friend of Malan, Oliaro, was going to publish the journal. His son, Alberto, is now the managing editor. They drew up a contract which initially said that the associate regional editor for Europe had to be approved by the publisher, so that lasted a little while. But every two years the contract was changed slightly until it was dropped. Then Malan had an untimely death sometime around

1958. He had a heart operation down in Houston, did well and then didn't do well, and died down there. Cleland came in as the next European editor. The co–chief editors essentially represented the European areas and the North American area included South America. I became the regional editor for North America.

Around 1961 we were meeting in Dublin, and there was a move underway to unseat Henry, because Gerbode and Shumacker and a number of others of the university type thought that he had become a little proprietary. You can see that happen in some societies. If a guy has been there too long, he feels that he is the only one who calls the shots. I was supportive of Henry, but he was never loved much at home. The point is that Henry was no longer secretary-general and I became that; then later he no longer was co–chief editor and I became that. Yet I managed to maintain my friendship with him, because he knew I wasn't trying to boot him to get the job myself.

Dale: What is your idea of the future of that journal?

Deterling: It is a tough journal to support fiscally, because you have such dynamism and backing of vascular surgery in the United States, and it has become so well controlled from the quality control standpoint that I think all the rest of the world appropriately looks at United States as a standard. The *Journal of Vascular Surgery* is the journal of the North American chapter, because the members were never told that they had to put their papers in the green journal. That is a good thing, because it helped the green journal survive. After the *Journal of Vascular Surgery* was formed, DeBakey himself said that he respected the green journal as providing a link between the different parts of the world, which it has done. But it is not a journal that is going to get huge numbers of subscriptions. I don't know if it ever went much beyond four or five thousand, and it is probably going to maintain that role, depending on the effectiveness of its management. That worried me so many times when I was editor that about every three or four years I would look at other publishers, and that second look still goes on

Dale: What are you doing now?

Deterling: My wife became ill about 1985. During the summer I detected what seemed to be signs of colonic cancer; she was up at

Lake Winnepesaukee with her mother. I hauled her right down. She also had a breast lump, so she had a double cancer. The colonic thing that I feared most was taken care of effectively. The breast cancer, however, had one node, I think in the axilla. She had radiation and chemo and was fine for about a year and a half. I started to take Fridays off when she got her blood count and her chemo; she recovered during the weekend. She died in 1986.

In October 1985 I stopped doing clinical work because it was coincidental with our medical center developing an insurance company. They wanted a risk management department, so I became the medical director of risk management, which I still am. From that time, they have grown exponentially and actually have a corporation called Liability Limited, which I don't have any part of, since I am chairman of the Board of Registration in Medicine. I didn't want any conflict of interest showing up in the *Boston Globe*.

Dale: Where is your office?

Deterling: My office is in an administrative building in the medical center, on the floor where the legal department and Liability Limited are located. It is very convenient, as it is three blocks from the Board of Registration.

Dale: Are you there every day?

Deterling: No. My secretary gave me a list of about fourteen committees and boards that I was on, and we got it down to Tuesdays and Wednesdays. And so I spend from about 7:30 or 8:00 a.m. until maybe 8:00 or 9:00 p.m. those two days. I'm the chairman of the Quality Assurance and Utilization Review Committees at the medical center, and also Medical Review chairman of the company that does review. So I'm more than busy; that's why I can't get to this wonderful book that I'm trying to get through. But I think that the work that I'm in now is rewarding enough in terms of its contributing something. This October I hope to drop my hospital work completely, and might have some more time to get into more fun.

James DeWeese

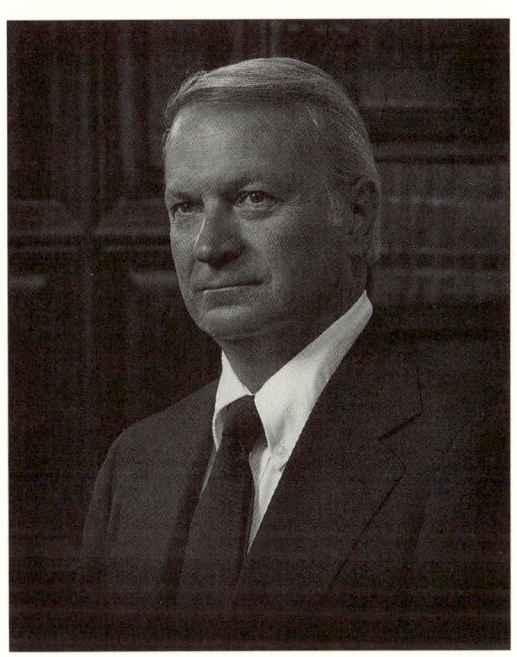

ACADEMICIAN, scholar, researcher, clinician, teacher, politician—Jim DeWeese is all of these. He and Andrew Dale were the closest of friends, and they had many overlapping interests—arterial bypass, venous disease, history, leadership, and golf. President of both vascular surgical societies, member of the American Board of Surgery, and secretary general of the International Society for Cardiovascular Surgery, DeWeese has been the respected guide for vascular surgery during the past few turbulent years. He was interviewed June 18, 1989.

Dale: Jim, tell me about your parents and where you were born.

DeWeese: I was born in Kent, Ohio, on April 5, 1925. My family came to Kent from southern Indiana two years before I was born. They had lived in Corydon and Byrneville. I had two brothers who were ten and twelve years older than I was, and a sister who was eight years older. My mother and father were teachers, and my father had become Harrison County superintendent of schools. During that period, he went to medical school at the University of Louisville. He then had an opportunity to come to Kent as the school physician, head of the Department of Physiology, director of physical education, and director of athletics. We lived across the street from the campus, and my brothers and sister and I went to the university school. I graduated in 1942 from Kent State High School.

Dale: What did you do in high school besides study? Did you play football?

DeWeese: It was a small school, so everyone did participate. I played on the football, basketball, and golf teams.

Dale: And then you went on to where?

DeWeese: I applied and got a scholarship to Harvard. I decided at that time I would try to go east, although the rest of the family had gone to midwestern schools. Dad really wasn't very happy that I was becoming an "easterner." Actually, I was only at Harvard for a year, from June 1942 to June 1943. During that time I received a year and a half of college credits. I applied and was accepted into the naval V-12 program. I was scheduled to return to Harvard in the program in June 1943. At that time, you could apply to medical school after completion of one and a half years of credit with the understanding that you would receive at least one more year of college credits. So in June 1943, on my way home from Boston, I stopped at the University of Rochester Medical School. I had interviews with Dean Whipple, Wallace Fenn, and George Packer Berry, who was the assistant dean and director of admissions. In a few days, I received a letter from the University of Rochester that I was accepted to medical school if I could complete the requirements. However, after returning home, I was chopping up the stump of a large chestnut tree in the front yard of the house when a chip flew up and hit me in the eye. It caused internal bleeding and a retinal detachment, so I spent the summer having operations at the Cleveland Clinic and being very quiet. The navy made periodic examinations of my eyes. In the meantime, I began taking some courses at Kent State College. During that year, I completed two and a half years of credit. Finally, the navy said that my eye had not improved enough for me to return to Harvard in the V-12 program, so I had to report to Great Lakes for induction into the navy. When Dr. Berry heard that this was going to happen, he called and said, "You'd better get up here to Rochester. I haven't lost anybody that I accepted to Rochester, and you're the only one left. So damn it, get up here, and we will get you into a school." I worked in the anatomy department and was classified as a student. Finally, I started in the fall of 1944 at the University of Rochester.

Dale: In the V-12 program?

DeWeese: No, when I had gone to Great Lakes I received a discharge from the service for medical reasons.

Dale: How did you decide to become a doctor? Because of your father?

DeWeese: I'm sure that had a lot to do with it, although my father had always told us, "Oh, you don't want to be a doctor—see how busy you are." My father was extremely busy. His activities at the college gradually decreased through the years; he finally ended up being the school physician, but while he was relinquishing these other activities he also had a busy general practice. He saw patients in the front room of our house, which had been turned into an office. Patients would sit in the living room, or they would come in and have a bite to eat with us while waiting. My mother, on the other hand, had told all of us, "You are capable of doing whatever you want to do." Despite the fact that Dad did not encourage any of us to go into medicine, my two older brothers became physicians, and my sister married a surgeon. My older brother, Bill, with whom I was particularly close, was becoming a surgeon, so there was never any question in my mind about what I was going to do from the time I was in high school.

Dale: How did he happen to be called Bill rather than his actual name of Marion?

DeWeese: His name is Marion Spencer DeWeese, but his older brother had a doll by the name of Bill, and when he saw the baby he said, "Oh, there's Billy." It was Bill from then on.

Dale: Getting back to Rochester, where you went to medical school—you entered in September 1944, which was the same time that I arrived as an intern.

DeWeese: During my first two years of medical school we were there continuously, but then the war ended and they gave us a summer vacation in 1946. I then returned in September 1946 to take a one-year student fellowship in pathology and bacteriology. I was invited to do this by George Packer Berry, who was chairman of bacteriology. It gave me an opportunity to do some research and also assist in teaching the bacteriology course. Dr. Berry left shortly after that to become dean of the medical school at Harvard.

Dale: What sort of man was he?

DeWeese: He was very brusque, but an excellent teacher. He made a great point of trying to stimulate young physicians, but he was best known for his organizational abilities.

Dale: What were your impressions of Nobel prizewinner Dr. George Whipple?

DeWeese: George Hoyt Whipple won his Nobel Prize for recognizing the cause of pernicious anemia and demonstrating that it could be treated successfully with liver extracts and vitamin B_{12}. He was a very quiet, staid downeasterner who had a gentle sense of humor. He was best known by the students for his weekly quizzes, during which everyone would sit around on stools in the big laboratory while he would sit in the middle of the group. He carried a list of the names of the students in the class, and after he would pick out a name, he would look over his glasses at you and ask a question concerning pathology. No one ever knew when the question would come, which prompted extensive preparation by each student for each class. He also usually gave the weekly pathologic demonstrations of the autopsy cases of the week, which were held in the autopsy room.

Dr. Whipple kept things very simple. He and George Eastman

were the ones who built the University of Rochester Medical School. Eastman had insisted that it be built like a factory, without all the fluff. It was a plain building, and inside the building, they left all the corridors and laboratories with just bricks for the wall. They wanted to put all of the money into building space and laboratories. It was years before the gray brick on the walls of the medical school was finally painted.

Dale: As I remember, it was called "late penitentiary style." Was Dr. Whipple still there when you were a resident in surgery?

DeWeese: Dr. Whipple was still there, but Bill Hawkins was the chief of surgical pathology.

Dale: I remember Dr. Whipple participating while Bill Hawkins ran the show. He acted like another student. He had that little old binocular microscope that was beat-up but that still enabled him to make remarkable observations. After the year as a fellow, you finished your last two years?

DeWeese: Yes, and I graduated in 1949.

Dale: And then you went into the surgical residency?

DeWeese: Yes. At that time, we didn't have a matching program. You interviewed in many places, and then the programs would send telegrams of acceptance to you in the late evening, which would be delivered to us in the large waiting room of Strong Memorial Hospital. The students would all gather there; each of us was expected to respond that night as to whether we would accept their program. I had interviewed, along with my brother, at Michigan, and my family was hoping I would return to the Midwest. I had also interviewed at Cleveland Western Reserve. They interviewed the students at Western Reserve by having the members of the staff sit at a big table, and you would go in and sit with them while they asked you questions. Dr. Holden's question to me was, "Well, I see you had an eye injury. Do you think this will affect your ability to be a surgeon?" I was aghast; no one had asked such a personal question in any of my other interviews, so the only thing I could think of was that I had noticed that when I was playing golf, I seemed to have depth perception enough to know where the hole was and where the ball was, so I said, "Well, it hasn't affected my ability to play golf." There was some snickering in the room, but Dr. Holden was a very stern man, and he just kind of looked at me. I was a visiting professor back there two years ago, and it was a day when they were interviewing students again. Dr. Holden had retired by then, but on Saturday mornings he attended grand rounds, just as he did when he was chairman. I was able to repeat the story of my interview, and I believe this time he did smile.

I was still quite interested in the University of Rochester, primarily because of Earle Mahoney. He was not the chairman, but to many of us he was the leader of the department. Dr. Mahoney had taken an interest in me during medical school. I had given a student seminar on congenital heart disease and had made pictures of the defects from Maude Abbott's book that very much impressed Dr. Samuel Clawson, who was chairman of the Department of Pediatrics. Apparently he had told Earle Mahoney about the conference. At that time Dr. Mahoney was just getting things started with cardiac surgery, always doing the first of the new operations. I never called him Earle; I never called him anything other than Dr. Mahoney.

As an aside, it is interesting that, earlier on, Dr. Clawson had not been as supportive of surgery. Dr. Mahoney actually had to do the first successful ligation of a patent ductus while Dr. Clawson was out of town. Dr. Max Garber, one of the younger pediatricians, found the case, they sneaked him up to the OR, and Dr. Mahoney performed a successful operation. That would have been in 1944 or 1945.

Dr. Mahoney stayed in his office the night of the intern selections to talk to people if they had any further questions or decided what they wanted to do. We were milling around this large room about eleven o'clock at night, and I had had some acceptances, including Michigan, Chicago, and Western Reserve. We all suspected that Hopkins was going to take one or two of us because Jim Maloney was there at the time and was doing an excellent job. The top man in our class, Bill Robertson, received an acceptance telegram from Hopkins, but had already decided to go into pediatrics. The second man in our class was also accepted, and he did call Hopkins and accept them. Bill Robertson had told them, "I'm not coming—I'm going into pediatrics—but Jim DeWeese and another of the applicants

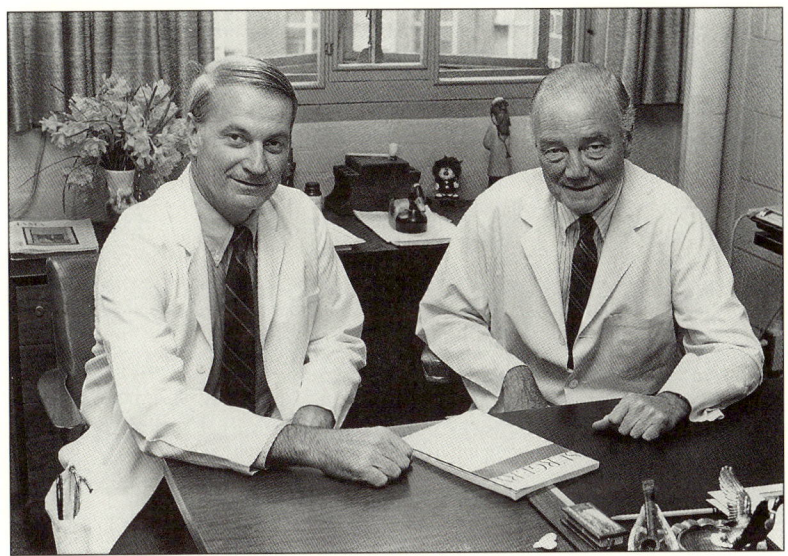

Jim with Earle Mahoney in Rochester, 1971.

from here haven't signed up yet." They indicated that one of us should call back. By then I had decided that I wanted to go to Rochester, so Fred Golomb called and accepted Hopkins, and I told Dr. Mahoney that I wanted to stay in Rochester.

Dale: John Morton was chairman of the department then. What were your impressions of him?

DeWeese: Dr. Morton was a gentle yet very particular person. At that stage, he was certainly a person we all admired for what he had accomplished. His lectures were outstanding. Those were days when attending surgeons gave a lecture every week; I still have notes and remember well the talks that they gave. I think it is a shame that this is no longer carried out, because it is the only opportunity for many students and residents to hear the professors who are giving talks in many other places. Frequently, students and residents have contact with the leaders in surgery on a one-to-one basis only in the operating room or at conferences. Dr. Morton was an excellent teacher. In the operating room, he taught by first assisting; he had gotten to the stage where he did not do many of his own operations, but we all learned from him and considered him an outstanding individual.

Dale: What about Merle Scott?

DeWeese: He had more of a flair; he had shown evidence, both as a part-time and full-time surgeon at the university, of continuing to be interested in the newer things. At that time, he was interested in the esophagus and achalasia and was doing the new procedures being performed at that time. He was also very interested in peripheral vascular disease and had established a constant temperature room to study the effects of sympathectomy or epidural and spinal anesthesias for dilating the peripheral blood vessels and increasing the temperature of the feet. He and Dr. Morton thought they were able to ascertain which patients might respond to a sympathectomy by measuring the effect of a paravertebral block on the skin temperature of the feet. Lumbar sympathectomy was pretty much the only vascular operation performed at that time. It meant, however, that all of the vascular problems were referred to surgery, so that as soon as direct vascular reconstructions were possible in the 1950s, the cases were already coming to the surgeons for treatment. He and Dr. Mahoney provided the impetus to proceed with the new areas of surgery at the University of Rochester and Strong Memorial Hospital.

Dale: My recollection is that when Merle Scott was chairman of the department, he agreed to sponsor a policy of sympathectomy for all patients who were candidates, and a large number were done under that program before it was recognized that it was essentially useless—correct?

DeWeese: That's true. Every patient with gangrene or other evidence of severe peripheral vascular disease had an emergency sympathectomy the day of admission to the hospital. It is interesting that we did a similar type of study when Dr. Rob came to Strong. We took all stroke cases from the emergency room to the operating room and explored them for carotid occlusion and did carotid endarterectomy if there was a lesion. That also proved to be the wrong way of managing patients.

Another excellent teacher at Strong Memorial Hospital in the early phases of my training was Herm Pearse, who had pretty much retired during my senior years of training. He was in charge of the training program, however, and as the fifth year approached, he asked me, "Well, are you going back to Kent, Ohio, to practice?" I said, "No, I am going to stay on and try to do the things that Dr. Mahoney is doing." Dr. Mahoney was really my mentor at that time. On the other hand, Merle Scott gave both Sy Schwartz, who finished a year after me, and me the opportunity to stay on in the Department of Surgery for at least one year after finishing residency. This was in 1956.

Dale: Was there a hiatus when you were in the service?

DeWeese: Yes, I was in the army from 1952 to 1954. I was assigned to Germany and later to Carlisle Barracks in Pennsylvania.

Dale: So then you had your two years?

DeWeese: Two years during which time many things were getting started in both vascular and cardiac surgery. You were in the laboratory as a young professor, and Dr. Mahoney was still very active in the clinical development of cardiac surgery as well as doing some laboratory research on arterial and venous procedures.

Dale: Was Merle Scott chief at the time?

DeWeese: Yes, Merle was instrumental in making things happen at Rochester. He initiated the process of allowing the senior residents interested in research and an academic future to spend a year as a junior attending surgeon in the laboratory and also doing clinical surgery. Mike Radakovich, you, me, and later Sy Schwartz took this opportunity.

Dale: Let's talk a little bit about your laboratory experience.

DeWeese: My first year was primarily working with a project that Mahoney and Mavor had initiated. They were working on hypothermia and the effect of fibrillation and then defibrillation of the heart with potassium. The defibrillators at that time were not always effective; Mahoney and Mavor demonstrated that potassium could be used to stop the heart of hypothermic animals, later dogs, and that then, with gentle massage, the heart could be revived. I know you went on and carried this out on a patient as an emergency at one time, which was worthy of a clinical report. During that time, electric defibrillators became better, but there was still an impetus to continue to do some basic evaluation of the effect of hypothermia on cardiac metabolism, which was the subject of my first experiments.

In addition, I continued an interest in the development of grafts for vascular surgery. When Dr. Frank Bauer was a senior resident and I was the associate resident in general surgery, we had started a homograft bank. We would get permission to obtain arteries at autopsies and we would then place them in antibiotic solution for a brief period, freeze-dry them, and store them at −30°. They could then be reconstituted with saline for human use.

It was an exciting period. People frequently ask me, "If you wanted to be a vascular or cardiac surgeon, why didn't you go somewhere else to learn it?" The answer was simple. Everyone was going to meetings and coming back and trying something new. We would copy others' experiences in some cases, but we were also developing our own techniques and presenting them at meetings. There was no place to go that was doing much more than we were at that particular time.

Dale: What is the policy for the residents today? Do they have any specific time in the laboratory?

DeWeese: Through the early years, it was certainly the feeling of younger people, starting with you, Dr. Schwartz, and me, that it was very important that the residents spend a year in the laboratory after their second year of general surgical residency. There finally came a time, however, when it was decided that we would try it the other way and only have the individuals who really wanted to do it stay for one or even two years in the laboratory after their second or third year of residency.

Dale: Let's talk a little bit about the vascular societies in which you have taken great interest and played a great part. What has been the role of the vascular societies through the years?

DeWeese: My first involvement with the vascular societies was attending the meetings—I was influenced to do so by Dr. Mahoney, you, and, later, Dr. Rob. I know that, from the late 1950s through the present time, there have been very few years that members of our group have not had at least one paper on the program of both the Society for Vascular Surgery [SVS] and the North American Chapter of the International Society for Cardiovascular Surgery [NA/ISCVS]. All of our group were interested in these young societies. Morton, Scott, and Pearse were charter members of the SVS and also of the ISCVS, so the idea of the importance of these societies was inbred in me. After I started going to the meetings, I attended them yearly. My first organizational involvement occurred after I had been appointed to a committee with Dr. Blaisdell and Dr. Foster of the Inter-Society Commission on Heart Disease Resources. I was asked to chair the committee and answer the question: "What are the optimal resources for the treatment of patients with vascular disease?" The first report was completed in 1971. The committee came up with some recommendations, the major one being that the most important resource for vascular surgery was a well-trained vascular surgeon. In the paper, we made a recommendation that the American Board of Surgery and the American Board of Thoracic Surgery might find it appropriate to find the means to certify well-trained vascular surgeons, since this would be the most important part of providing the optimal management of the patients. We had gotten input from fifty of the most active and well-known vascular surgeons in the country at that time, and their comments made it easier for us to prepare the document. It was really a combination of many people's ideas. We submitted the paper for presentation to both of the societies, and it was accepted for presentation by the ISCVS. Although the report was not uniformly appreciated, at least it was what was needed at the time. I think as a result of my work on this project and my presentation at the vascular meeting at Monterey, I was elected secretary of the Society for Vascular Surgery. I have been involved as an officer of either one or both of the societies and therefore as a member of the joint councils of the two societies almost constantly since then, so I have had the opportunity of living with them and growing up with them through the years.

Dale: When and how did the vascular societies cease to be completely honorary and become activist?

DeWeese: I think it was a year or two before I was president of the Society for Vascular Surgery. However, as the secretary of the society, I remember finding a letter in the files from one of the previous presidents to one of the previous secretaries, stating that he did not think it a good idea that the society take part in advocating that vascular surgeons be credentialed, since the Society for Vascular Surgery was really an honorary society.

Dale: As I remember it, there was considerable discussion as to whether the society should continue as an honorary one or if they should become active. They are now active.

DeWeese: This has been a slow transition, particularly for the Society for Vascular Surgery. The ISCVS was more quick to become activist. It is interesting that some of the leaders who were initially slow to accept activism as the responsibility of the societies have now become leaders in activism.

Dale: Jim, tell me about your relationship to Charles Rob.

DeWeese: I guess I have always been a team player, and I always supported whoever was chairman of the department. At the time Dr. Rob came, I was doing much of what vascular surgery was being done at the university, since you had already left. I remember being told by someone that one of the orthopedic surgeons had told him, wasn't it too bad that I was through doing vascular surgery since Dr. Rob was joining the faculty. I went to the man who started the rumor and carefully explained to him that, as far as I was concerned, this was the best thing that could happen to me, because I felt Dr. Rob would come in and attract new patients and referrals and probably not take many of my referrals away. Even more important, he would recognize the need for getting more operating room time and space for the development of vascular surgery, and I thought it would be the best thing.

Dale: This was before he arrived. How did it work?

DeWeese: It worked out just that way. Once it was obvious to Dr. Rob that I was a team player, he gave me the opportunity to help build the department and the ability for me to grow. I remember that his advice to me at one point was, "Jim, what you need to do is find a young man about fifteen years younger than you and let him be your 'sucker.'" It was then that I realized that I myself was Dr. Rob's "sucker" at Rochester. He is just thirteen years older than I am.

Dale: What was the main thrust of Charles Rob's chairmanship?

DeWeese: He provided much stature to the department because of the things that he had accomplished and because of his extraordinary ability to speak and to teach. He was an excellent surgeon, an innovator, yet he was still able to learn from others to provide improved techniques for the management of vascular patients.

I think one of Dr. Rob's contributions, and one that was particularly advantageous to me, was that he allowed us to develop a Division of Cardiothoracic Surgery. It was at a time when there never seemed to be enough operating time or space for new programs, and frequently the chairman of surgery was hesitant to support them. Dr. Rob wrote a letter to Dr. Mahoney before he came to assure him that he recognized Dr. Mahoney's contributions in cardiac surgery and did not intend to interfere with him, except possibly with "coronary artery surgery." He also said when he came he would do thoracic aneurysms. He did thoracic aortic aneurysms, and I believe he did one ventricular aneurysm. However, he allowed cardiac surgery to develop. Dr. Mahoney and I began a cardiothoracic training program in 1972. One of Dr. Rob's last official acts was to make me chairman of a new Division of Cardiothoracic Surgery.

Dale: Did Charles do general surgery as well as vascular?

DeWeese: Superbly. It was only a small part of his practice, but he would lay it out like Earle Mahoney and Herm Pearse, who I believe were mentors for both you and me. He demonstrated a beautiful anatomic approach to all operations.

Dale: Then Bill Drucker came on as chairman?

DeWeese: Dr. Drucker came July 1, 1977. I was also able to work with Dr. Drucker very well.

Dale: What did Bill Drucker bring with him? What was his thrust?

DeWeese: He brought a renewed interest in teaching, particularly of medical students. He provided in the department something that we had missed a little prior to his arrival. He had a very good relationship with the students and was named Teacher of the Year for two or three years. During the years he was there, he inspired a lot of young students to go into surgery. In addition, he provided a lot of help to the residents in their research activities and in seeking experience in other research programs. He also allowed the development of both the Vascular Section and the Division of Cardiothoracic Surgery.

During those years, I was very involved nationally with the vascular societies, and they were continuing to work toward the accreditation of vascular surgical training programs and the certification of vascular surgeons. We had ups and downs and mixed support from the general surgical community during those years. Finally, when Bill Blaisdell was a member of the American Board of Surgery (ABS) and the Residency Review Committee (RRC), they agreed to the accreditation of vascular surgical training programs and the certification of vascular surgeons. However, the parent bodies of these two organizations disapproved it. He reported to our joint council meeting that the only thing that some members of the board could recommend was for us to accredit programs ourselves. Therefore, the joint vascular societies did start to accredit programs themselves, and for three years did just that. When finally the Residency Review Committee, with the permission of the ACGME [Accreditation Council for Graduate Medical Education], began to accredit official residency training programs in vascular surgery in 1984, Dr. Drucker was very helpful to us in obtaining an approved program. One of his last actions was to allow a separate section of vascular surgery to be formed within the Department of Surgery in 1987. I became chief during that time, so I was chief of both vascular and cardiothoracic surgery.

Dale: Does it appear to you that vascular surgery has now become rather standardized, with little room for technical improvement?

DeWeese: No, it does not. I am now on the Board of Surgery and chairman of the vascular committee. It is amazing to us how difficult it is to make a question that seven of us, who all are vascular surgeons, can agree upon as having one correct answer. This also applies to what technique should be used for a particular operation. There is still not a standardized approach to how to perform many operations. I do not believe that the same standard approach can be used for all abdominal aneurysmectomies.

Dale: Well, standardized along with standard variations is what I am asking, which is just what a young man told me this morning in talking about standardization.

DeWeese: Yes. Fortunately, much of vascular surgery is standardized, but I would still hope that technical improvements in the future would make it better.

Harry Hubert Grayson Eastcott

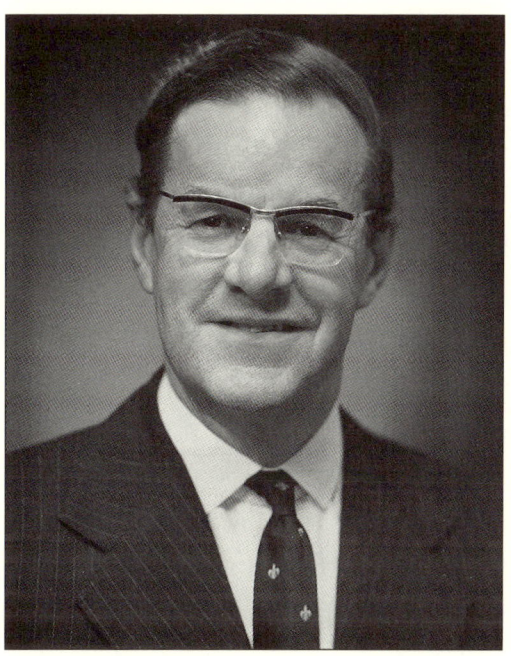

"FELIX" EASTCOTT seems to have been forever on center stage in the world of vascular surgery. Although his home base is in London, he is a familiar figure the world over. He has published many articles, chapters, and books, and his numerous visiting professorships in universities all over the world explain his wide group of friends. Urbane, witty, and friendly, Eastcott is an encyclopedia of knowledge. His career includes not only surgical experience, but administrative and teaching responsibilities allowed to few surgeons.

Eastcott's early carotid repair showed him to be a rising star. Later, high positions in the Royal College of Surgeons confirmed his early promise. It is very important when a person leads a rapidly evolving field; it is more so when contributions continue over several decades. Eastcott remains bright and active, spirited and interesting, still the fabled traveler. He was interviewed January 19, 1987.

Dale: What was your early background?

Eastcott: I was born in 1917 in Montreal, where my father, a West Country Englishman, was working as a civil engineer with the Canadian Pacific Railroad, so I may be called a citizen of both countries. My mother, also a Plymouth woman, accompanied him in his railcar on many distant trips to inspect the lines and construct new ones. During the long evenings the men often played cards. My mother, too, became an expert at poker, far surpassing my father as a card player. In 1922 the family returned to Plymouth, England, moving to London in 1929 during the Great Depression.

Dale: Did you have an unusual record in high school?

Eastcott: I did attend good schools—Plymouth Hoe Grammar, Enfield Preparatory, and the Latymer School in north London. I was an interested but rather lazy boy until about fifteen years of age, but recovered in time to attain three distinctions in languages by seventeen and a couple of scholarships that enabled me to convert to science at sixth form level and move on to my preclinical study at St. Mary's Hospital Medical School. There I was fortunate to obtain the Primary Certificate of the Royal College of Surgeons of England while still an undergraduate, as one could in those days.

The war began for us in 1939, at which time a dozen of us clinical students were assigned to the Hammersmith Hospital, where we filled sandbags around the operating room and later helped in the care of the air raid casualties of the first two big blitzes of 1940 and 1941. The first research on crush kidney arose out of those patients who had been pinned under fallen masonry for many hours before rescue. All this was good for our clinical education, and we also had some really good teachers, most of whom were, or would soon become, household names in medicine—men such as Paul Wood, John McMichael, Sharpey Schafer, and Eric Bywaters. I qualified in 1941 (my last oral examination, in gynecology, took place during an air raid, and the examiner was in Royal Air Force uniform and wearing pilot's wings). Somehow I reached honors in surgery, and was soon appointed to be one of Professor Grey Turner's house surgeons, so I was able to remain at the Hammersmith. During this time my chief himself became a surgical patient, with an obstructed ectopic pelvic kidney which had to be removed between raids by his old friend, the famous Gordon Taylor, then a surgeon rear admiral. I remember, during a brief etiquette visit to my convalescent chief, shyly asking him if he was getting over his operation, and his reply, "No, Eastcott, I'm benefiting from it!" It was during that time that I first met Gordon Taylor, who strongly advised me to join the Royal Navy rather than the Army Medical Corps; he had served in both in two wars and much preferred the navy.

Dale: Was there time for any extracurricular activities?

Eastcott: During the last years of peace, most Saturday afternoons were spent on the rugger field. At night I played the tenor saxophone in the students' band. It was during that time at Hammersmith that I found and later married Bobbie, who was a theater (OR) nurse for Grey Turner's unit. Incidentally, she never saw me operate (perhaps just as well) until the last case, a carotid endarterectomy, done at the time of my retirement from the hospital service.

Dale: Who were your other teachers?

Eastcott: Sir Zachary Cope was one of my surgical godfathers. Early on, he helped me to decide what to do with myself, and later he again supported me for the staff appointment at St. Mary's. A few years after this, in 1960, when I still wasn't really set on a career, he remarked, "Eastcott, that's interesting work you're doing on the arteries." I replied, "Thank you, sir. You've helped me get on with it." Cope responded, "I want you to write a book about it." So I did that, and my affairs prospered from then on.

Dale: What did you do during the remainder of the war?

Eastcott: I did a chest residency under Sir Thomas Holmes Sellors and Vernon Thompson, and then a spell in general surgery at King Edward VII Hospital at Windsor. But by then I wanted to get onto active duty, so I volunteered for the Royal Navy in 1943. I served at first in naval air stations in Britain, and later on carriers in the Pacific and Australia. It was a good exposure to the wider world of life outside medicine and involved a lot of travel. Also I learned to fly, as I'd always wanted to. It was a great experience.

Dale: Do you still fly?

Eastcott: Not now. I went on sporadically for about twelve years after the war, but then my four daughters and other responsibilities decided me to give it up as being a damn foolishness for an amateur in the busy skies 'round London. But I still love to fly as a passenger, and happily get a good deal of that.

Dale: What happened after the war ended?

Eastcott: After demobilization several of us attended a tutorial course that Ronald Raven used to give, mostly for ex-service candidates for the final FRCS [Fellow of the Royal College of Surgeons]. I passed the exam and returned to St. Mary's, working under Arthur Dickson Wright, a brilliant operator in just about every field of surgery. From him one learned the highest technical standards, though he was an absolute terror in the operating room. Helping him with aortic coarctations and other early peripheral vascular cases stimulated my interest in what already seemed a promising specialty. Then I had an inspiring year with Sir Arthur Porritt, whose qualities of character and leadership have always made him a role model to me. It was he who arranged for me to go to the United States for a unique year of graduate education at Harvard Medical School and the Peter Bent Brigham Hospital in Boston. There I worked in Dr. Francis Moore's unit, with Charles Hufnagel on artificial heart valves and frozen arterial homografts, and with David Hume, who was about to begin his great work on kidney transplants.

Dale: What other surgeons did you meet in Boston?

Eastcott: There were many, each with a message of real value for my professional improvement. Francis Moore taught me to respect the scientific method, Bert Dunphy opened up new horizons in clinical surgery, and Carl Walter showed me the importance of bio-

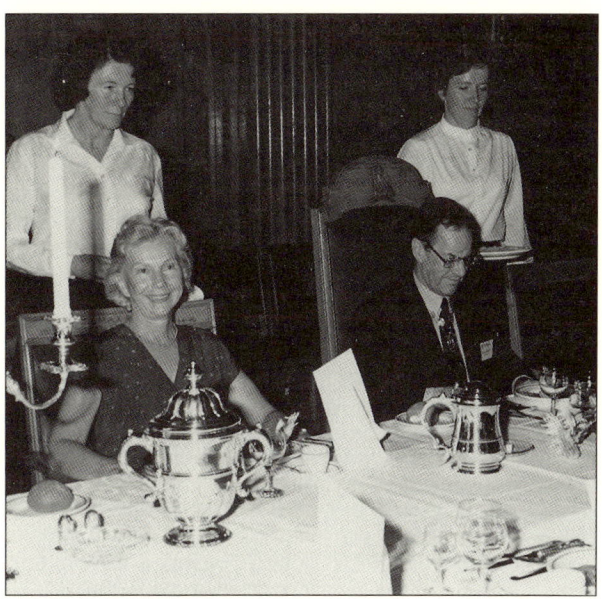

Corrine Dale and Eastcott in London

engineering know-how. All three became our lifelong friends, and their families, too. I did also meet other great men who worked at hospitals other than the Brigham. Richard Cattell at the Lahey Clinic made a third-time bile repair duct look so easy; we later came to know him socially, too, through some good mutual friends. I first met Robert Linton in the ocean surf at Atlantic City. I had become tired and hot during a long afternoon at the American College of Surgeons Clinical Congress, which in those days visited there every third year. There in the ocean I saw what looked like a billiard ball or perhaps a dolphin bobbing up and down between the waves, but it was Dr. Linton's completely bald head. He came up out of the water and said something like, "Hi there, you're from England, aren't you?" We had a lively talk there between the breakers.

Dale: Did you meet John Homans?

Eastcott: Yes, I remember him very well. He used to limp in on his cane to Brigham Grand Rounds and say, "The worst thing I ever did was to describe Homans' sign."

Dale: Then you returned to London?

Eastcott: Yes, that was in the fall of 1950, when Charles Rob, I suspect at the suggestion of Sir Arthur Porritt, suggested that I apply for the post of assistant director of the surgical unit at St. Mary's Hospital in London, where he had just been appointed to the chair when Professor C. A. Pannett retired. The strength and informality of Charles Rob's guidance over the next four years proved invaluable to my progress in general surgery, as well as in the early clinical application of my research work in arterial grafting. During our close association we recorded several first-time operations, the best known of which was the repair of the internal carotid artery for atherosclerotic stenosis associated with transient ischemic attacks. It is safe to say that, without the inspiration of Sir George Pickering and the confident support of Charles Rob, I would never have dared to clamp that woman's carotid on May 19, 1954.

Dale: So that was your first one?

Eastcott: My very first carotid operation was done on a dog, and it was Dave Hume, in the Harvard surgical lab, who showed me how to do it. My first human carotid resection was in 1952, when I resected part of the common carotid in an old gentleman of eighty-two. It had become densely adherent to a mass of secondary carcinomatous lymph nodes. The anastomosis was completed in twenty minutes, and the patient did well. The operation for stenosis that you mentioned took place on a day when we had with us a distinguished group of visiting American surgeons, among whom were Mike DeBakey and Jack Wylie, who is reported to have suggested an endarterectomy, as Charles Rob also had. I felt, since my experience at that time was practically limited to resection and repair, that I had better do that than embark on another method of which I had a much smaller experience. At any rate, the operation went smoothly, the anastomosis remained patent, and the patient lived another twenty years to die at age eighty-six of a heart problem. There followed, many years after this operation, an interesting sequel, now the basis of a warm personal reminiscence. One of the visitors on the day in question had taken a color photograph of the operative scene. About twenty years later, the slide was shown by Jesse Thompson in his address to the Society for Vascular Surgery. He revealed that the photographer had been George Dunlop, who many years later in 1977 became the president of the American College of Surgeons and presented me with my certificate as Honorary Fellow of the College.

Dale: How long did you continue to do general surgery?

Eastcott: I still do a bit. I like to do breast work and hernias, or an emergency gastrectomy or obstruction in a vascular patient.

Dale: At the height of your career, what percent of your work was in the vascular field?

Eastcott: I don't really know when the height of my career occurred. My biggest years of operating were in the late sixties and early seventies, when I was doing a lot of general surgery. Then I became increasingly involved with the Royal College of Surgeons and the time for clinical work became more restricted. Soon there was time only for vascular work, so that it came to be about 85 percent of my operations from then on.

Dale: You travel a great deal. How much of the time are you in London?

Eastcott: I am no longer traveling as much. I've only been to America once this year. In the past, it could be five or six times.

Dale: Did you ever travel by ship, or always by plane?

Eastcott: Only three times by ship. In 1949, with Bobbie and the first two little girls, I went over by sea. There were no transatlantic planes then. The second time was in 1953, when Charles Rob released me for a month's naval reserve training, during which I crossed to Norfolk, Virginia, in an aircraft carrier. They gave us shore leave there, so I was able to go up to Boston by rail and see some old Brigham friends and find out what had been happening. The last time was in October 1982, the day after that last carotid at St. Mary's, when Bobbie and I decided to make a sort of retirement cruise and sailed from Southampton on the *Queen Elizabeth II* for New York. There were several old friends aboard, including Rodney and Sue Smith. Rodney and I had been very close during some difficult times at the College during his presidency, when the government of the day had been more than usually tough with the doctors.

Dale: When did you become the president of the Royal College of Surgeons?

Eastcott: I had been vice president for two years, and it was during that 1982 visit to the States that I found myself, as first reserve, in the chief office. One morning soon after we had arrived in Chicago for your College Congress, there came a phone call from London. It was Ronnie Johnson-Gilbert, the secretary of the Royal College, with some dreadful news. I said, "Is it about Alan?" He said, "Yes, they have little hope of his recovery." Sir Alan Parks was a wonderful person, a leader of the profession, and a fine president. He was dying after cardiac surgery for a massive myocardial infarct. So I became acting president for a few weeks while they sorted things out. Eventually, thank goodness, we elected Geoff Slaney, which was a great relief to everyone, especially me.

Dale: What is the future of vascular surgery?

Eastcott: I believe it may diminish. For one thing, the noninvasive tests and the interventional radiologists will, between them, probably reduce the number of open operations needed for occlusive disease. Though aneurysms, carotid problems, and vascular trauma should continue, I suspect that most other conditions may decline in response to preventive measures that are already widely accepted by the public. Already, we see the effects of this in advanced countries such as the United States, Australia, and Finland, where previously very high prevalence and mortality figures are now subsiding. Vascular surgery certainly won't disappear, but it may be less common than it is today.

Dale: What about criticism that too much carotid surgery is being done, more so in the States than in Great Britain?

Eastcott: That's something that must be decided by science, not by a hunch. It needs a controlled trial. It's good to know that such a trial is already being organized in North America by Dr. Henry Barnett. We already have one underway in Britain that now includes many other European countries and is in its fifth year, though ours was designed for a "gray area" and deals only with those patients in whom the decision for or against surgery is not clear. This, as you will know, is a larger group in Europe than in the United States. We could not mount a trial in which present clinical indications appear clearly to favor operation or nonoperative treatment.

Dale: Is it similar to the situation in coronary artery bypass surgery?

Eastcott: Yes, it is, though coronary surgery relieves symptoms;

carotid endarterectomy only tries to prevent something that may or may not happen without it. There is, of course, a difference in the general approach to patient management in our two countries. In the States, if something seems to be needed, it gets done one way or another. In Britain, we are more conservative, particularly if it comes to spending money. Yet cost is not the main constraint in carotid surgery, because it's not that expensive. It's a simple operation that can be done in any unit equipped for vascular surgery.

Dale: Did the limitation on animal surgery influence the development of vascular surgery in Britain?

Eastcott: Well, yes, I suppose it helped in some ways, because instead of having to learn in the dog lab, we had the opportunity to treat many patients. So several of us younger surgeons could do these new operations and develop our methods in approved hospital practice.

Dale: What of the future of today's young men and women?

Eastcott: They're able, widely and well trained. But the field is highly competitive in Britain. The prospects for even the best of them are uncertain in terms of waiting so long for an opportunity of doing on their own what they have learned. I became a consultant early, at age thirty-two. But the average now is thirty-seven to forty years old. It has been proposed that a "subconsultant grade" should be created to create more vacancies, though so far our conservatism has resisted that idea. The solution is not clear, but something must be done attract the better quality young people and to sustain their confidence for the future.

Dale: Tell me more about Charles Rob.

Eastcott: Charles did more for me personally than almost anyone, with the exception of Lord Porritt and Sir Zachary Cope. He fostered my career by helping me overcome some gaps in my surgical training. He taught me how to do pancreatectomy, esophagectomy, and other operations that I had either not seen or had only assisted with. He made a major surgeon of me. I was the one who deputized for him when he needed to be away, which was often. Charles helped me get started in vascular surgery. He had done quite a bit during his war service, and knew a lot about the clinical side. The reconstructive work we learned together.

Dale: One more question before we conclude—did you know Mike DeBakey?

Eastcott: I first met him in 1949 outside the Hilton in Chicago, to which I had driven one thousand miles overnight from Boston with Charlie Hufnagel and some others, including the owner of the car, Tom Donovan. Charlie introduced me to Mike, who paused with interest and inquired, "How is Sir Russell Brock?" We had a most cordial conversation. I took to him at once and we have been friends ever since. There has been nothing but warmth and kindness from him in all the years I've known him, though he certainly does scare me silly when he drives me in his Maserati.

Sterling Edwards

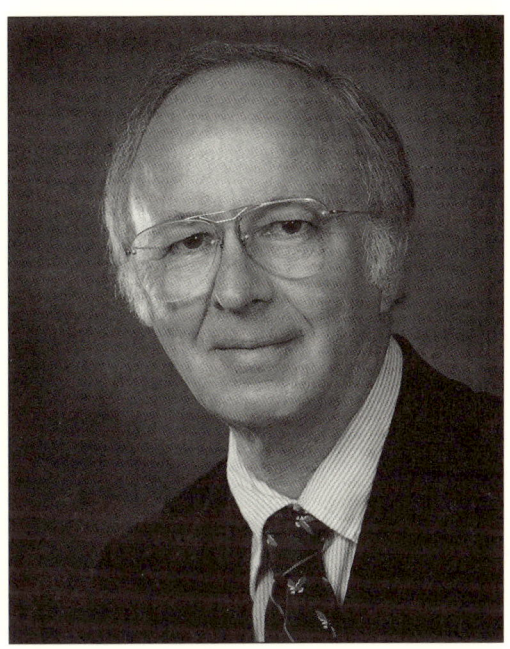

I F IT IS DIFFICULT to be top-notch, it is more so to be first-rate at everything attempted. Sterling Edwards comes close to it (although by his own admission he was too small for football). Early in his career, Edwards left his home in Birmingham to learn what else there might be in Philadelphia and Boston, but returned home to build an innovative and original laboratory and service. He later moved west to Albuquerque with a vision of a different kind of Department of Surgery, one dedicated chiefly to the patient rather than to the laboratory. In each stage of a long career in surgery, he has been successful. A pleasant person whose inner drive is concealed, he has an open, friendly personality yet can be firm when it counts. The appreciation, love, and respect of his students, staff, and patients are understandable.

Edwards was interviewed December 8, 1986.

Dale: Tell us about your parents and early schooling.

Edwards: I was born July 23, 1920, and I grew up in Birmingham, Alabama, living with my mother and father in my grandparents' home. Grandfather was a doctor—one of the early psychiatrists who used things like hot water baths for therapy, as modern-day people use tranquilizers. My father was the first Chevrolet dealer in Alabama. But I was always more attracted to medicine than to salesmanship.

I attended high school in Birmingham and tried desperately to make the football team, but I was too small. I chose college at Virginia Military Institute primarily because in 1938 it was obvious that there was going to be a second world war, and I could take pre-med but also get a commission in case the war started and prevented med school.

Dale: You thought as long ago as 1938 that there would be a war? A lot of people didn't know that.

Edwards: There was a war in Europe already. It looked as though we might get into it.

Dale: What did you do at VMI besides study? Weren't you a wrestler?

Edwards: Yes. I found a sport where my size didn't matter so much, and so I went out for wrestling and enjoyed that very much.

Dale: At what weight did you wrestle? Weren't you captain?

Edwards: I wrestled at 145 pounds. My senior year I won the Southern Conference Championship. In the conference finals I defeated a man from Chapel Hill who had beaten me in the regular season. I had learned his tricks.

Dale: And so you got him back. Also you graduated first in your class.

Edwards: I graduated "with stars," which meant that I was in the above-ninety-average group.

Dale: That is the equivalent of Phi Beta Kappa. Where did you go to medical school?

Edwards: Six months after the Japanese struck Pearl Harbor, I graduated from VMI. By that time, there was a federal program to continue medical schools during the war. They placed me in the ASTP [Army Specialized Training Program], as a private first class, to go to medical school at the University of Pennsylvania. My monthly pay was fifty-four dollars.

Dale: Who was your best teacher in medical school?

Edwards: During the war most of the academic professors were away in service—at least all the surgeons were. Dr. I. S. Ravdin, the departmental chairman, was serving as commanding general of the Twentieth General Hospital in the China-Burma-India theater. Dr. Eliason, who was too old for the military, became the chief of surgery. He was a good surgeon and a strict disciplinarian.

Dale: What happened after medical school?

Edwards: I interned for nine months at Massachusetts General Hospital. Then I entered active duty at Valley Forge General Hospital outside Philadelphia. It was a plastic and reconstructive surgery center. I assisted four older plastic men for one year. When they were discharged, several young surgeons like me, with very little training, had to take over that thousand-bed hospital.

Dale: Who were the senior surgeons there?

Edwards: Brad Cannon was one. Two of those in the same position as I were Joe Murray, who later did the first kidney transplant, and Milt Edgerton, who is now chief of plastic surgery at the University of Virginia. They stayed in plastic surgery and became world leaders in that field.

Dale: So you were thrown into a position of serious responsibility quite early. Did it help you?

Edwards: It was great. We did a lot of surgery. I learned the meticulous techniques that plastic surgery required, which certainly helped later on.

Then I returned to Boston to finish my residency in general surgery at the Massachusetts General Hospital. Dr. Edward D. Churchill was the chief. He was just back from the war, where they called him "Pete." He was a quiet person with whom I found it a little hard to communicate. I never really came to know him, but he was a good chief, and in later years I followed some of his teaching as far as administration was concerned.

Dale: Was he a good technical surgeon?

Edwards: He didn't do a whole lot of surgery after he returned. Dr. Richard Sweet and Dr. Robert Linton were my surgical heroes at the Mass General.

Dale: Tell me about the vascular surgeons at the Mass General.

Edwards: Vascular surgery consisted chiefly of sympathectomies and amputations. There were also efforts to remove emboli from arteries, but that was about it at that time. Arthur Allen was there, but I was on the other surgical service, so I didn't know him. I admired Robert Linton because he was forward-looking. He visualized the future of vascular surgery, and he inspired me to do the same. Dr. Linton was a quite careful surgeon. He would take all the time that was required.

Dale: You returned to Birmingham after you finished there. In fact, you came on there just as I left in 1952. I recall that Champ Lyons, who was chief, said, "Sterling wants to do a fellowship, but we need him here now to help with the load." What was your relationship with Champ Lyons?

Edwards: Dr. Lyons was an interesting fellow. He was quite intelligent. The main thing he did for me was to let me develop an animal lab. He let me go my own way in the development of vascular surgery.

Dale: He was a great speaker.

Edwards: Yes, he was. He was great in the use of words, but if you analyzed what he had said, I sometimes thought he was speaking more to impress than to teach.

Dale: Was Tinsley Harrison there?

Edwards: Tinsley was a much better teacher. He had held a lot of different academic positions—he'd been dean at Bowman Gray, at Southwestern in Dallas, and was chairman of the Department of

Medicine in Birmingham. He was very conservative from the surgical standpoint. When coronary artery operations came along, he resisted them for quite a while.

Dale: I have always believed that there were three great technical discoveries that undergirded and fostered the development of vascular surgery. They were the discovery by Arthur Voorhees that a cloth tube could be used to replace an artery, your demonstration that crimping the tube would allow it to bend within the body, and Tom Fogarty's balloon endoarterial catheter. Tell us about your development of the crimp principle for grafts.

Edwards: I asked Dr. Lyons if I could develop a homograft artery bank. Jim Pate had just come to us from the Naval Medical Institute in Washington, D.C., where he had been involved in the development of freeze-dried techniques to preserve homografts. He helped me set up a homograft bank in Birmingham. Jim later became chief at the University of Tennessee, in Memphis. We set up the bank and it was my responsibility to take the arteries by autopsy. I sure lost a lot of sleep doing that.

I sent an abstract on arterial homografts to the American Surgical Association in 1954. They accepted it and there I was, two years out of training, giving a paper in Cleveland to the American Surgical Association. The paper just before mine was by Voorhees, Jaretzki, and Blakemore, reporting their use of a cloth tube to replace an artery. It was tremendously exciting. I saw a chance to avoid getting up every night and harvesting those autopsy arteries. I also saw that there was a better future for something off a shelf rather than a graft that you had to obtain from another human being.

I went home after the meeting and began to try nylon cloth (which came from Anne's slips) as a tube graft. We prefabricated grafts with cuffs and seams of nylon, as Voorhees had described, but it was awkward as the dickens to sew those things. Alabama is a textile state, so I began to look around for some textile manufacturing outlets that might work with me to develop textile tubes without all those seams and cuffs. I found a company called Chemstrand in Decatur, Alabama, ninety miles north of Birmingham. It was a branch of Monsanto.

Chemstrand assigned a man named Jim Tapp, a physical chemist, to work with me. They entered this strictly on a public relations basis; they didn't think they would make anything out of it but they saw a medical need, so they assigned him to spend whatever time was necessary. Two or three months after the meeting in Cleveland, Jim and I decided to develop a prefabricated graft that you could take off the shelf and use in a human being.

We figured that we needed to get rid of the seams and cuffs, to reduce the porosity of the cloth so the patient wouldn't bleed to death, and to do something to prevent kinking of the tube after it was placed. Jim Tapp solved all these problems except the last in two months. He used a shoelace braiding machine to form a nylon tube. At the time I didn't even know that a shoelace was a tube!

We started with nylon because the Chemstrand people knew more about it than any other synthetic. We formed a braided tube whose porosity could be reduced by dipping it in formic acid, which caused the fibers to swell and stick to each other. That also reduced fraying of the ends. After three months we had tubes that would nicely replace the abdominal aorta of a dog, but they were straight and stiff and would surely kink if flexed or bent.

Jim Tapp was making this tube by braiding it over a glass rod and then dipping it in formic acid. One day, as he forced the tube off the glass rod, it came off in a corrugated form. He realized that the corrugations prevented all kinks!

He sent one of these to me by mail, saying, "Hey, I think we have solved the kinking problem." I said, "No, Jim, it won't work. Everybody working in this field is absolute in believing that you need a smooth tube. This one is rough on both the inside and the outside." But I did place some in the abdominal aortas of dogs. When we autopsied them later, we found that the cavities of the crimp in the grafts were leveled out by a thin layer of blood clot; they became a smooth tube after a few hours. They worked!

Dale: So that is how crimping was discovered? It was one of the great inventions of our time, because it allowed synthetic tubes to bend without buckling.

Edwards: It was before the days of the Food and Drug Administration—so different from now. In the fall of 1954 the police brought in a man who had been shot while robbing a grocery store.

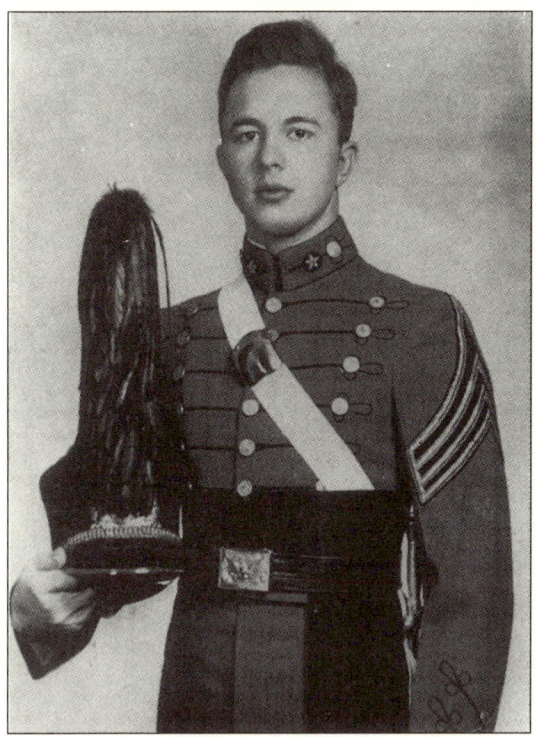

Sterling at the Virginia Military Institute

His femoral artery was injured in the groin. We didn't have a homo-graft of the proper size. Herschel Graves, our senior resident, said, "Why don't we use that tube from the dog lab that you've been telling me about?"

I told the patient, "This has never been used before. I can't save your leg otherwise, because there is a three-inch gap in your femoral artery." We placed the corrugated nylon graft into his femoral artery. It worked. After he recuperated he became a star on the prison foot-ball team, which was a pretty good indication that the graft was worthwhile.

Dale: Why did you leave Birmingham and go to Albuquerque?

Edwards: I remained on the surgical faculty of the University of Alabama for seventeen years, 1952 to 1969. Champ Lyons died of a brain tumor in 1965, and John Kirklin, from the Mayo Clinic, was appointed chairman of surgery. John was very good to me and didn't interfere with what I was doing, so I worked under him for several years.

Dale: Sterling, did you want that position yourself?

Edwards: No, I was a candidate for it, for self-protection, but I didn't seriously want it. John Kirklin did cardiac surgery, so peripheral vascular wasn't his main interest. At that time, I was doing cardiac also. John let me continue that in the same room I had had before. But it did set a limit on what I could do there. Meanwhile, one of my students at Alabama had become the chairman of surgery at Albuquerque, at a very young age. He asked me to come and start a cardiothoracic program there, so I moved in 1969. But he soon decided that he didn't like being chairman; he didn't like administration. Four years later, in 1974, I took over the whole department.

Dale: What sort of administrative policies did you try to develop?

Edwards: When I took over in New Mexico, the National Institutes of Health were less able to afford surgical research. In the old days at Alabama, you could write them a letter and get $100,000 to do research with almost no trouble. But that was changing. I decided that instead of trying to make an academic research department, I would try to train practicing surgeons of high caliber. The second thing, which is now common but wasn't then, was to appoint residents for five years instead of having a pyramidal system where several were cut each year to make the residents compete with each other.

There was trouble talking the faculty into abolishing the pyramid. But every year we take the best people we can get and commit ourselves to the completion of their training five years later. The results have been amazing. The program has done so well that for the last five years we have not taken anyone who wasn't absolutely top-notch, Alpha Omega Alpha, at his or her medical school. We've been able to obtain fine residents with a commitment to finish. We tell them, "We are going to train you to be the best clinical surgeons we can. If you want to go into research later, that's fine, but the first requirement of an academician is to be a good clinical surgeon." You can let them learn research on top of that, but don't try to take a primary researcher and make an academic surgeon out of him when he's not already a good surgeon.

Dale: I do agree with that concept, but it is still widely ignored. How do the subspecialties fit in? Some people after a year or so will want to be a urologist or an orthopedist—how do you work that out?

Edwards: We take six interns every year, three of whom have already decided that they want two years of general surgery and then go into urology or neurosurgery or something else. People do change their minds, and sometimes we can allow them to trade, but our system is not very flexible. We do have rotations in general surgery for those residents. They have a four-month gynecology rotation in a private hospital where there aren't any other gynecology residents. Each of our residents will have done about fifty hysterectomies and about ten or twelve caesarian sections before he or she finishes. So if they go to a town where they have to do those things, they are prepared. I am really pleased with the broad training that these young men and women have had when they finish.

Dale: Where do most of them practice?

Edwards: We encourage them to go places where they are needed, which are medium-sized towns, rather than to stay in the big cities. About 50 percent of them have done that.

Dale: You've been interested in a good many other things too, such as popliteal aneurysms.

Edwards: I was trained to do the usual things, so I tried to think of alternatives. I thought, in the case of the popliteal aneurysm, Do we really need to take the aneurysm sac out? Why not bypass it and ligate it, because the real problem is embolization of a clot from within the aneurysm down into the leg and foot.

Dale: You were the first to advocate the bypass approach. What other firsts do you recall?

Edwards: While at Alabama, I was the first to use Teflon patches to close intracardiac defects, and in New Mexico, we were the first to use intra-abdominal arteries—the splenic and the left gastroepiploic arteries brought through the diaphragm for coronary bypass when no veins were available. We have tried all kinds of things. I could be the editor of the "Journal of Negative Results." In fact I've thought about starting one so people wouldn't repeat all my mistakes.

Another problem to be solved was why femoral artery reconstructions stay open less well than iliac artery endarterectomies or reconstructions. Iliac endarterectomies stay open indefinitely, but femoral endarterectomies close rapidly, so I thought maybe it was the size of the vessel. I thought, Let's make the femoral artery bigger, and I used the saphenous vein as a long patch after endarterectomy to make the femoral artery as big as the iliac artery. That didn't work, because it still didn't stay open as well as the iliac. Sometimes it made the femoral artery too large, and it clotted. The same thing occurred when we used vein patches in the carotid. They don't do any better, as far as preventing recurrent stenosis.

Dale: Is there too much carotid surgery being done?

Edwards: The carotid endarterectomy is a prophylactic procedure. If you do it after someone has had a stroke, you're not going to help them. You've got to time this operation properly. When is prophylaxis best done? We know it's helpful after people begin to have transient ischemic attacks. The question is, should you start the prophylaxis whenever you find any stenosis? We don't have the answer yet. I don't think there's too much carotid surgery being done in good institutions. But the prophylactic surgery being done by general surgeons who've had two to three months' experience on a vascular rotation and think they can do the job often leads to too high a morbidity and mortality rate. That's where the problem lies, not in the hands of real vascular surgeons.

Dale: What do you mean by a "real vascular surgeon"? What sort of background has he had?

Edwards: A trained vascular surgeon is one who has had a year's special training. Vascular surgery is and should be a specialty. The main thing I'm against is the surgeon who does an operation occasionally. Doing an occasional colon operation is just as bad as taking on an occasional aneurysm.

The pride of some surgeons bothers me. They're not willing to say, "I don't know how." Not long ago, I sent a thoracoabdominal aneurysm to Stanley Crawford in Houston. I said, "Stanley, I've not done one of these in a while. I want you to do it." And Stanley did a beautiful job. I had to swallow my pride to do that, because Stanley and I were roommates at MGH, but I will not do an "occasional" operation if there is somebody who can do it better.

Dale: Do you think that the patient's family puts pressure on the surgeon to go ahead and do it?

Edwards: Partially. The surgeon dislikes telling the family that someone else can do it better, because he thinks that this will hurt his reputation. But it helps develop respect and fosters the belief by patients and their families that this surgeon is interested in what's best for the patient and not just his own ego.

Dale: What is your idea about the talented young man or woman who has finished a general surgery residency program that includes some vascular surgery? Should they be doing any vascular surgery? In other words, this is a young man or woman who has not had a specific fellowship or residency as a vascular surgeon. What's his or her role?

Edwards: I have mixed feelings. We don't have a fellowship. We have only enough cases to train our general senior residents well. Two of our own residents, who are excellent technicians, have gone to a city in New Mexico, and they are doing vascular as well as general surgery and are doing it well. They call me up frequently when they have an unusual problem. I can't say it can't be done by a general surgeon who is capable. If these surgeons had stayed in Albuquerque and they had only an occasional vascular patient referred to them, I'd say they ought not to be doing it. But there they have a lot of it, so it's not just training but how much exposure or how much opportunity you have to continue it. It is an individual matter.

Dale: What other problems do you have with residents?

Edwards: One of the things that has always bothered me is surgical residents who have excellent judgment and technical skills, but are poor communicators—they relate poorly to their peers. They are going to be failures, because they are not going to get referrals. These are the kind of residents who are always arguing with the nurses or the medical or pediatric residents. We try to counsel these people, but usually there is not much change. We're concerned about what else can we do about such a personality problem.

Next, there are all kinds of new ethical problems that we are having to face: when to turn off the ventilator; when to operate on somebody who is senile; should you operate upon an abdominal aneurysm in an old senile patient in a nursing home? We haven't yet done enough thinking about it. But in the last year I was able to talk the faculty of our medical school into letting us start a course for third year medical students on "Physicians' Responsibility." Every two weeks the third-year medical students meet for two hours with us. We present a trigger event, some problem such as when to turn off the ventilator in a specific situation. The students divide into small groups of about ten, each with two faculty members. Not only are we trying to talk about ethics, but also communication skills. We do role-playing. Somebody will take the part of a terminally ill patient and another will come in as a physician and talk to that patient while the others sit there and listen. The simulated patient gives feedback. Another thing we do in this course and in these sessions is to encourage the students to bring up their own emotional problems, such as, "I lost a patient last week. How did I feel when that happened?" We hope that the faculty that we select will be open enough to talk about their own feelings about it. The conference has been going for a year now. It has been received with tremendous enthusiasm.

Dale: What are your plans for the future?

Edwards: After thirty-five years of surgery, I'm reaching a point where I think I'd like to do something else. The thing that attracts me most is the effect of diet and exercise in preventing and even in treating things that I have been operating on all these years. Low fat, low cholesterol, low sugar, and low salt diets can help people with claudication. I've seen it happen. It happens to people with angina. I've seen them improve. I think there's beginning to be some evidence that we can regress arteriosclerosis in humans if we treat them effectively to get cholesterol levels down.

Dale: What part does exercise play in that?

Edwards: It helps build collateral circulation. Whether it has anything to do with the prevention of plaque deposition, I don't know.

Dale: Is it your plan to open a center for this?

Edwards: I'm going to try to develop a residential center where we place people for two to four weeks at a time on a healthy, low-fat, low-cholesterol diet along with an exercise program. I want to make it a research institute because I really want to get some documented evidence, which has not been available yet.

Dale: What sort of exercise do you particularly favor?

Edwards: It has to be aerobic to do any good. But it's important to let people decide what kind they like best—walking, treadmill, or other kinds.

Dale: What kind do you personally like best?

Edwards: I'm jogging every day, two miles, about thirty minutes. Fast walking may be better, because there are not so many joints to be damaged. A lot of people will do that when they won't jog or swim.

Dale: Do you have any success in persuading postsurgical patients to diet and exercise?

Edwards: That's an area I would like to concentrate on. The time after the shock of an operative event or a heart attack is when people are most motivated to change. But you can't do it by giving them a book. They won't do it. A residential exposure for two or three weeks is necessary. I went to one myself, and my blood pressure came down without any medication.

Dale: What thoughts do you have about your career so far?

Edwards: You and I may have been tremendously fortunate to have lived through the most exciting era in surgery that there has ever been. To be a part of it was great good fortune.

Thomas Fogarty

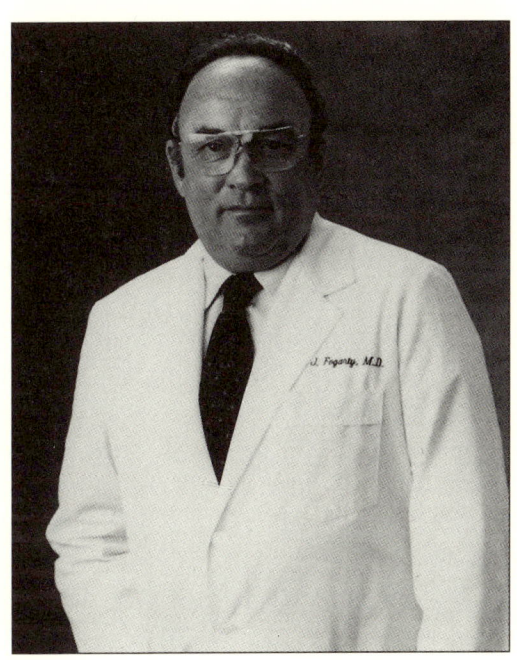

Tom Fogarty was, is, and always will be a maverick. Analogous to Albert Einstein failing elementary arithmetic, he was declared by his early teachers to be a poor risk for college. Later, he seemed a better fisherman than scholar.

This interview reveals a warm, humble man who claims no fame nor seeks position or honor from his colleagues but who has achieved them because of his talent and skill as a surgical pioneer. One who, because his research interests were stymied, left academia to develop a successful surgical group in which his innovative mind could roam freely, Fogarty invented the Fogarty balloon catheter, the first effective endovascular tool, which has saved countless limbs and lives. Interestingly, the origin of the concept arose from the seed of daily clinical practice, and lacked academic and standard institutional support. Individual entrepreneurial effort gave birth to the endovascular techniques and instruments that are emerging today. He was interviewed December 8, 1986.

Dale: Tom, let's begin chronologically with your parents and your early education.

Fogarty: I was born February 25, 1934. My father was a railroad mechanic. We lived in Cincinnati, where I went to a Catholic grade school and Roger Bacon High School. I then went to a Jesuit College, Xavier of Ohio.

Dale: When did you become interested in medicine?

Fogarty: My dad died when I was young. We had a difficult time with finances, so I started working at an early age. My first jobs were delivering newspapers and mowing lawns. Then I worked at a hospital. At that time, hospitals hired a lot of children because, as charitable institutions, they were not subject to child labor laws. They could pay what they wanted.

When I was in the eighth grade, I worked in central supply at the Good Samaritan Hospital, in Cincinnati, Ohio. I worked there all through high school and college and became a scrub technician in the operating room. So I worked in the hospital from the eighth grade on into college.

Dale: Do I recall that you developed a carburetor or something of the sort?

Fogarty: My friend, Bill Linferd, had a Cushman motor scooter. His dad was a dentist and he was one of the more wealthy kids in the parish. He was somewhat shunned because he was so bright; it wasn't popular to be bright. The motor scooter had a problem mechanism. The problem was that when you shifted from a high gear to a low gear going up a hill, all of a sudden the thing would take off and the guy in the rear would find himself lying in the street. We started messing around with the clutch mechanism and developed a type of centrifugal clutch to be used in middle speeds.

Dale: Did you patent it?

Fogarty: No, but we should have. It ended up in the hands of the scooter manufacturer, Cushman. So I learned to patent things when I was sixteen years old.

Dale: Where did you go to medical school?

Fogarty: At the University of Cincinnati, but I nearly didn't get into college. In high school I wasn't much of a student, so I had a hard time getting a recommendation to college. In fact, the principal said it would be the biggest waste of money he ever saw for any college to accept me. I actually started college on probation.

Dale: Were you on academic probation?

Fogarty: Yes, I had never studied before, so I was concerned about what the results would be. But it turned out well and I was able to get the grades.

Dale: In college you became motivated?

Fogarty: Sometimes deprivation can be a significant motivation. If you don't want to go through life without some reward, you come to recognize that if you are going to get a reward, you are going to have to do something. At seventeen or eighteen, I finally figured out that I had better start doing something.

Dale: So you made it through college, and you went on to Cincinnati Medical School. Is that where you met Jack Cranley?

Fogarty: Actually, I met Jack Cranley when I was a scrub technician while in high school. He hired me as his private scrub technician, and I worked for him part-time through high school and college. He encouraged and helped me in many ways. The jobs and fiscal support he provided helped pay my way through school.

Dale: Tell us the story about how the catheter was developed.

Fogarty: It seemed like embolectomies to remove clots never worked. As you know, when something doesn't work, it's everybody's fault but the surgeon's. I got to thinking that there must be a better way of doing this. But it didn't come to me for a long time— many years, in fact. The observation was made in high school.

I made a balloon catheter in medical school, but did not have a chance to use it until my fellowship year.

In Ohio, after you graduated from medical school you were not required to take an internship in order to be licensed. You could practice medicine without an internship. But I was interested in a good rotating internship, and I wanted to go to Oregon for it. After my experience in Oregon, I decided I wanted to pursue surgery. I applied for a surgical residency and was accepted. But, during the middle portion of my internship year, I received a draft notice with an enclosed bus ticket back to Ohio to report for military duty.

Dale: What year was that?

Fogarty: It was 1961. Dr. Engelbert Dunphy was professor of surgery at the University of Oregon at that time and interceded. They allowed me to complete my internship year, but after that I would be drafted. I decided to go back to Cincinnati, where Dr. John Cranley engaged me for a fellowship year. Somehow the draft board lost me.

Dale: Lost you? Lost your records?

Fogarty: That's right. I never heard any more from them. I called Dr. Dunphy and he said, "Keep your mouth shut; let me do some checking." He did that and repeated to me, "Keep your mouth shut and come back here." So I completed a full year with Dr. Cranley and his group. It was during that year that we clinically evaluated the new balloon embolectomy catheters.

Dale: It must have been immediately obvious that this was a worthwhile device. Did you have any trouble with the balloons? When I worked with similar balloons, they were always breaking. There were problems getting the rubber just right.

Fogarty: Yes, there were many problems.

Dale: No doubt you left the new Fogarty catheters with Jack Cranley when you went back to Oregon. Did you take some out there and did you use them?

Fogarty: Yes. At that point in time, I was making all of them, so I spent a lot of time making them for Dr. Cranley's practice. For about a year or so I made them all.

Dale: How long was it before the Edwards organization began to get into it to make them for public sale?

Fogarty: I couldn't get any manufacturer to make them. They gave me the runaround; I guess they thought I was some stooge fooling around. I didn't have any credibility. Dr. Starr was the head of the cardiothoracic division at the University of Oregon. He had developed a relationship with Lowell Edwards, who actually was an aeronautical engineer. Dr. Starr asked Edwards if the company that he had started would be interested in making them. He thought it was a good idea, so that's how we finally obtained a catheter manufacturer in 1963.

Dale: You've been inventive beyond that. Tell us about some of the other things that you have pioneered.

Fogarty: I had always been interested in trauma produced by clamping a blood vessel. I made a lot of different instruments back when I was in college, trying to diminish the damage, and actually convinced Dr. Ray Krause to use some of them. But they were pretty cumbersome and Dr. Krause didn't have very much patience, so I had to wait some years before I could reinitiate that interest and finalize the Fogarty vascular clamp.

Dale: What about the Fogarty dilating device?

Fogarty: When I returned to Oregon, I found that Charles Dotter had begun to dilate arteries with a series of intraluminal dilators. I think he did his first in 1963. I owe a lot to Dr. Dotter, because he gave me more experience with complicated arterial thrombolectomies due to his dilation attempts. Dr. Dotter wanted me to make balloon catheters for him that would dilate. But Dr. Dunphy made it clear if I was interested in a surgical career, I had better steer clear of Dr. Charles Dotter, so I did. I did learn from my experience that there were some situations where dilation worked. So I maintained an interest in that over the years.

The extrusion catheter that I later developed was an effort to improve over the standard present-day systems that radiologists still use.

Dale: What was the reason that Bert Dunphy was antagonistic toward Dotter? Was it because he was a radiologist, or was there some personal problem?

Fogarty: I think Dunphy thought that Dotter was crazy as a loon for believing that you could forcefully separate the walls of an artery and have it stay open. He didn't have any animosity toward him. He just didn't want one of his students associated with a crazy man. It was as simple as that.

Dale: That's not a good concept for a teacher, is it?

Fogarty: No, I don't think it is either, but unfortunately a lot of surgery is based upon tradition, where innovative ideas are poorly accepted. It's not conducive to progress. It's one of the problems of the surgical approach to disease.

Dale: Inertia encourages continuation of current dogma while resisting change. How long did you stay at Oregon, Tom?

Fogarty: Through my internship and four years of surgical residency. But for two years, between 1965 and 1967, I went to the National Heart Institute. The origin of that was that I decided I wanted to take out a year to do some research in cardiovascular physiology. I discussed this with Dunphy and told him I'd like to go to Washington for that. I meant the University of Washington, on the West Coast, but he thought I meant to the NIH in Washington, in the District of Columbia.

The next thing I knew, I heard him on the phone talking to Glenn Morrow at the NIH. I ran in and said, "Dr. Dunphy, I said the *state* of Washington!" He replied, "This is where you are going." So I was interviewed there and felt fortunate because it was a highly sought position. They must have interviewed in excess of two hundred people, and they took five.

Dale: So that was fortunate. What was your relationship with Glenn Morrow?

Fogarty: Mostly a fishing one. We were good friends, and we spent a lot of time fishing together on the Pocomoke River in Snow Hill. We remained close friends after I left NIH.

Dale: Was it a trout stream?

Fogarty: No, we fished for largemouth bass, standing in a boat rowed by our guide, Dusty, casting to the banks of the stream.

Dale: What was your favorite plug?

Fogarty: "Rapala." It ended up in my nose on one of those trips. Dr. Morrow surgically extracted it.

Dale: Getting back to the NIH—you were there for a year?

Fogarty: Two years. It was partly clinical and partly research.

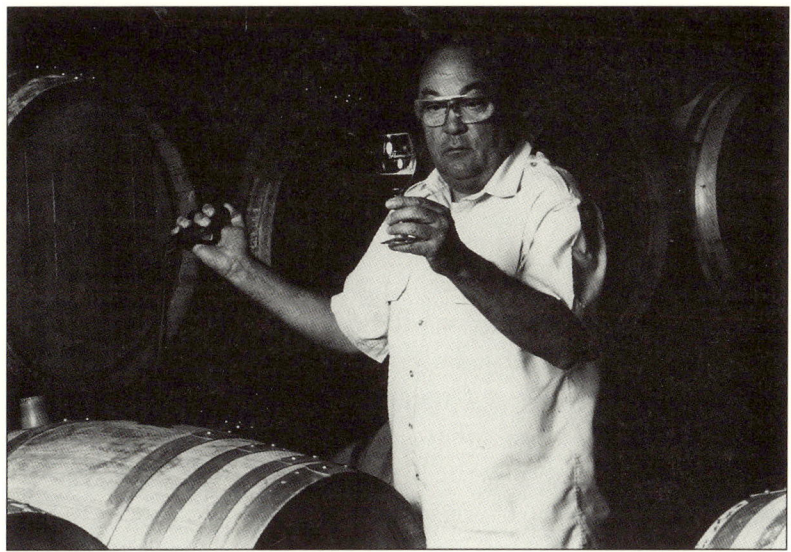
Tom the wine vigneron.

Dale: I've thought of Glenn Morrow as primarily a research man. Was he a good technical surgeon?

Fogarty: He was sound but not flashy. He didn't make many mistakes, but he was not adventuresome. He recognized that technical prowess can get you where you don't want to be.

Dale: What happened to Glenn?

Fogarty: He didn't like to see people suffer and that applied to himself. When he developed a series of problems that would leave him significantly compromised neurologically, he did himself in. I was so sure he was going to do it that I made it a point to visit him before he did it. He had a progressive neurologic disease.

Dale: Did you ever talk to Bert Dunphy about death? I recall that he came to Vanderbilt and while lecturing on something else, he fell into a fifteen-minute ad lib discussion of his philosophy of death.

Fogarty: Yes. He really thought that physicians had many responsibilities to patients. One is to recognize limitations as to what can and cannot be done. He was always saying, "Let's think about what we are doing here."

Dale: What happened after the NIH?

Fogarty: I went back to Oregon to finish my last year of surgical training. From there I went to Stanford for my cardiac training with Norman Shumway. I stayed on as a full-time faculty member. Shumway was a terrific teacher, but at the same time gave me enough independence. The time spent with him was enjoyable, and he significantly contributed to my career. After the full-time faculty experience, I ended up in private practice at Stanford.

Dale: What occasioned that transition?

Fogarty: I was operating eighteen hours a day, which I didn't mind, but I had no chance to do any research or to write papers. Meanwhile, Dr. Morrow had offered me a position at the NIH in Washington. They were developing a cardiovascular institute, which encompassed all of the cardiovascular province and included lipid specialists, hypertensive specialists, cardiologists, surgeons, physiologists, and pathologists. I was to head that team. It was something I wanted to do.

Pat Daily was the other surgeon on Shumway's staff at that time. When he learned that I was leaving, he said, "Well, I'm leaving also." Then both Pat and Norm Shumway approached me, asking, "Why don't you enter private practice right here at Stanford?" My wife wasn't anxious to leave the area, so after we talked it over, Shumway assured me that I would have the opportunity to do some research and the lab would still be available. That's how I ended up in private practice. It wasn't my original intent. Ironically, I saw private practice as an opportunity to do research that I couldn't achieve as a full-time faculty member!

Pat Daily and I worked together for about four years; then he went down to the University of San Diego as department head of cardiac surgery. He also ultimately ended up in private practice.

Dale: That left you without a partner. What did you do?

Fogarty: It wasn't difficult. There were people graduating from a number of programs. We now have Wally Buch, Perry Shoor, Jim Zimmerman, Vince Gaudiani, Neil Olcott, Duncan Mason, and me. We have two interventional radiologists in our group, Bill Hayden and Paul Cipriano. We do about 60 percent cardiac and about 40 percent peripheral vascular work, usually 1,100 cases per year.

Dale: Tom, it is said that too many carotid operations are being done.

Fogarty: That's an easy and probably accurate statement, but it requires qualification. If somebody does a thousand procedures, you can probably find two that shouldn't have been done. So that would mean there were too many. The statement is therefore correct, but the sense of it is not. Whether or not that procedure was correctly timed is another matter.

Dale: Another current question is how long we can continue to pour money toward elderly people with difficult problems; for example, the eighty-five-year-old man with a ruptured aneurysm, which is perhaps going to cost $50,000 and will return a man to gardening or something of that sort. Can we continue to do this sort of thing, or must we follow the Russians, who don't do it, or the English, who already limit such treatment?

Fogarty: I hope that it never occurs. I have seen eighty-five-year-old people with severe illnesses who were enjoying life and could still do things of interest to them. They have their wits about them. Those people should not be denied the benefits of modern medicine just because they are eighty-five. It is dangerous to think of such change without looking at each case on an individual basis.

Dale: Is there a place for euthanasia decided by a committee, representing the patient, his family, the legal authorities, the church, and medicine? Should a patient with terminal cancer be allowed to have euthanasia?

Fogarty: It depends on how you define euthanasia: There lies the problem. I think there are ways that people can gracefully exit, which by some definition would be considered euthanasia. Another definition would be to let nature take its course, perhaps with minimal deprivation. But it's dangerous to put that terminal event in the hands of humans.

Dale: Is euthanasia an issue which should be addressed openly among physicians and surgeons, or is it best left alone, as it is now?

Fogarty: It most certainly needs to be addressed. A lot of pressure is being brought because of cost containment programs.

Dale: What do you think of the idea that the technical part of surgery has achieved its zenith—that there are few, if any, frontiers left for the nimble fingers of the surgeon. Is it true?

Fogarty: No, I don't think that is true. But I do think that the tools of the surgeon are going to have to improve. Surgeons have been trained to cut and sew, but they are going to have to realize that there are ways of doing things that do not involve cutting and sewing. Surgeons are not accepting new technologies as rapidly as they should. It is a reflection of the way they have been trained in the past.

Dale: Another question: Should the young man or woman who has finished a general surgery program with the average small content of vascular surgery be doing vascular surgery? Or should those patients be referred to a person who to a considerable extent limits his or her practice to vascular problems?

Fogarty: At this point in time, it depends on the circumstances. I don't think you can automatically eliminate the general surgeon from involvement in vascular surgical procedures, because the primary concept is that they have the technical talent and the basic knowledge to do some of the common procedures. There are other situations where even some people who are totally dedicated to doing peripheral vascular surgery should not be doing some components of peripheral vascular surgery that are very complicated. There need not be a total separation of the general surgeon from the vascular system.

Dale: Is medicine today as attractive as it once was to the youth of America?

Fogarty: When I chose to go into medicine, I did so because I would enjoy it. I wasn't thinking about the monetary return or the lifestyle. I just thought that it was something I would like to do. But now, young people don't think that way as much. They seem to choose the lifestyle that they want and then look for a field that will provide that lifestyle. That's the wrong way to go about it. By that approach, medicine is not as attractive as it once was. But as a way of deriving satisfaction, it's there. You get as much satisfaction, or probably more, than twenty years ago. The reason that's true is that there is more social awareness. We don't have just mechanical or technical problems to deal with. From that standpoint, it's even more challenging, and can be more rewarding. It also can be a lot more frustrating.

Dale: Tom, tell me about your personal life.

Fogarty: I met my wife, Rosa Lee Brennan, at the University of Oregon. She was working in the record room in between college semesters. I started dating her during my residency at Oregon. She returned to college, and I went to the NIH in Washington, D.C. Shortly after I got there, we married. We had our first child in 1968—and now have four. Tom Jr. has just finished his first year of college.

Dale: How did you get into the wine business?

Fogarty: Everybody drinks wine in California. One of the individuals I met at Stanford was a fellow named George Burteness. He had a small winery in the town that I lived in, in the foothills of the Santa Cruz mountains. It's only about fifteen minutes from Stanford. He had a vineyard and a winery. I started making wine as a hobby. Later, I began to see it as a retirement plan, so I got it started. Success in the wine industry requires some consistency and perseverance. The customer must recognize that you make wines that they perceive are consistently good. We started in 1975 and became serious about it in 1981.

Dale: How much do you make?

Fogarty: About eight thousand cases last year. We sell a lot of it directly from the winery. Last year we started distributing to certain states outside of California.

Dale: What label does it bear?

Fogarty: It's very original: Thomas Fogarty.

Henry Haimovici

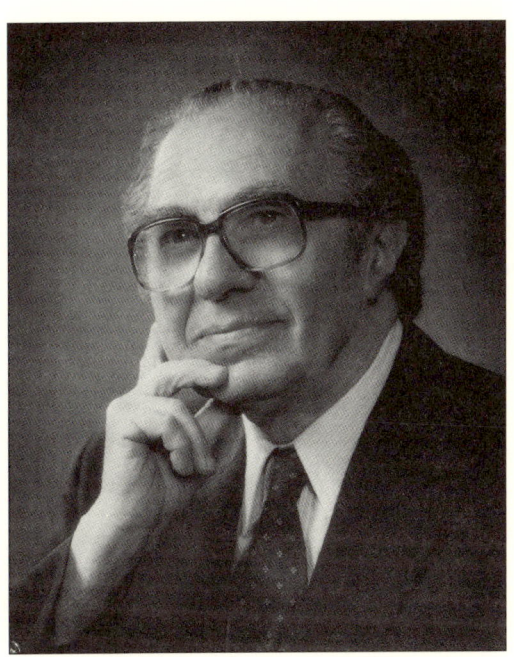

HENRY HAIMOVICI is a true international surgeon. Born in Romania on the Danube, he attended university in Bucharest and completed his medical and surgical studies in Marseilles, France. He published his first book, with a preface by René Leriche, in Paris. As a Rockefeller scholar, he studied in Boston with Walter B. Cannon. After serving in the French army during World War II, he went to New York and was a longtime attending in vascular surgery at Montefiore Hospital. A founding member of the International Society of Cardiovascular Surgery, he served as its secretary general and as editor of its *Journal of Cardiovascular Surgery*. He has been elected an honorary member of medical societies in over ten countries. He was interviewed June 11, 1991.

DeWeese: Henry, where were you born?

Haimovici: I was born in Romania on the banks of the beautiful blue Danube, close to the origin of its delta and not far from the Black Sea.

DeWeese: When was that?

Haimovici: September 27, 1907.

DeWeese: What do you remember of your early childhood? Who were your parents? What did they do?

Haimovici: My father had a wholesale business of manufactured goods. My mother (her born name was Lenobel) was primarily taking care of the household and the children. There were four of us—three brothers and one sister.

DeWeese: Where did you attend school?

Haimovici: Kindergarten, high school, and college were all in Tulcea, the capital city.

DeWeese: This is outside of Bucharest?

Haimovici: Yes, it's on the banks of the Danube, not far from the Black Sea. Bucharest is inland.

DeWeese: What ages would you have been at the various schools?

Haimovici: I started college at the age of thirteen and finished at the age of twenty. The lyceum includes eight years, which are divided into two stages, first four years (junior) and then the other four (senior). To accelerate the first four years, I took two classes in one year during the first stage, so that I passed the first in three years, while the second took the usual four years; thus the total college education took seven years. At the end of the seven years I took the examination for the baccalaureate. The year was 1927.

The educational curriculum in Romania, during my time, was

based on the French system. After I passed the baccalaureate, I decided to go to France for my university studies.

DeWeese: What school did you go to in France?

Haimovici: To the medical school in Marseilles. Medical studies in France are preceded by one year of study at the faculty of sciences, where one had to take physics, chemistry, botany, and zoology.

After my year at the faculty of sciences, I got my diploma of PCN, which stands for physics, chemistry, and natural sciences. After that I applied to the medical school. The Marseilles faculty of medicine is a component of the Aix-en-Provence University. Aix is twenty-eight kilometers from Marseilles.

DeWeese: How old were you then?

Haimovici: I was twenty-one. In France the system is quite different from here. Concomitantly with the studies at the medical school, one could apply for internship, which is called externship in France. After the first year of medicine, I started studying for the externship, which was based on a competitive examination accessible to a limited number of available positions. I passed this competition after one year of medical school.

Thus, while taking courses at the medical school, one is involved as an extern in care of patients in hospitals. I then prepared for examination of internship, the French equivalent of residency. After two years of preparation, I took that examination for internship, which is a most difficult competitive test. When I took this examination in 1932, only ten out of sixty candidates were accepted.

DeWeese: And this is how many years after you had started?

Haimovici: The first year was taken at the medical school, the next year I became an extern, and after two more years of that I became an intern (resident), called *Interne des Hospitaux*, an important title in France. Now, I was assigned on a rotating internship. I went through everything—medicine, surgery, and all subspecialties, including obstetrics. During the training in the Department of Medicine, the professor asked me to write an article for the *Journal of Gastroenterology* on early dyspepsia, a paper which is listed in my curriculum vitae. This was my first paper.

DeWeese: Is that period similar to our last two years of medical school?

Haimovici: It was a general rotating residency, but after two years it became specialized. This was concurrent with my courses at the medical school. After I finished the five years at medical school I did not receive the M.D. degree, because that was obtained only after completion of the five years of the internship. At that point I had to present a thesis in order to get the M.D. degree. So in 1937 I finished the internship and obtained my M.D. degree.

DeWeese: And how old were you then?

Haimovici: I was thirty. The title of my thesis was "Les Embolies Arterielles des Membres." This work reflected my early interest in vascular surgery. My orientation to the vascular field was stimulated by one of my chiefs, Robert de Vernejoul, who, incidentally, just celebrated his one-hundredth birthday in March of this year. I have his picture in my office inscribed to me. He was one of the chiefs of surgery that I admired most. The other, equally admired, was Jean Fiolle. Both were professors at the medical school, Fiolle being the chairman of the department.

After I passed my thesis, Professor Fiolle said to me, "Your work should be published in a separate book." On his advice I went to Paris and presented it to Masson, considered the best medical publisher in France and one of the best in Europe. After reviewing the manuscript and the illustrations, they accepted it readily. The book is 336 pages long and was prefaced by René Leriche and Jean Fiolle. After Leriche read the galleys, I received a letter from him congratulating me in a most flattering way.

The *JAMA* of July 9, 1938, had a review of the book which started as follows: "This monograph should be translated into English. It is such a splendid piece of work in every detail that it ought to be available to everyone." Incidentally, I found out from Geza de Takats much later (in 1951) that he was the reviewer of my book in *JAMA*.

DeWeese: Was this book written in French?

Haimovici: Yes. May I add that in 1938 the French Academy of Surgery awarded me the Duval-Marjolin Prize, given for the best thesis presented by an intern in surgery in the country.

With your permission, let me turn back for a moment, since you wished to know what led me to vascular surgery. I was stimulated by Robert de Vernejoul. This event took place in 1935 when I was his resident, during which time he had two cases of embolectomies. As you know, Labey was the French surgeon who did the first successful embolectomy in 1911. The French surgeons were aware of this procedure. As a novice, I was quite impressed by this first experience of embolectomy, which seemed like a simple procedure by the fact that one opened the artery, removed the blood clot, and closed it, and it resulted in good flow restoration. I learned later, of course, that this procedure may be more complex.

Besides arterial embolectomy, my early interest in vascular surgery was further stimulated by other vascular problems which occurred during my training. Toward the end of my surgery training, I was involved in another vascular problem. I was on call on Christmas Eve in 1937 when I got a call to see a female patient in medicine who had just developed a cold, blue leg that was quite painful. She was in heart failure. At first I thought that she had an arterial embolism. The surgeon on call was alerted and with his assistance I proceeded under local anesthesia to expose the femoral triangle. The femoral artery was spastic and small, but I found no clot in it. So I did only what we were doing in France at the time—a periarterial stripping that Leriche called a periarterial sympathectomy. Following this, the artery expanded to normal size. Looking at the vein next to the artery, I could see that it was enlarged and full of blood clots. But I could not understand the relationship between the clinical picture and blood clots in the vein. The puzzle became more pronounced a few days later when the patient developed gangrene of the foot and, shortly after that, an amputation below the knee became unavoidable. The cause of the gangrene remained a puzzle. The question was, how could thrombosis of a vein cause gangrene? An answer was obviously needed, so I wrapped up the amputated leg, took it under my arm, and went to the anatomy department of the medical faculty, where at the time I was a prosector teaching. The purpose of my visit to the laboratory was to examine the amputated leg. We had an x-ray machine that Professor Salmon used in his work on arteriography of arteries on cadavers in which he had been studying the arterial supply to the muscles and skin, a classic work. We used a mixture of minium-turpentine injected into the popliteal artery. All leg and foot arteries to the minute branches were visualized. The reproduction of the arteriogram appears in my publications. So the gangrene could not be of arterial origin. I dissected the veins of the amputated limb and found them to be all thrombosed. Nevertheless, nobody could explain the cause or the mechanism of the gangrene unless it was due to the venous thrombosis. To find out about this possible mechanism, I went to the library of the medical school. I found that a few publications of the eighteenth and nineteenth centuries reported a few isolated cases of gangrene associated with venous thrombosis.

I wrote up the findings, and at the urging of my chief I presented the case to the Marseilles Surgical Society in January 1938, and it appeared in their journal. Later, this case was reported in the *Presse Medicale.* The title of this paper was "Les Gangrenes des Membres d'Origine Veineuse." Historically, it is interesting to note that Gregoire published a similar case under the title "Phlegmasia Cerulea Dolens" in the *Presse Medicale* three weeks before our contribution.

DeWeese: Who was first?

Haimovici: I didn't know Gregoire's paper, since the two papers were published in the same journal three weeks apart. His case was also gangrene of the leg. My presentation at the Marseilles Surgical Society antedated that of Gregoire. My priority or his is immaterial in this matter. Gregoire's case caught the interest of the vascular fraternity. However, after my return to the United States, I published another case of venous gangrene, which appeared in the American literature in 1948. This was the first detailed publication of a case seen in this country. My subsequent contributions and my 1971 monograph on the subject, "Ischemic Forms of Venous Thrombosis," have covered the subject quite comprehensively. I introduced for this condition the term *ischemic* venous thrombosis, which indicates the pathogenic mechanism of this entity.

Another phase of research during my residency related to arterial embolism. As I was preparing my thesis, it occurred to me that some information about the role of the arterial wall in arterial embolism was indicated. The professor of physiology, Jean Malmejac, and I undertook a work on the dynamics related to arterial embolism. The papers in this phase dealt with the sympathetic contribution to the symptoms of arterial occlusion. Our experiments showed that the occlusion in itself is not the only factor responsible for the ischemic changes, but that they are due also to the reflex of the autonomic nervous system, irritated by the pressure brought about on the arterial wall and adventitia by the embolus. A diagram in my book on arterial embolism deals with the isolated, perfused limb using cross-circulation from a normal leg. It was called the Delezenne Cross-Circulation Method. The conclusion was that in arterial embolism it is not only the mechanical blockage but also additional spasm that together are responsible for the acute ischemia.

DeWeese: Before we go on, what period of time was this?

Haimovici: It was between 1935 and 1937, when I was working on my thesis. In addition, I wanted to know the influence of the embolus in situ on the arterial wall changes. For that phase, I worked in the Department of Pathology, which was headed by Professor Lucien Cornil, who was also the dean of the medical school. The reaction of the arterial wall to an aseptic and septic embolus was undertaken in experimentally induced arterial emboli in the dog. A chronological study of the various stages of the lesions was carried out. Collaboration with members of the pathology department appeared in publication and my thesis as a detailed description of the findings.

About one year after I finished my internship, I was appointed head of a surgical OPD clinic, which kept me attached to the medical school and to the hospital, where Professor Fiolle was the chief of the Department of Surgery.

Early in 1938, shortly after the above appointment, I received a call from Professor Cornil, who wished to see me at his home, since he was unable, due to illness, to go to his office. What Professor Cornil had to tell me was a total surprise to me. The latest council of the medical faculty had decided to set up an Institute of Neurology and Neurosurgery like the one in Paris headed by Clovis Vincent. How did I come into that? This is how things unfolded. "We've had," he said, "to make a few decisions for the immediate future concerning a chief for this institute, and we selected you to be trained in the various aspects of neurophysiology, neuropathology, and neurosurgery. The Rockefeller Foundation has offered to build the institute, as they did in Paris, and, of course, the medical school had to contribute part of it. You are going to be in charge of that institute." I was almost speechless. Having just finished my residency, I hardly was qualified for such a position, even after the contemplated training. "We know," he said, "but we think you have potential for that. First of all, listen to what I still have to tell you. You will have to go to the United States to study neurophysiology and get acquainted with the present level of neurosurgery. In the meantime, you will have to go to Paris to meet Dr. O'Brien, the director of the Rockefeller Foundation." During my interview, Dr. O'Brien, who was informed about my scholastic background by Professor Cornil, asked whether I had given some thought to with whom I would like to study neurophysiology. I said I would like to work with Professor Cannon at Harvard. He responded, "Well, you could not have chosen better than that, since Cannon is the most prestigious physiologist in America. But there may be some difficulty here, because Professor Cannon is about to retire, so there is a question of whether he may be willing or able to accept a new fellow. I will have to inquire about this with Professor Cannon and find out. In the meantime, you may have to wait a few days in Paris and return to the office for us to advise you about the results." Fortunately, Professor Cannon was able and glad to accept me. These arrangements were planned in August 1938, during the time of a potentially serious international situation due to the occupation of part of Czechoslovakia by Germany. As a result, my plans to leave for America had to be postponed until the situation cleared up. So, I left Paris on October 20, 1938.

One day after my arrival in Boston, I met Dr. Cannon in his laboratory. He suggested that I first work with him personally. The investigation to which I was assigned was on a neurophysiologic concept that he called the law of denervation.

I was assigned to determine whether the motor neurons innervating skeletal muscles became sensitized to various stimuli after partial denervation, the same way as did the autonomic-innervated structures after partial denervation of ganglia, shown by Cannon and several of his associates. The denervation of the muscles of the hind leg of the cat was achieved by semisection of the spinal cord. The partial denervation of the spinal nerves resulted in sensitization to a number of chemical agents. Thus, like the smooth muscle, the skeletal muscles obeyed the general law of denervation of Cannon.

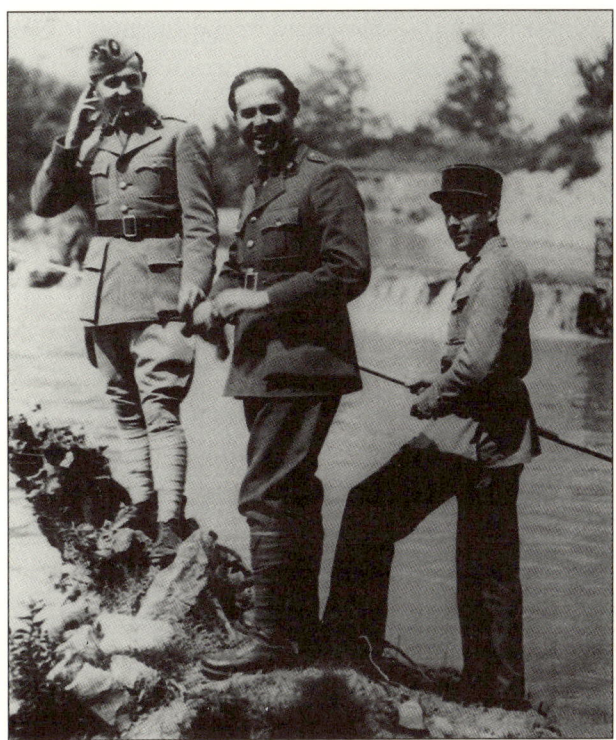

Henry in the French Army in 1940.

At the end of several months, this work was completed and published in the *American Journal of Physiology.*

At this point, the nerve cells of the brain remained to be tested. Thus, preliminary experiments in the motor area of the brain were carried out, which yielded similar evidence of supersensitivity of the disconnected pyramidal tract. This study was not completed before I left Harvard. However, after my return to France, Cannon wrote to me on December 15, 1939, stating that "a further development of work which we did together has shown that when the motor area is isolated on one side of the brain, leaving the pyramidal tract, that area becomes sensitive to a number of stimuli, so that the opposite legs go into marked extension, whereas the legs innervated from the normal hemisphere remained flaccid."

In addition, he suggested another subject for me to work on by myself. It sounded like an esoteric problem. It was whether basal metabolism of proteins is influenced by the autonomic nervous system, as had been claimed by some investigators. Their opinion did not fit into Cannon's concept of this problem. These investigators used pharmacologic means to block the sympathetic system. Contrary to that, Cannon suggested that I block the sympathetic by doing total sympathectomies "from stellate to pelvic ganglia" and then study the basal metabolism.

Next, still in Cannon's department, I investigated sympathetic regeneration after complete ablation of the sympathetic ganglia and chains. Most previous investigators have studied regeneration after section of nerves or partial sympathectomy, but not by total sympathectomy. I used the cats who had had total sympathectomies from the previous project and found out that preganglionic regeneration of fibers occurred in two areas. The first dealt with the adrenal gland, its medulla playing the role of a postganglionic synapse. The second site of regeneration was of new fibers joining the cervical ganglia, which affected the pupil and nictitating membrane.

By the end of this period I had completed three investigations and was prepared to continue, had the war in Europe not changed my plans.

My year with Cannon was a most productive period of research, which opened a new door for me to an exciting field. But above all, I was fortunate to have had the opportunity to work with a man exceptional both as a scientist and human being. His stature as a physiologist was and still is considered today to be that of the "American Claude Bernard."

Besides training in neurophysiology, my program of studies included neurosurgery, to be carried out after my return to France. While I was in the United States, the Rockefeller Foundation made arrangements for me to visit a few of the important neurosurgical centers there and in Canada during April 1939. In order to get acquainted with the state of the neurosurgical specialty, I visited institutions in Philadelphia, Baltimore, St. Louis, Chicago, and Montreal. I also tried to obtain an appointment with H. Cushing, but he had just moved from Boston to New Haven. These visits were most educational and pleasant. Meeting the leaders in neurosurgery at these centers offered a memorable opportunity to discuss and witness this specialty, which I was looking forward to in my future training.

By September 1939, war broke out in Europe. France started mobilizing. I went to the French consulate to inquire whether I would have to return to France. The answer was no. However, I felt it my obligation to go back. Cannon said the Rockefeller Foundation would be very happy to continue to sponsor me. In spite of that, I decided to leave.

I was drafted into the French Army early in 1940. I was assigned to Montpelier, where a large base hospital was located for wounded soldiers coming from the northern front of France. The general in charge of the hospital was Professor Jean Delmas, a friend of Professor Fiolle. I was put in charge of a two-hundred-patient section. We had hardly any surgery to perform. Also, the war between France and Germany ended rather quickly, France having signed an armistice on June 25, 1940. After my return to Marseilles on July 25, 1940, I decided, if possible, to return to the United States and resume my position with Dr. Cannon. As a matter of fact, I received letters from him encouraging me to make every effort to return to Boston. I needed two visas, one for exit from France and the other the re-entry visa for the United States. These documents were difficult to obtain during the war. It took two years before the U.S. State Department issued my visa for re-entry into the United States. I returned on October 12, 1942; by that time, Cannon was retired. I was assigned to Beth Israel Hospital, which was affiliated with Harvard Medical School, and became involved in two investigation projects, one on infectious toxic shock and the second on the use of gelatin as a plasma substitute.

For the first project, I obtained bacterial toxins from Dr. René Dubos, who was from the Rockefeller Institute but was temporarily working at Harvard in the bacteriology department. The toxins were used to induce shock, and these studies resulted in two papers, "Cardiovascular Dynamics in Fever and Shock Following Injections of Bacterial Toxins" and "The Cardiovascular Dynamics of Shock Due To Infection." Dr. A. S. Freedberg and I presented one of the papers to the New England Heart Association; the second paper was published in the *Journal of Clinical Investigation*. This work on shock had been suggested by Cannon, who at the time was the national chairman of the section on shock and had advised me to join that group. It was quite an interesting investigation, both from a pathologic point of view and in view of the cardiovascular hemo-dynamics.

The investigation on gelatin dealt primarily with its antithrom-botic action. When given prophylactically in a single injection, gelatin exhibited a definite antithrombotic action, but no beneficial effect was obtained when given after injury to the vein. This paper as a preliminary report was published in the *New England Journal of Medicine,* and was coauthored with J. Fine.

After two years, 1942 to 1944, in Boston, I had offers in New York. I had married, and my wife and I were planning to live in New York, so in September 1944 I moved. My wife, Nelicia Maier, M.D., Ph.D., was primarily a biochemist whose special interest was enzymology of cancer tissue. Later, we joined our interests in arterial tissue metabolism of atherosclerotic arteries. At that time, my wife obtained a fellowship at Memorial Hospital for cancer research.

I was appointed at Mount Sinai shortly after my arrival in New York and became a member of the vascular clinic. In addition, I received a Dazian Foundation Fellowship and was given laboratory space to continue with my investigations.

In the vascular clinic, patients with Buerger's disease represented a substantial group. Since smoking was considered an important etiologic factor, nicotine was felt to play a significant role. This was one of the reasons that I decided to investigate the site of action of nicotine using the Laewen-Trendelenburg (L-T) preparation in the frog, which consists of the perfusion of the isolated vascular bed of the hind legs. We showed that in addition to its known sites of action on ganglion cells and adrenal medulla, nicotine may also act directly on the neuroeffector cells of the blood vessels.

Using the L-T preparation, I have studied the action of several substances (Dibenamine, curare, and thiamine), some in combina-tion, and their interaction.

A few months after my appointment to Mount Sinai, I was also appointed to Montefiore Hospital as an associate attending on the vascular service. There was limited activity in this service consisting primarily of management of occlusive arterial disease needing amputations and of varicose veins.

In addition, I was interested in research on a new substance, Dibenamine, an adrenergic blocking agent. In 1947 I received a call from Dr. Louis Goodman, previously from Yale and coauthor with Alfred Gilman of the classic book on pharmacology and professor of pharmacology at the University of Utah in Salt Lake City, who was just finishing with M. Nickerson the investigation of the pharmacologic properties of this substance. He wondered whether I would be interested in undertaking it in my clinical work in arterial hypertension and vascular disease, such as Raynaud's disease. After some preliminary use of Dibenamine was encouraging, I requested that Smith, Kline, & French prepare an oral form. Eventually, it achieved a capsule easy to handle, originally under the name of 688A, which later became known as Dibenzyline and is still on the market today. Dibenzyline was a definite progress of this medication, since it was given orally. The published results stimulated several investigations for treating arterial hypertension with Dibenzyline. This was the first pharmacologic agent for treating hypertension.

During these studies, I observed that the patient who received Dibenamine or Dibenzyline developed complete suppression of sweating in the palms of the hands. After controlled studies, I demonstrated that man has a dual innervation of the sweat glands, contrary to the classical concept of its strictly cholinergic characteristic. I called Dr. Otto Loewi, formerly of Vienna, who had won the Nobel Prize for studies of autonomic problems and who at this time was at New York University. After reviewing all my data, he agreed that they were well documented. So I presented a paper to the American Physiological Society Meeting in Atlantic City in 1949. As a result of this presentation, I was elected a member of the American Physiological Society in 1950.

In 1954 I started to carry out experimental work focused on atherogenesis. This involved Dr. Nelicia Maier as the biochemist. The primary scope was to investigate the metabolism of the arterial tissue and the fate of aortic homografts in experimental canine atherosclerosis using abdominal and thoracic segments, in situ and transposed. This was carried out in aortic tissue of man, the rabbit, and the dog, with special reference to a number of specific enzymes. This experiment led to the concept of susceptibility of certain arterial segments. Classification of arterial lesions encompassed the peripheral, abdominal visceral, coronaries, and cerebral vessels. The investigation was supported by the National Heart Institute for twenty-two years.

In 1966 I organized an international symposium on recent advances in atherosclerosis, sponsored by the New York Academy of Sciences. I also assumed the role of consulting editor of a volume published by the New York Academy of Sciences. My personal experience, published in 1960, was confirmed by further observations as well as by a review of the world literature in a monograph entitled "Metabolic Complications of Acute Ischemia and Reperfusion of Ischemic Skeletal Muscle" published in 1988. The concept of arteriovenous shunting in varicose veins led to a revision of the pathogenesis and treatment of primary varicose veins. A review of my findings appeared in *Surgery* in the May 1987 issue, as the leading article.

A symposium on vascular diseases was organized in 1969. The proceedings of this symposium were published in a volume entitled *The Surgical Management of Vascular Diseases.* Among the faculty members of this first symposium were Allan Callow, Charles Hufnagel, Robert Linton, Jerry Lord, Fiorindo Simeone, Frank Spencer, Richard Warren, Irving Wright, and many other well-known cardiovascular specialists. I chaired this symposium annually until 1979. Frank Veith became co-chairman from 1980 until 1986, and thereafter I was honorary chairman.

DeWeese: Tell me about the International Society for Cardiovascular Surgery as we conclude our interview.

Haimovici: This being a lengthy story, I suggest the best way to answer your questions concerning the early formative organization of the ICVS, which later became the ISCVS, is to refer to the history of the society published in 1977 in the *Journal of Cardiovascular Surgery.* The following are a few excerpts from its history.

In March 1950 I organized the International Society of Angiology. I had obtained the support of René Leriche, who felt that an international society was an excellent idea and agreed to be its first president. Shortly after that, Emile Holman of San Francisco; A. Michael Boyd of Manchester, England; and Fernando Martorell of Barcelona, Spain, agreed to be its vice presidents. A list of charter members was then rapidly established through contacts with the leading surgeons in the United States, Europe, and South America.

The first meeting of the International Society of Angiology was held in Atlantic City on June 9, 1951. The congress held in Lisbon September 18–20, 1953, represented an important landmark in the society's history: It was at this congress that precedents were established concerning the patterns of the scientific programs and the constitution and by-laws. At the executive session of the society held on October 18, 1957, with Dogliotti presiding, the society voted to have its name officially changed to the "International Cardiovascular Society." The central organization at the Munich Congress in 1959 voted to publish the *Journal of Cardiovascular Surgery* as the official organ of the society. E. Malan and I were appointed co–chief editors, and were backed up by an international editorial board selected from members of all three chapters.

C. Rollins Hanlon

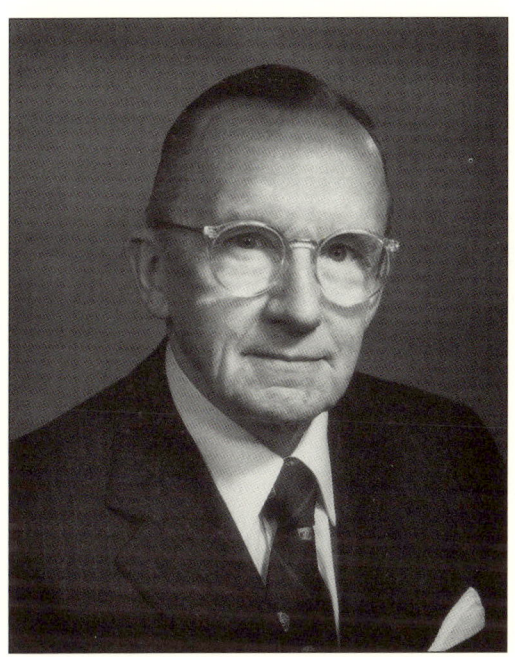

KNOWN BY EVERYONE AS ROLLO, Hanlon has had an enormous impact on surgery nationally, through his association with St. Louis University, and internationally, as executive director of the American College of Surgeons, which he has developed into an organization that has had a tremendous impact on the continued education of physicians, has improved the health care system, and is responsive to the concerns of surgeons. His memory for names and events makes him a friend of all who meet him, and he is eloquent in speech and writing. Hanlon has truly been a leader for American surgeons over the decades. He was interviewed December 12, 1986.

⇒

Dale: What did you do in your early years?

Hanlon: My father was a salesman with seven children. I was the next to last, born on February 8, 1915, in Baltimore, the only child who became a doctor. Living in Baltimore, I developed early on a knowledge and an interest in Johns Hopkins, but not as an undergraduate school. I received my early education from the Jesuits at Loyola High School, and later at Loyola College, which was a small, nonboarding school on the outskirts of Baltimore. I was taking a classics course at Loyola and, in about the second year, I decided that I was going to medical school and that I would apply to Hopkins. In 1931 there was only one previous graduate from Loyola who had been admitted to Hopkins.

Loyola was a small college where I could combine a classics curriculum with a hand-tailored course of sciences. I would do the laboratory work during holiday periods, Christmas holidays, and so forth, and in that fashion I managed to combine the courses.

Dale: What else did you do in college?

Hanlon: I was editor of the newspaper, which was called *The Greyhound.* It was a weekly; every Friday I had to deliver it to the printer, made up with two personal editorials. That was an early disciplinary test of meeting deadlines, getting it to the printer come what may. Also, I wrote occasional pieces for various literary quarterlies. Then, too, I was manager of the football team.

Dale: Was your football team successful?

Hanlon: We were obviously overmatched in almost every game. We would play teams like Boston College, which had a large number of big coal miners' sons from Scranton and Wilkes Barre and such places. We had a 134-pound halfback on our team. After a game with Boston College, he was so badly beaten up that he couldn't bend over to tie his shoes the next day. I had to tie them for him. Frequently, our team would play the same eleven men from start to finish because we couldn't afford to take a large squad to out-of-town games.

Dale: What year did you graduate from college?

Hanlon: I finished college in 1934. That summer, before going to medical school, I traveled to Europe on a freighter as a sailor. I was what you called in those days a "work away," a category that received a penny a trip. As soon as they "dropped the hook"—the anchor went down—you were free. So as soon as we landed in Rotterdam, or Antwerp, or wherever it was, I was free to travel until they weighed anchor again. I could travel around Europe as long as I made it back to the ship by the time that it left. The unions blocked out that program after 1934.

Dale: What actual work did you do on the ship?

Hanlon: I chipped paint, painted the decks and superstructure, and cleaned out the deep tanks and the hold, just like the other sailors. I was nineteen years old and weighed only 135 pounds, but I was wiry and hard. It was good work and I saw a lot of interesting things on the voyage, and met sailors from all over the world.

Dale: Then you entered the Hopkins Medical School?

Hanlon: I was recommended to Hopkins because I had done biological research with a Jesuit scientist who was well known for his work on protozoa. My first paper was on the relation between the hydrogen ion concentration of the medium and the contractility of the paramecium. My interest in research continued during medical school, working with Philip Bard in physiology, another summer in pathology with W. G. McCallum, and with Arnold Rich.

Bill Longmire and I worked together. We were two of the eight interns chosen for the surgical services after graduation. After that year, Bill and I spent a year in the old Hunterian Laboratory working on shock. With Phil Price, Bill was working primarily on blood volume using the Evans blue dye T1824, and I was working on various other physiological aspects of shock. We were aware of Blalock's work at that time, although I didn't know him personally. I first became interested in cardiac tamponade, learning that after a period of time it could produce irreversible shock.

Dale: Who was the chief of surgery when you were in medical school?

Hanlon: Dean Lewis. He had come from Arthur Bevan and the Chicago school of surgery. He was the antithesis of the Halsted school, famed for meticulous work. Lewis was quick; it would take him twenty minutes to do a gastroenterostomy. He would just reach into the abdomen and pick up a loop of bowel and put it to the stomach. He would never explain how he knew that it was the proper loop. No one dared to ask him any questions.

Dale: He was authoritarian?

Hanlon: He was. But he had an incredible mastery of the literature. His phenomenal memory allowed him not only to recall a reference but to remember where it was in the library. He would say, "Go down to my office and ask my secretary, Miss Baker, to get out such and such a reference, and that's where you will find it." On an obscure thing like a sarcomas of the sternomastoid muscle, you wouldn't think that anybody had ever heard of it, but he had filed it all away in his memory and could bring it back. He conducted things in the "pit," where he taught students in the way that European surgeons did. Barney Brooks did the same thing.

If you wanted an internship, you didn't make a formal application; as a fourth-year student, you just stayed down front to expose yourself to his questioning. Much of it concerned historical things in surgery. If you performed well, he was aware that you were interested. One day, walking out of the elevator in the lobby of the Halsted Building, he looked at me and said, "Do you want an internship?" I responded, "Yes, sir." He said, "See Miss Baker" and that was all the negotiation that it took. No interviews or formal application.

Dale: What were the financial provisions for a house officer?

Hanlon: The first year, you got six white suits and board and lodging. That was the total extent of it. To that was added all of the experience that you could wish. Since I lived in the hospital and was single, it was a marvelous opportunity. We worked unmercifully hard. By modern standards, it was not appropriate, but we didn't feel put-upon or underprivileged. In fact, those were very happy times. Today, people would say, with justification, that we worked too hard and should have had more time off, but we were basically interested in learning all we could about surgery. It was a marvelous experience!

Dale: It was an initiation into the band of brothers. One hates, and at the same time, loves the search for Galahad's grail! How long were you at Hopkins?

Hanlon: The next year, two of us from among the eight were selected to stay on and we both went into the lab, Bill Longmire as one fellow and I as the other. Later, Bill left to take his father's practice in Oklahoma, after his father had a stroke. Then Dean Lewis, who had followed Halsted as chief, became ill, and W. M. Firor became acting chief of surgery at Hopkins. While we were in the lab, Evarts Graham had come to look at the position and had decided not to take it. Also, Mont Reid had come from Cincinnati to consider it. Ultimately, Dr. Alfred Blalock from Vanderbilt accepted the chair. Before that, I had gone to Cincinnati, where Reid, a Halsted resident, was chief of surgery, succeeding George Heuer.

I worked at Hopkins for two years and then in Cincinnati for a total of four years before entering the navy. One of those years I spent as an exchange fellow at the University of California at San Francisco. The arrangement was that we sent a resident from Cincinnati to work under Howard C. Naffziger at California. Actually, you spent six months with Naffziger in neurological surgery (he would never call it neurosurgery any more than he or any other native San Franciscan would refer to San Francisco as "Frisco"), and six months in general surgery with H. Glenn Bell.

Then came Pearl Harbor in 1941. Like many other people, I wanted to join the Johns Hopkins unit, which was going overseas. I couldn't work that out, so I tried to enlist in the navy but was turned down in San Francisco on the day after Pearl Harbor.

Dale: Why were you rejected?

Hanlon: They said I had a hallux valgus, a history of sinusitis, and an enlarged inguinal ring (which twenty years later became a hernia). That was in 1941. By 1944, when I actually entered service, they were less picky about doctors.

Dale: So you returned to a resident's position with Mont Reid at Cincinnati? Tell me about the steel wire wound closure.

Hanlon: In Cincinnati we closed abdominal wounds with steel wires placed through all layers, two and a half inches from the edge of the wound. Serum oozed from between the wire sutures and made a miserable looking wound, but it was simple and unbreakable. Not pretty, but people got well!

Dale: I like the bottom line of that—people got well. Forget the theoretic discussion. Get 'em well!

Hanlon: There were no skin sutures. Many young surgeons had the tendency to try to pretty it up and put skin sutures in. But if you placed skin sutures you lost one of the advantages, namely that the serum and secretions could leak out.

Dale: That type closure was used for civilians in Vietnam. They were closed and then sent home to live or die.

Hanlon: That closure also was used at Dunkirk. Later, steel wire gave way to new synthetics.

Mont Reid had become interested in arteriovenous fistulas at Hopkins. That continued when he moved to Cincinnati. Patients came to him from all over the country with difficult, challenging lesions. He was a cool, meticulous, but swift operator; an impressive person. Unhappily, he died at an early age, in his fifties, of a coronary. Three of us—Frank Hinman, Jr.; Ed Gibbs; and I—were house officers when he had his ultimately fatal coronary. He had an oxygen tent in his bedroom at home. The three of us supplemented his nurses around the clock and spent eight hours each with him daily during the month that he survived. We checked that his oxygen was right and that any adverse signs were noted. That was in addition to doing our regular work at Cincinnati General. The three of us volunteered. I was on from midnight till 8:00 A.M., and then went back to the hospital, took a shower, and went about the day's work until the next evening. It wasn't considered a big deal, sort of taken for granted.

Dale: Was the system at Cincinnati different from that in Baltimore?

Hanlon: There were modifications. Josiah Smith was the resident; we didn't use the term chief resident. There was just a resident, while all the others were assistant residents or interns. Louis G. Hermann was there and had made the place famous for Pavaex, a passive exercise boot used for lower extremities with impaired circulation. You put the foot and leg into this boot in which there was alternating negative and positive pressure. It was an interesting concept, but not useful for advanced arteriosclerosis.

Dale: When did you enter the service?

Hanlon: In 1944 they had realized that doctors with small physical problems could be useful. I entered the navy without a full year of residency in Cincinnati.

I was ordered to the Naval Air Station at Memphis. After a short time there, I was given the opportunity to volunteer for "unspecified hazardous duty." Nobody knew what that meant. The alternative seemed to be the marines, who would be assaulting various islands. My duty turned out to be in an intelligence outfit attached to General Claire Chennault's Fourteenth Air Force in China. I was caring for people in that, as well as in secret units such as counterintelligence. I had an interesting time for two years in the interior of China, and then went back to Shanghai. After the war was over, I was assigned as the chief of surgery on the hospital ship *Repose*. I had a good experience up and down the China coast in that hospital ship for six months. Then I returned home with no prospects for a job.

Dale: The hospitals were full of returned veterans looking for further training. After V-J Day in August 1945, we all found scores of young doctors waiting in line, especially since there was a moral (at the least) commitment to provide a position for at least one year.

Hanlon: I went to visit John Alexander at the University of Michigan. He had become a good friend of Alfred Blalock during their time together at Saranac Lake for tuberculosis. Alexander continued to have tuberculosis in one or another organ until he died. He had a nephrostomy tube for renal tuberculosis. When I first saw him, he was in bed. He got up to take a walk with the tube draining into a gallon glass jug which he handed to me for transport. We walked up and down the corridor during the interview for a possible job, with me carrying the jug of urine and him speaking as we went along. It seemed absurd, but it was serious business for me. He gave me a tentative commitment for a position after the next change of house staff.

I returned to Baltimore, my home, where my mother still lived, and visited Hopkins, where I had spent so many happy times. I found that Bill Longmire was a sort of super-resident under Alfred Blalock in 1946.

Longmire said to me, "Why don't you come on the staff here?" and I said, "That's a marvelous idea, but I'm committed to John Alexander at Michigan and consider myself very fortunate. I couldn't go back on my word that I was going there." He replied, "I'll speak to Dr. Blalock." Dr. Blalock called John Alexander and told him that I was not coming. I was uneasy with that, but he seemed to have squared it with John. So I missed Alexander and Cameron Haight by returning to Baltimore.

Dale: How was your experience back at Hopkins?

Hanlon: I wanted to learn to perform bronchoscopy, but found that it was done by the nose and throat department, which so guarded that prerogative that it wasn't possible for me. The only place to learn was at the Henryton Sanatorium outside of Baltimore, on Saturdays at 7:00 a.m. I learned a bit about bronchoscopy that way, to go along with my developing thoracic surgical skill.

It had been customary to have two chief residents who would relieve each other, but for a brief period of time I was the only resident. That was a busy time. Friends used to tease me about having fallen asleep once while Dr. Blalock was talking to me. That was not strictly true. I was in his office with somebody else and when he wasn't talking to me I was sleeping. When he spoke to me, I was awake.

In any case, it was a marvelous time. After I finished this "retreaded" residency, Bill Scott and I had an office together and shared a secretary as assistant professors. In the animal laboratory at the National Institutes of Health, we were working on changing the vasculature of the lung in tuberculous monkeys. Every Wednesday, we would go over about 7 a.m. and operate all day on those monkeys. What we were trying to do was to see how the monkey lung behaved with a modified lung circulation. We would cause tuberculosis in the monkeys by exposing them to a room filled with vaporized tubercle bacilli. That certainly was a dangerous occupation. Several technicians developed tuberculosis.

Dale: The high incidence and clinical importance of tuberculosis is largely forgotten today, since its control in industrialized countries by chemotherapy. The everyday presence of those patients in general hospitals as well as sanatoriums in the 1930s to the 1950s strongly suggested research such as you describe. How long did it last?

Hanlon: In 1950 Bill Scott moved to Vanderbilt in Nashville and I to St. Louis University. But for a time we would fly back to Bethesda to operate for a day or two. The entire project went for six years.

Dale: Flying was not so commonplace then.

Hanlon: No, but we did it. The project ended after Oveta Culp Hobby became Secretary of Health, Education, and Welfare. There was a national polio scare to which she didn't react as vigorously as some people thought she should. When she finally realized that it had become a political issue, she preempted the building where we worked. She literally moved us out into the exterior darkness. Goodbye, tuberculosis!

Dale: What was the main thrust of your time at St. Louis from 1950 to 1969?

Hanlon: I was the first full-time person. You might think that they would start with the Department of Medicine, but they used part-time people in every clinical department. They were trying to change St. Louis University to fit the modern medical pattern.

Dale: How did you become director of the American College of Surgeons in 1969?

Hanlon: I had been a governor of the College and then was elected as a regent in 1967. A search committee looking for a successor to John Paul North asked if I would be interested in becoming full-time director of the College. Frankly, the thought had never entered my mind.

Desirous of a new challenge, after considering leaving St. Louis after nineteen years, which Sir William Osler would have thought was too long in one position, and recognizing my age of fifty-four, I enthusiastically accepted.

Dale: What was the challenge of an administrative position?

Hanlon: A lot of people did consider it retirement. But I thought I saw a coming revolution in medical and surgical care, in which the American College of Surgeons should participate.

Dale: Have you missed clinical surgery?

Hanlon: Being a clinical surgeon is a stimulating thing. It's wonderful to get people well. But when you open some doors to enter something new, you can't keep all the old doors open.

Dale: So you opened other doors? And through some of those doors came the politicians with whom the College of Surgeons must deal.

Hanlon: The basic thrust of the College had been nonpecuniary. It was designed to improve the care of surgical patients and to encourage high standards of competence and ethical practice. It was definitely not set up to improve the financial lot of the fellows. On the other hand, we had become a part of the Joint Commission on Accreditation of Hospitals, which the college had helped set up long before my time. The standards of the joint commission were being used by our government to fill in the law, so that it was becoming a quasi-governmental body.

The American Medical Association did not always agree with the College's ideas of what was important or needed, and at times we vigorously disagreed. I found that we had a very limited operation to deal with Washington on socioeconomic matters. The money was set aside to do that for some time before we actually decided that it was time to do it. I think we have moved into it in a very responsible and gradual way, making sure that we don't so politicize our operations that we lose the respect of the people in Washington and elsewhere. We have tried to advocate responsible and effective polices, although sometimes not as politically as some would wish.

Dale: What is your estimate of the malpractice crisis?

Hanlon: It disappoints everyone, ourselves included, that we haven't solved it. It is now being recognized that our litigious citizenry is not solely a medical problem. It is frustrating both to the fellows of the College and to the officers. I think that, although it is disappointing, it's not just a matter of throwing more money at it to solve the matter. The trial lawyers have a vested interest in maintaining the system, and that's not just the trial lawyers on the plaintiff's side, but also lawyers on the defendant's side.

The doctrine of responsibility has been extended so that inordinate awards are made. It is simply not feasible to continue having a half-million physicians, not all of whom are in practice, subsidize the misadventures of all the people who are having medical care in this country today. Until the public perceives that the present arrangements can't go on, we have to make do with stopgap measures, such as some degree of tort reform, limitation of pain and suffering awards, and other such piecemeal approaches.

Dale: Now let me turn the emphasis to your family just a bit before we close. Your wife, Peg, is a pediatrician. Tell me about how you met her.

Hanlon: When I came back from the war and visited one of my friends, Richard Varco, in Minnesota, he said, "What you ought to do is give my love to my favorite pediatrician in Baltimore, who is Peg Hammond." I replied, "Richard, I will do that." The next time I saw Dick, I told him that I had followed his advice and that we had progressed famously and were engaged to be married!

It happened that I was working with Dr. Blalock, while Peg was working with Dr. Helen Taussig, who had a particular interest in congenital heart disease. Peg had spent a year at the University of Minnesota, which is how she knew Dick Varco.

The first time that I met her was when, as a pediatric resident, she called me to put a yarn truss on a baby with a hernia. I was overworked and probably a bit brusque. I don't think I made a very good impression on her. Our first date was to a football game and then to dinner, after which we went to a party with the Hopkins staff. During that time we had discussed, not always on the same side, the relationship between Dr. Blalock and Dr. Taussig, who would care for the cardiac patients postoperatively. By the end of that time, I was convinced that she was the woman for me and I've never varied from that. We had our first date in 1948; announced our engagement on March 20, 1949; and were married on May 28th, 1949, and I celebrate those three anniversaries every year.

Dale: Did you have children?

Hanlon: We have eight children—four boys and four girls. We had three boys in rapid succession each year after we were married. The oldest is the only one who is a physician. He's an anesthesiologist and assistant professor at South Alabama School of Medicine in Mobile. There are four grandchildren at present.

Dale: What are your plans after the approaching retirement from the College, which you have announced?

Hanlon: I don't like the word retirement. I come to the office between seven and seven-thirty every morning, as an executive consultant to the College.

Anthony Imparato

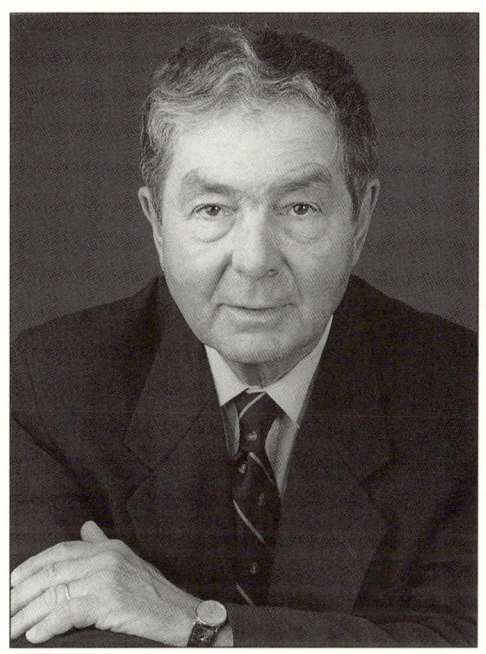

TONY IMPARATO was born, raised, educated, and has made his career in New York City. Innovative and persistent, he has contributed greatly to vascular surgery and to the training of vascular surgeons. His contributions to our understanding of atherosclerotic disease of the carotid artery result from careful observation and analytical thought. Tony is also an avid and skilled fisherman. He was interviewed December 8, 1986.

Dale: When and where were you born?

Imparato: In 1922, on July 29, in a part of Brooklyn where there was still farmland. It would now be called suburban, I suppose. I went to the local public school until I was eight, after which I was sent to my father's ancestral home on an island in the Bay of Naples. There were Bronze Age artifacts on the island as well.

Dale: What is the name of it?

Imparato: Ventotene. One of Caesar's wives was banished there, and one can still see the remains of a Roman town. My father remembers that the remains of Roman centurions were uncovered by farmers when they dug to plant their vines. I was sent there because my folks decided I didn't eat enough.

Dale: Didn't eat enough?

Imparato: I was a skinny little kid, and they were quite concerned that their only son might be a feeding problem. This was an interesting time in my life for a number of reasons. I lived an outdoor life, went to the local public school in the morning, had a tutor at home in the afternoon, learned about birds and fish, but mainly learned the language and learned early in life about a culture that was new to me. This, in retrospect, was very valuable intellectually. I came back to the United States at the age of ten having almost forgotten the English language and needing to relearn it in a few months. Thereafter, I completed my elementary education in the local public school, where I did reasonably well, earning the American Legion History Medal and the honor of being the salutatorian. I went to the local high school, which had the distinction of having probably the largest student enrollment in the country. I'm not sure how many, but there were thousands of us.

Dale: What was the name?

Imparato: New Utrecht, a Dutch name—as was the name of the borough, Brooklyn, corrupted from "Bruekelein."

Dale: Was it a Catholic school?

Imparato: No, it is a public school, and I would say that nearly half the youngsters were of Jewish extraction, the other half were probably Italians, and the remainder reflected the New York City melting pot.

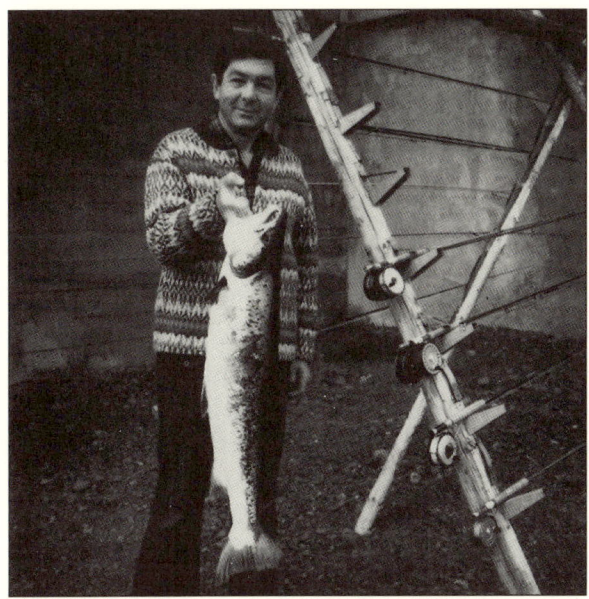

Tony and a 20-pound salmon caught on the Grimsa River, Julano, 1976.

I received a New York State Regents Scholarship, based upon grades received on statewide examinations. I can remember very clearly that the man who came to announce that I was the recipient had been my seventh grade teacher, John Gonoud. He was a very fine man. He literally came running over to our house, since he lived in the neighborhood, to let us know he had read the results of the Regents examinations in the *New York Times*.

I then went to Columbia College in the city of New York. Columbia was a great school because of the content and organization of its curriculum. It was based upon the ideas of a number of the ivory tower scholars at Columbia, who had served in World War I and had not understood the causes of that war, although they knew history, philosophy, the humanities, and economics. They designed their curriculum with the idea of attempting to understand the causes of that war. In a very short time, it became apparent that the curriculum had to encompass all of recorded human history. Starting in antiquity, an exhaustive history course called Contemporary Civilization complemented a humanities course that surveyed most of our Western literature. This curriculum outlined the plan of study for the entire four years. This, too, has had a profound influence on my life. With that background, it has been possible to develop a number of interests outside medicine.

I don't know when I got interested in going to medical school. There was never any question in our family that one went to school as one's primary mission in life. If one had the wit to successfully complete one's courses, one continued on. There was no formal announcement as to where you were going or what you were to do. You were just to work at your job as a student.

Dale: What did your father do?

Imparato: He pressed clothes in a clothing factory. He was a very intelligent man. I grew up with his drawing all kinds of schemes for desalinating sea water. He was from an island where there was no fresh water, yet conceived the idea that since it was a windy island, one could use wind to raise sea water to the highest point of the island and use sunlight to evaporate the water from the salt. Using gravity feed, the water would be brought down to the village. This was based on his observation of how sea water evaporated to dryness in a font that the Romans had built to keep the fish they had caught alive. He had gone into business with an uncle during the Depression, manufacturing women's suits and cloaks. He and my uncle "lost their shirts," so he went back to pressing.

Dale: What were your other interests in high school and college?

Imparato: In high school I played football, but I was never on a varsity team. We played football and baseball. Basketball was almost unheard of. We did lots of roller skating. In those days you could play roller hockey right in the streets. It was a pretty rough game. We did lots of ice skating, so much ice skating that I developed knee problems from it. I had two cousins who were very active in sports as well and who were very good golfers.

Dale: Were you interested in music?

Imparato: I sang in school choral clubs and acted on the stage. That is how my wife tells me she first became aware of my existence.

Dale: Tell me about that.

Imparato: I was in a play and she was in the audience with a mutual friend. It was during my junior year in high school.

Dale: What was her name?

Imparato: Agatha Petriccione. She is of mixed ancestry; her mother is Swedish and her father was Italian, which is an interesting combination. I met her formally several months after the play performance. Her father was a businessman who designed and manufactured women's handbags and liked to travel. In the spring he usually took his family on auto trips. Agatha had come back in early summer from a cross-country trip to California. She had missed some school as a result of the trip and was going to summer school to make up what she had missed. On the day that the *Normandy* first sailed into New York Harbor, a group of us were at the beach when a mutual friend who had known her from childhood brought her to the beach. That is how I first met her, the day of the *Normandy*'s maiden voyage. It has been a long relationship. We were married about five years later in 1943, after my first year of medical school at New York University.

New York University Medical School proved to be a happy choice for me, since it complemented my experience at Columbia. Many questions were asked. Students were referred to source material rather than to textbooks. There was an attitude of skepticism, sometimes bordering upon therapeutic nihilism. There was, however, no nepotism. If you worked, you were respected for it.

I fully intended to go into internal medicine. When the chief of surgery, Arthur Wright, who was the Stewart Professor of Surgery and who was about to retire, asked me if I wanted a surgical internship, I was highly insulted since local folklore was that no reasonably good student would accept a surgical internship. At that time the war was still on. Agatha and I had been married, didn't have any children, and needed to make decisions about internship and about future active military duty. It was late 1944. I was in the Naval Reserve V-12 program.

Dale: Is that when you graduated?

Imparato: I graduated in 1946, the final surrender in World War II having been in December of 1945. But applications for internships were made earlier, in 1944, when it looked as though the war was going to go on for a long time. We felt very keenly about what was going on, and so upon graduation I went directly into the navy and served a rotating naval internship, right out of medical school.

Dale: Where were you stationed?

Imparato: I was stationed within probably one hundred miles of New York for my entire tour of duty, which amounted to more than forty months. I was at the old Brooklyn Naval Hospital in St. Albans, I was with the commandant of the Third Naval District Office, and I was at the Naval Hospital at Sampson. I never went overseas. Finally, about a year before I was to get out, I decided that I needed more training. Dr. Sam Standard, a surgeon on the faculty at New York University, had asked me to see him and talk to him about my plans after I was released from military duty. I told him that I would probably go into internal medicine. He said, "No, I think you ought to be a surgeon." Well, you know, he convinced me to go into surgery. By the time I was released from active duty in April 1949, the rush for residencies was tremendous. I went to the places he recommended, received a few tentative offers, including one from Lester Dragstedt, who wanted me to work for him for a year or two in the lab before being considered for clinical surgical residency. Since I wanted a clinical appointment, I did not accept that offer. When no other was offered, I decided to reapply the following year and do a year of physiology in the meantime. I went to see Dr. Homer Smith, of kidney fame, at NYU.

Dale: Oh yes, he was a great man. He was based where?

Imparato: New York University Medical School. He was chairman of the Department of Physiology. So I talked to him and said that I wanted to become a surgeon, and that I wanted to spend a year in physiology waiting to get a job in surgery. He said, "Well, if you want to be a surgeon, you really ought to spend a year in anatomy." At that, I thought he was trying to get rid of me. He told me to talk to Donald Sheen, an Englishman who ran the anatomy department and was an excellent teacher. I went to speak to him and he practically jumped out of his shoes. He said in his rather proper English accent, "It has been my contention that surgeons don't know where they're at, anatomically speaking, when they are in the operating room, and I think that every surgeon ought to spend a year in anatomy before going into clinical surgery."

My year in the anatomy department as a teaching fellow probably was one of the best years I spent in surgical training. I spent the entire summer up in the attic of the anatomy lab, doing cadaver dissections with one of the professors, a Viennese neuroanatomist named Dr. Joseph Pick, coming to look over my shoulder. I would dissect from about eight o'clock in the morning until noon, then leave to pick up Agatha and our daughter, Maria, and go out to the beach, spend the afternoon at the beach, and come back home. By the time the school year started in September, we had a lot of postgraduate students as well as undergraduate students who were taking refresher courses in anatomy. Doctors who had trained in many of the surgical disciplines before entering military service were coming out of the services. I don't know how many cadaver dissections I finally did, but many of the students were loath to dissect, and I became sufficiently proficient to do most of the major regional dissections in very short order, a hand or an axilla in probably thirty or forty minutes. It was a valuable year.

Dale: Let me interrupt you to get something more about Homer Smith. He has always been a fascinating figure to me. What sort of man was he?

Imparato: He was a skeptic, as many were at NYU. He was a little opinionated. I will give you a specific story about that. During residency, the group immediately senior to me operated on a man with full-blown Leriche's syndrome and performed an aortic endarterectomy. Apparently, an embolus was liberated into the left renal artery and the patient, previously normotensive, became markedly hypertensive. Homer Smith was contacted about this, but would not concede that hypertension could be due to a Goldblatt phenomenon. That was in the days before anybody had much experience with renovascular hypertension. Anyway, the patient had a nephrectomy, which restored his blood pressure to normal—indeed, so precipitously that he developed a stroke. Dr. Smith was a super expert in his field, probably too far ahead of his students, and I don't think anybody, certainly not anybody in our group of medical students, got to know him very well.

Dale: Did you read his book *Man and His Gods*?
Imparato: No.
Dale: Well, you must. It is a masterpiece.
Imparato: Yes, I am sure of it. I know of it. I did read the book he

wrote on kidney physiology. We knew a little bit about his personal life, but that is another story and really nothing firsthand.

Time came, while I was in the anatomy department, to apply for surgical residency. The professor of surgery of the undergraduate division was John Mulholland, who had succeeded his father-in-law, Arthur Wright, as chairman. By this time, he had ceased to be a clinical surgeon, having become intrigued with educational and research concepts. I talked to him about a position on his service, but in spite of my having been elected to Alpha Omega Alpha, he demurred. Some of the most active clinical surgeons in the metropolitan area of New York, formerly affiliated with Columbia at the postgraduate medical school, became affiliated with NYU at the urging of Dr. J. William Hinton, who was a very active general surgeon. They took over one of the divisions at Bellevue Hospital.

I would say that Hinton was active on that service for about twelve years. It became an outstanding service not only for training residents, but for its academic achievements as well. Dr. Hinton was one of the most astute surgeons and surgical thinkers I have ever met, but he couldn't speak well. He couldn't put his ideas into easily understood words. Careful listening, however, proved highly rewarding. He ran a very active service. He brought Jerry Lord down from Columbia, where he had worked with Blakemore to run the vascular service. He brought in the postgraduate group of surgeons, many of whom he had trained. They became actively involved in the teaching of general surgery at Bellevue and at the postgraduate hospital. Thoracic surgeons were invited to join the staff. An active research laboratory program developed. A heart-lung machine was in the lab by 1954. Unfortunately, Hinton took over the service late in life. He must have been about fifty-five when he became chairman, but he organized a very impressive service in a very short period of time. I was about halfway into my internship when Dr. Hinton called me in one day and told me that he was intrigued with the question of why infradiaphragmatic vagectomy failed to permanently abolish gastric vagal effect. Dr. Joseph Pick of the anatomy department had suggested that there might be cholinergic nerves in the sympathetic splanchnic whose presence might be detected by doing cross-nerve anastomoses, vagus to splanchnic and splanchnic to vagus in the chest of dogs. I worked on that project through the entire six year clinical residency, doing cross-nerve anastomoses and gastric secretory studies. The professor of neurosurgery, Tom Hoen, came to the dog lab and showed me how to do the anastomoses. I was able to satisfy Koch's postulates translated to apply to a physiology experiment. I tested the animals for gastric secretory response to vagal and splanchnic stimulation, and ablated the function by cutting the nerves and doing the anastomoses. Then I was able to show physiologic return by response to insulin, which was then confirmed with a technique that Arthur Vineberg described. Prolonged stimulation of the vagus nerves in the neck for nine hours depleted pepsinogen granules from the gastric mucosa. When I cut out the anastomoses, vagal response again disappeared. Our interpretation of these findings was that vagal fibers in the vago-splanchnic anastomoses reached the stomach via the splanchnic nerve sheaths.

In 1954 I was slated to become the chief surgical resident at Bellevue the following year. I became well acquainted with Dr. Jerry Lord, who was in charge of peripheral vascular and cardiac surgery. He and Dr. Peter Stone did the first endarterectomy at Bellevue Hospital while I was still a junior. It must have been about 1952.

Dale: Soon after João Cid dos Santos?

Imparato: Oh, yes. Jerry kept up with what was going on. He was very active. We were doing portasystemic shunts and closed mitral commisurotomies, so that by the time I got to be chief resident in 1955, I had been groomed to do the cardiac and vascular procedures. The year before becoming chief resident, I followed Jerry around wherever he was doing a vascular procedure. By the time I got to be chief resident in 1955, we did the full gamut of peripheral vascular and closed heart operations, as well as portasystemic shunts. As a matter of fact, we even got to wrap some thoracic aneurysms with reactive polyethylene.

Dale: You were wrapping with the plastic?

Imparato: Yes, wrapping it with plastic to try to create fibrosis, and it worked. It produced intense fibrosis.

Dale: That was what Herm Pearse was doing. He was taking cellophane from packs of Camel cigarettes, autoclaving it, and putting it in a patient. I remember it very well.

Imparato: That's interesting. Anyway, in the interim, I was reactivated for the Korean business at the very start of my internship in 1950, but I was only gone for about eight months.

Dale: How did that happen when you had so much time already?

Imparato: I was in the organized naval reserve and was called up to replace those fellows who got shifted into the army. That was a short time. I went to chemical warfare and radiologic defense school in Edgewood, Maryland, to receive training in planning for nuclear disasters. When I was released from active duty I went back to work as an intern at Bellevue Hospital.

Dale: What year was that?

Imparato: I was on active duty from September 1950 to April 1951. By the time I returned, there were only two interns left for a 150-bed surgical service. I was number three. It made me realize why I was welcomed back with open arms. It was good, however, since as interns older than most, our small group got to do a lot of work. We were taught many operations ordinarily reserved from more senior trainees: lumbar sympathectomies, cholecystectomies, bowel anastomoses, unusual hernias, varicose veins, and amputations were commonplace. Anyway, before I finished my surgical training, Dr. Hinton had organized a plan for creating a practice group within the university and invited me to join him. I had accepted the invitation, but by the time my training was completed, the whole plan fell apart. I was going to work as a GI person and continue the work I was doing in the laboratory, in spite of the fact that I had done so much vascular surgery during my training. In California I did a number of pediatric surgical cases, because there was no pediatric surgeon in town, and my training had included considerable pediatric surgery. One of them was a portacaval shunt on a youngster with Gaucher's disease with severe ascites. The procedure stopped his ascites at once. I have a fifteen-year follow-up on him. He never had a recurrence. The other was a child with congenital jejunal atresia whose jejunojejunostomy never worked, even though it remained open. She recovered when I did a duodenojejunostomy. When I came back and was bent on doing pediatric surgery, I told the professor and he said, "Fine, go work with Jerry in the open heart program." So I went to work with Jerry doing open hearts.

Open heart surgery in the early days was a very painful experience, as we all know. The pump problems had only been partially solved. Besides the open heart surgery, there was another encounter that influenced me greatly, and that was meeting Meyer Texon, who worked in the medical examiner's office with Dr. Milton Helpern.

Texon had been doing autopsies in the medical examiner's office and rediscovered what had been noticed many times before—that atherosclerosis occurred at certain sites in the arterial system: at branches, bifurcations, curvatures, and sites of abrupt taper of arteries. He went to a hydraulic engineer called Skalak at Columbia and together they decided that this meant that the lesions were hemodynamically induced and that the critical factor was diminished lateral pressure, the Bernoulli effect. Texon had gone to Hinton, who had referred him to Jerry Lord for collaboration in setting up experimental models to test their ideas. Jerry conceived the idea of simply creating curvatures in vessels by transecting the femoral arteries and interposing long segments of carotids between the cut ends. Although I had my hands full working in the open heart program, I went to work as well in the lab and did these preparations in dogs. We indeed found that intimal hyperplasia could be produced at curvatures, but one couldn't predict precisely at which curvature. It might occur at one curve or two curves or skip curves. It appeared capricious, but indicated to me at least that the flow conditions which were associated with lesions were probably quite specific.

Dale: Were you feeding a special diet?

Imparato: No special diet. This gave me some insight into what atherosclerosis probably represented. I accepted Texon's idea of a primary hemodynamic etiology as early as 1960. It was difficult to get grants from the NIH, because that was the heyday of the cholesterol inhibition theory. We had animals to whom we fed Kendall diets. We also fed thiouracil orally, which resulted in marked hypercholesterolemia. This, however, did not markedly influence the development of the intimal hyperplastic lesion. Basically, I have continued to do this work, studying the evolution of lesions by electron microscopy, which made it possible to trace the migration of smooth muscle cells from the media through the internal elastic lamella to the intimal location. We recorded the desquamation of the endothelial cells. I think most significantly we were able to show that this happened without alteration of diet in hemodynamic models without the intervention of platelets. There was no carpet of platelets in our hemodynamic models, as is found in balloon trauma models, indicating that myointimal hyperplasia does not need to be mediated by the platelets. We now have rather sophisticated equipment built for us by Craig Hartley in Houston, which permits us to get velocity profiles and flow curves across the vessel lumen. We are attempting to correlate the occurrence of lesions with specific flow abnormalities. We have tried all kinds of things to prevent lesion formation: mitotic inhibitors, antimetabolites, corticosteroids, 5-fluorouracil. Nothing that we have done has predictably and totally prevented lesion formation. The most exciting recent development in our work is that we now have a stain that strikingly defines the relationships of the cells of the vascular wall and the organized matrix elements elastin and collagen. The early degradation of elastic elements that occurs within hours after abnormal flow conditions are created suggests that the matrix of the vascular wall may hold the key to intimal hyperplasia and atherosclerosis.

Dale: You are still working at it?

Imparato: Yes, we are still working at it. Additionally, based on the laboratory experiments in the early and middle sixties, I became suspicious that the lesions that we found at operation doing carotid endarterectomies were not evolving as our pathologists said they were. We decided to examine plaques, both grossly in situ and microscopically, to try to deduce how they evolved.

We started to do this in the late sixties. To backtrack a little bit, as a participant in the Joint Study of Extracranial Arterial Occlusion, I had done some carotids already, based on our own angiographic studies since we had no angiographers then.

Dale: Which hospital was this?

Imparato: NYU and Bellevue. Joe Ransahoff had come down from Columbia's Neurologic Institute, where he had been doing some carotids, to be the professor and chairman of neurosurgery. He decided that not one of his neurosurgeons could match the performance of a vascular surgeon in doing carotid endarterectomies, in spite of the fact that he himself felt quite confident in doing "a simple carotid." He voiced the opinion that if there were anything complicated about it, a vascular surgeon could do much better than a neurosurgeon in taking care of the problem. He invited Roy Clauss and me to participate in the joint study, in which he had already established a foothold. The groups met in workshops about three or four times a year, each time in a different institution, so we traveled all over the country. This was very valuable experience for a young surgeon, since we discussed our experiences frequently.

It was striking that experienced surgeons talking to one another about what was being observed at the carotid bifurcation sounded as though they each were talking about a different part of the anatomy or entirely different pathology. I felt that the only way to compare notes, as it were, was to photograph plaques in situ. The photograph would also help the pathologist analyze his findings without the artifacts created by surgical manipulations. These studies led us to conclude that intraplaque hemorrhage was a primary, or at least an earlier, step in the degradation of plaques from a simple fibromuscular stage to a complex compound stage with atheromatous debris, ulceration, and eventual thrombosis. It appeared that the presence of encysted fat in the plaque occurred after the breakdown of intrafibrous plaque hemorrhage, as opposed to the more commonly held notion that hemorrhage followed cholesterol abscess formation. Also at that time, we began to investigate the mechanisms of our failures of arterial reconstructions. It is amazing how much seems to occur purely by chance. I happened to read in a textbook of pathology that for a hundred years it was known that the difference between a gray- or salmon-colored thrombus and the red- or mahogany-colored clot was not age, but rather the difference in the conditions in the vessel in which each formed. If the thrombus is salmon-colored, it forms by the lamination of platelets and fibrin trapping a few blood cells, occurring in an actively flowing system. The red clot occurs after the fact, after the vessel becomes completely occluded and flow stops, resulting in the stasis clot. So I began to explore my failed arterial reconstructions, looking for this flow thrombus. Based on this approach, we were able to convince ourselves that at the sites where we found the flow thrombus we found areas of thickening of the vascular wall. Some of these areas looked exactly like the sites of spontaneously occurring atherosclerosis. Some were at curvatures; others were at a point of attachment. Some were at sites of anastomosis where there seemed to be a taper or something of that sort. Our experimental models in the lab became more varied as we tried to test each of our observations.

Our experimental preparations were based on clinical observations. In 1967 we sent an abstract on intimal hyperplasia to the Society for Vascular Surgery. I guess Jerry sponsored it. Jim DeWeese wrote me back and said, "Well, we won't accept this for presentation at the U.S. meeting, but why don't you go to Vienna and present it to the ISCVS." The title of the paper was "Intimal and Neointimal Hyperplasia as the Cause of Failure of Arterial Reconstructions." It was presented there the same day Charles Dotter appeared. Dotter presented his paper immediately before mine and described graded catheter dilatation of atherosclerotic lesions. They tore him apart. I presented immediately afterwards and there wasn't a single comment. Nobody said a word. I was so discouraged I never published that paper, but Phil Sawyer quoted the presentation in one of his own some years later. It wasn't until 1972 that we published the paper with that title.

Dale: Tell me, what do you think is the place for a young person who has had a good general surgical residency with some vascular experience, but hasn't had a fellowship and wants to do vascular surgery?

Imparato: I think he ought to get himself a fellowship. Also, I think that a year's clinical training is probably cutting it very thin. I think the field is sufficiently complicated and demanding that a year's training at a clinical level is the minimum. I have had them for a year, a year and a half, and two years, and there is no question that by the second year a maturation has occurred that is quite apparent.

Dale: How many cases do they do, or are they exposed to, in a year?

Imparato: I can tell you what the fellow did this year. He did about 160 or 175 major cases and probably scrubbed on another 200 or 300. We have to provide cases for the general surgical residents as well. We've got usually seven, sometimes eight, general surgical residents that come through, and we have to provide them a minimum of forty cases each. Some of the residents get to do sixty, seventy, or eighty cases, but even then they don't have the polish that the fellows acquire.

Dale: What accounts for the drop in the number of applicants to the medical schools today?

Imparato: I think Stanley Crawford summarized it very nicely. For one thing, physicians themselves apparently are counseling their youngsters not to go into medicine, because of the outside pressures being exerted on physicians by bureaucrats. The other reason may be that there seems to be a change in the attitude of our youngsters, who regard the rigors of medical training as unnecessary. When I applied to medical school, the classic answer to the question, "Why do you want to become a doctor?" was unrealistically, idealistically, "Oh, I want to save humanity." Although unrealistic, it indicated the state of mind of many applicants. But an answer which is considered realistic now is that one wants to earn a living or pursue career goals or some such. Medicine has lost its appeal as a profession and is looked on more as a business. I think that turns off a certain number of highly motivated youngsters who may have an unrealistic but idealistic aspiration about medicine. You know, the ones who are idealistic may get turned off. Medical training has also become very expensive and continues relatively late into adult life.

Dale: Would you go into it again today?

Imparato: Oh, sure, I would go into it today and would hope that I would be directed into vascular surgery as well. What I have found fascinating about working with the arteries is that one can see what is inside the blood vessel. I could see it for myself, in a living patient, and this has been a tremendous stimulus to thought.

George Johnson

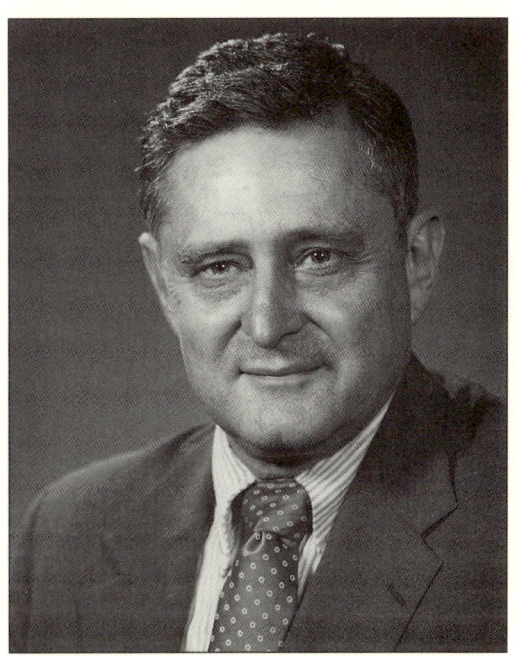

GEORGE JOHNSON may be the most unsung hero in vascular surgery. He is a quiet, considerate, and humble person whose country-boy manner of speaking underplays his achievements. He assisted his father with operations as a teenager and was a respected student at a topnotch university and medical school. Honored for his teaching abilities, applauded for his scientific contributions, and selected to lead many organizations, he also initiated a vascular surgical service at the University of North Carolina at Chapel Hill and established one of the first vascular surgical residency programs. Typical of Johnson's humility is that the honors he cherishes most are the appreciation his patients have expressed to him and his being named one of North Carolina's "Best Doctors." He was interviewed June 18, 1989.

DeWeese: George, tell us about where you were born, your family, and what happened during the first few years of your life.

Johnson: My life began in southeastern North Carolina, in Wilmington, on April 6, 1926. My father was a doctor who started off as a family practitioner and subsequently concentrated on surgery and obstetrics. His family was Scotch-Irish farmers from southeastern North Carolina. My mother was from south Georgia.

My early life was during the Depression. We had no money. My paternal grandfather was a farmer, and my maternal grandfather had lost all his wealth in the automobile business. Daddy was paid for his services with rabbit, deer, or collards, but little money.

In my early life, ages six to sixteen, I was surrounded by numerous friends. My life was epitomized by the title of the book, *Where Did You Go? Out; What Did You Do? Nothing.* Because Wilmington was a quiet, historical, safe town, we had the nearby woods and streets all to ourselves. Our mothers never knew where we were; we always returned for meals. My father had to work all the time to support my mother and her parents; sometimes it would be several weeks before I would see him. His presence was always felt, however.

I had many great teachers during that period who tried to teach me; I got through grammar and high school with roughly a C average. I made a D– in Latin, and the only reason I got a D– instead of an E was because Miss Lathrop and my mother were very close friends. But I think I had a good education. During high school I was in the Reserve Officers Training Corps. I became a company captain, which was a great thrill. We would march down the streets of Wilmington every Friday morning with a band playing and I would be at the front of my company.

I never graduated from high school but went on to the University of North Carolina at Chapel Hill through a special program whereby you could enter college after your junior year in high school and get your high school diploma after completing the first year of college.

DeWeese: Was that because you were so smart?

Johnson: No, it had nothing to do with intelligence, although you had to pass a test to get in. Actually, I tried to get into the air force and navy instead of going to college. They wouldn't take me because at that time I stuttered and I could not say words with "r" in them. Nobody could understand me. So I went on to Chapel Hill and joined a fraternity where they made me repeat "The red, red rabbit ran around the ragged roof rapidly" several times a day. They still call me the "Gweek." I think that helped me to overcome my speech impediment.

I was drafted into the infantry after my freshman year. I was sent to Camp Croft, South Carolina. We were drilling one day with about one thousand soldiers when a general stopped his car, got out, and came up to me and said, "Son, you've had training somewhere, haven't you?" I guess my years in Junior ROTC paid off. The next thing I knew, I was sent to Officers' Candidate School at Fort Benning, Georgia. I became a second lieutenant and was sent overseas, supposedly to invade Japan, but the atomic bomb dropped while we were in Pearl Harbor. So I was sent to Leyte and assigned to a quartermaster bakery, and guarded Japanese prisoners. I subsequently went to headquarters AFWESPAC—Armed Forces Western Pacific —in Manila and became a first lieutenant in the Information and Education Division. I was headed for a career in the army. They even tried to make me a captain, but after thirteen months in the Philippines I resigned. I went back to college for two years and then on to medical school. Just like high school, I did not really graduate from college until after I had finished one year of medical school at the University of North Carolina at Chapel Hill.

DeWeese: Why did you choose medicine as your career?

Johnson: I really don't know. I never talked to anyone about it and my father never asked me. I just always assumed I was going to be a doctor. I had never thought of anything different. I saw my first operation when I was eleven or twelve years old. It was a radical mastectomy, and I passed out. I helped my father operate when I was sixteen. I was helping him deliver babies and take out appendices, even giving anesthesia at times at night. I never will forget one time I was giving anesthesia and Daddy was delivering the baby and had to do an episiotomy. I was giving open drop ether, Daddy started the episiotomy, and the lady very nicely and very sweetly said, "Doctor, are you going to give me an anesthetic?" Of course, I thought she was asleep.

DeWeese: Where was this?

Johnson: It was a little community hospital in Wilmington by the name of James Walker Hospital. My Daddy was always there. I did my first hysterectomy with his help when I was about eighteen. I am only talking about four or five patients. He always did the hard part, and we never had any complications.

Back to Chapel Hill. After two years of medical school, I had to decide where I would transfer, since UNC was only a two-year medical school at that time. Every doctor in the state knew my father. He did more deliveries during the war than any other doctor in the state. They tried to get him to come to Duke at one time and join the full-time faculty, but he wouldn't do it. They tried to give him his boards in obstetrics and gynecology and he replied, "If I do that I might be restricted in what I do, and I want to do everything." So at Chapel Hill it had been "Little George this and Little George that." I guess I was proud of it, but on the other hand, I wanted to do something on my own. The only person who didn't know my father was the anatomy professor, a Dr. Van Cleave. I made almost straight A's in college and became a Phi Beta Kappa my junior year, so I thought I was doing pretty well. When I got to medical school and took my first anatomy exam, my grade was an E. Dr. Van Cleave wrote, "Whatever I can't read must be wrong." He couldn't read my writing. Even now, nobody can read my writing. He must have thought I was worth something, however; he later asked me to repair his hernia.

So I had to make a decision as to where I would finish medical school. I had my eye set on going to Harvard and applied. I was about fifth in the class and they usually took three or four at Harvard. The first three all were accepted. I became nervous and decided to also apply to Cornell in New York City. They accepted me the next week. At the deadline, I wired them back and told them I would take it. The very next day I received a letter of acceptance from Harvard. I didn't have any idea that once you had committed yourself to go to a school you could break that commitment, so I went to Cornell. I never was unhappy with that decision.

I married Marian that summer, before I went to New York City. Both of us were from a pretty rural setting in North Carolina and we were concerned about going to the Big Apple, but the Big Apple was very nice to both of us and we stayed there for about ten years.

DeWeese: After completing medical school, you stayed at Cornell for your general surgical residency. Did you look at other programs?

Johnson: I looked at the University of North Carolina at Chapel Hill. We didn't have much money in those days to travel around and look at places like students do now. They tried to get me to come back to Chapel Hill, which had just opened a residency training program, and Dr. Womack offered me a job. But I wanted to stay in New York. I was very pleased with what I saw there and it looked like a very good experience for me. It was a seven-year program, and it was a Halsted pyramidal system. Every year one or two people were cut out of the program, but I figured if you were good you could make it and if you weren't, you wouldn't. So I stayed there.

DeWeese: Who were the teachers there that you remember best?

Johnson: In my internship year, Herb Conway and I wrote a paper on "Congenital Absence of the Skull and Scalp." Bronson Ray was head of neurosurgery. When I was a junior resident on neuro-surgery, a little child who had fallen down the steps and was losing consciousness came to the emergency room. The chief neurosurgery resident, Henry Wood, was off. Dr. Ray and I did burr holes on this little kid and I guess we saved his life. He and I were both scared. So he and I hit it off really well. I also related well with Pep Wade, who was subsequently president of the American College of Surgeons. The one who supported me the rest of his life was Frank Glenn, who was head of the Department of Surgery. He and I wrote about fifteen papers together. I spent one year in the lab with John Beal, and we created Keefer-Martin and Mann-Williamson pouches, to study the control of gastric acid secretion. We lined the pig stomach with skin, but that didn't work. We also created an aortic flutter valve by an ingenious method that never was used in humans but worked in dogs. We would tear the aortic valve by inserting a crochet hook through a stab ventriculotomy so that they would get aortic insufficiency. Then we would invaginate the proximal aorta into the distal aorta so that the blood would flow one way but not flow back. I'm surprised they didn't all thrombose, but it did work. We measured pressures and showed that it prevented the dog from having marked aortic regurgitation.

DeWeese: Have people ever tried to use that in the venous system?

Johnson: No, I don't think it would work, because I think it would thrombose. My main interest in the laboratory was in doing metabolic research. I worked with the clinical arm of a metabolic team that was studying nitrogen balance and respiratory quotients in humans. We were trying to show that with hyperalimentation you could maintain nitrogen equilibrium. Dudrick later demonstrated this could be done in puppies.

DeWeese: Was anyone doing cardiovascular research at that time at Cornell?

Johnson: Yes. As a matter of fact, George Holswade and Frank Redo were trying to repeat Lillihei's work in perfecting a blood oxygenator so they could do open heart surgery.

DeWeese: Were they doing aneurysm surgery?

Johnson: Sam Moore and George Holswade, who had just come on as an attending, were doing some. There was a fellow named Ed Keefer who was "chasing ambulances" throughout New York City, obtaining aortas and freezing them. We were using some of these. I helped on a few aneurysms and some other vascular cases during my chief year. I had taken a liking to cardiac surgery and I had done some open hearts with Dr. Glenn. He let me do a few mitral valve fractures.

DeWeese: I remember Dr. Glenn writing a paper on the association of gallbladder disease and patients who require mitral valve operations.

Johnson: I did not write that one, but I did write a number of papers on gallbladder disease, on which Dr. Glenn had a tremen-

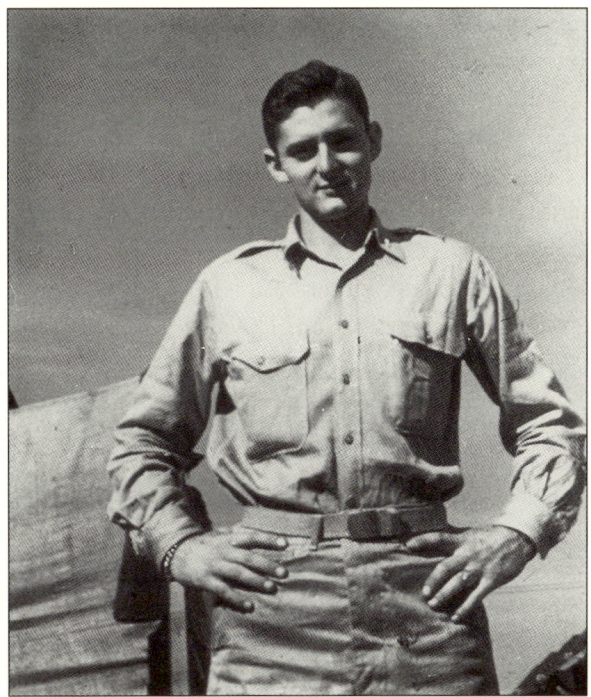

George, 1st Lt. Infantry, the Philippines, 1945.

dous file. When I was chief resident, my service did more operations than had ever been done before at New York Hospital, primarily because I had Charlie Pearce as an assistant chief. Charlie would go to the emergency room and find patients with gallstones who needed an operation as an emergency. We would do cholecystectomies at night and the other things all day.

Another great teacher was Victor Marshall in urology. Everybody treated me nicely. I guess it was because I was a southerner. I wasn't looked upon as a vascular surgeon when I finished my training. All the papers I had written had been on gastric and biliary surgery. You might say I finished primarily with training in gastrointestinal operations but with an interest in vascular surgery.

In my last year, 1958 to 1959, Claire Booth Luce, who was a friend of Dr. Glenn, said she was going to write a series of articles in *Life* magazine on health care in the United States, and one of them was going to be on the training of a surgeon. She said she would like to use one of Dr. Glenn's residents. Dr. Glenn was president of the American College of Surgeons at that time, and he thought it would be nice if somebody at New York Hospital did this. He asked me to do it. A *Life* reporter, Alix Kerr, spent about three weeks with us. They took about eleven hundred pictures and used eleven of them.

We had three children then and didn't think New York City was a great place to raise them, so we went back to North Carolina. I did not want to go in with my father because I didn't want to be known as "Little George." I talked to Dr. Howard Bradshaw at Bowman-Gray, Dr. Deryl Hart at Duke, and Dr. Nathan Womack at Chapel Hill to see if they would give me a job in academic surgery. Each of them wanted me to spend another year learning how to do cardio-thoracic surgery and spend a year in the lab; they would pay me $5,000 a year to do that. That wasn't much money. I'd had seven years of training and thought I was pretty good in thoracic and open heart surgery already, so I decided that I would go into private practice, but I didn't want to go back to Wilmington. I could have gone to Greensboro, Charlotte, Rocky Mount, or other places, but I chose to go to Durham, primarily because it was close to Duke and the University of North Carolina. I thought maybe the intellectual atmosphere in that area might rub off on me. I started by myself in private practice at Watts Hospital. I was on call all the time. We had no beepers in those days. I went to a football game after a year in practice and, of course, it would be my luck that they announced my name over a loudspeaker. Everyone accused me of getting free advertising. It was during that same period of time that Glenn Young, who was at Duke, and I became friends. He asked me to go to my first vascular meeting at the Biltmore Hotel in New York City. It was the first time I had been out of Durham in about a year and a half.

DeWeese: What year was that?

Johnson: It was June 1961. Glenn and I had a room at the Biltmore, and we were watching the College All-Stars play football. He had bought a bottle of gin, so we had a great time drinking gin and watching football. We went out at about midnight to get some breakfast in this little old dingy place near the Biltmore. As we walked into the restaurant, somebody in a booth got up and said,

"Dr. Johnson, my doctor." So you never could get away. Anyway, I haven't missed a vascular meeting since then.

DeWeese: You said you were getting a lot of referrals for vascular problems. What type of problems were they?

Johnson: There were mostly aneurysms, aortoiliac occlusive disease, and arterial emboli.

DeWeese: When had you done your first aneurysm?

Johnson: I did one or two when I was in New York Hospital. I also saw some, but I was really self-trained.

DeWeese: Had you done bypass grafts in your residency?

Johnson: I think I had, one or two. I remember putting in a homograft at Cornell and also putting in Teflon bypass grafts when I was at Watts.

DeWeese: Where did you learn to do that? Had you worked in the laboratory anywhere?

Johnson: No, I watched it and did some myself at New York Hospital. I didn't feel uncomfortable doing it. In the two and a half years that I was at Watts, I built a pretty good referral base in vascular surgery. I had good results. I guess there were only two others in Durham doing it, except for those at Duke. I had a number of friends at Duke and they were always willing to give me advice. We would talk all the time and I benefited a great deal from that. I used to go to all of the Duke conferences. I also joined the clinical staff at the University of North Carolina in oncology. I was making $27,000 a year and enjoying my practice. It wasn't mammoth, but it was really beginning to pick up. I built a $60,000 office building and was all set to stay when Bob Zeppa, who had been helping Dick Peters over at Chapel Hill, decided that he did not want to do cardiac surgery and wanted to go back into general surgery. In fact, I think he was interested in trying to set up a vascular surgery service at Chapel Hill. For some reason, Dr. Womack had taken a liking to me and told Dick to come over and try to get me to come to Chapel Hill. Dick came over and asked if I would work with him. I had a difficult time deciding what to do. I knew Dick was very difficult to work with, but I also realized that he was a great teacher. I told my father about the offer and asked for his advice. I was doing so well in private practice that I thought I really should stay in Durham, but he said, "Naw, go to Chapel Hill." I finally decided that I could be more effective in Chapel Hill, because I enjoyed teaching and research. I'd already written four papers while I was in private practice at Watts, one on sequestration of the lung.

DeWeese: Were you doing thoracic surgery?

Johnson: I was doing everything. No open heart, but vascular, thoracic, general surgery, and everything that came along. When I decided to go with Dick, I told him I didn't have my thoracic boards. He said, "We'll help you get them." He asked the Board of Thoracic Surgery to allow me to be an attending and still get credit for thoracic training under him at the same time. He taught me how to do thoracic surgery. We did a lot of tuberculous lungs. We worked with Will Seeley and Glenn Young from Duke at the tuberculosis sanitarium in Wilson. I also helped Dick Peters do the cardiac cases. I did that for a couple of years, and then Ben Wilcox, who had been up at the NIH, came back to Chapel Hill, and Dick Peters was recruited out to San Diego. It left a dilemma for me because both Ben and I were there. Ben was enthusiastic about being a cardiothoracic surgeon and he wanted to be head of the Division of Cardiac Surgery, as I did. But I was still interested in, and trying to build, vascular surgery. In the cardiothoracic division, vascular was always put on the end of all the cardiac surgery cases. We were even doing elective aneurysms at night. I suggested to Dr. Womack that maybe it would be nice if I went back into general surgery as a vascular surgeon. Dr. Womack said, "Well, I'll never create a vascular surgery service, but you can have all of my patients." Although the rest of the general surgeons never gave up vascular surgery, they did send all of their vascular cases to me. One of them said, "You can have all of my patients requiring vascular surgery, including the amputations." Everyone recognized me as the vascular surgeon even though there never was a vascular surgery service.

During the first ten years after I joined UNC we were very active doing research. Dr. Womack and I studied his concept of arteriovenous communications as the etiology of portal hypertension. We had a grant that was funded for twenty years. I worked with Jim Tapp of Chemstrend, trying to perfect sutures made of nylon and a nylon mitral valve; neither succeeded. I subsequently looked at metabolic response to shock, red cell deformability, and viscosity.

DeWeese: Who were the other chairmen?

Johnson: After Dr. Womack came C. G. Thomas. Tim allowed vascular surgery to become stronger. We both recognized that vascular surgery took some special training. He allowed me to start an unofficial fellowship, and the first fellow was Drew Grice, who is now in private practice in eastern North Carolina. The next year Blair Keagy also asked to become a fellow. We have had continuous fellows since then. The program was first approved by the vascular societies and then by the Residency Review Committee. I believe we've had a good vascular training program. We've had an active research lab and have been involved with both clinical and basic research. We are fortunate that the University has Ph.D.s in both the basic science department and clinical faculty doing a lot of basic research; a lot are interested in vascular disease at the basic level and are a great resource. I have been fortunate in having good support from not only my colleagues but the dean and department chairmen. I was most honored when I received the first distinguished professorship in the department, excluding Dr. Womack.

DeWeese: Who do you think should be doing vascular surgery?

Johnson: I think the best vascular surgery is done by trained vascular surgeons. However, in North Carolina there are a number of people who do not have any certification in vascular surgery who are doing superb vascular surgery. Those doctors who have had good general surgery training in vascular surgery usually can do the operations fine. I don't see many vascular patients who have been mishandled. Occasionally the judgment surrounding the operation has not been appropriate, but that is seen in the certified vascular surgeon as well. The technical part of the operation does not seem to be that much of a problem, but I feel that sometimes the indications are. In North Carolina, operations for vascular problems are still being done primarily by noncertified vascular surgeons. I am concerned that it continues to be done by people who know what they can do and what they can't do. That's where the danger arises. North Carolina must be unique, from what I hear is done elsewhere. This state was one of the first states to have quality state organizations in surgery where ideas have been freely exchanged. I am naive about what's going on in the United States, but I just don't think at present too much bad vascular surgery is being done in North Carolina by noncertified vascular surgeons. Perhaps in the future, all vascular surgery will be done by certified vascular surgeons if there are enough of them, and if the general surgeons lose interest in these patients.

DeWeese: Do you think that anyone coming out of a general surgical program in the United States should be given the right to perform operations?

Johnson: I think the experience in vascular surgery for all general surgeons is getting worse, and it's because of a lack of interest in vascular surgery by a number of the general surgery trainees. I think as time goes on there is going to have to be more special training in vascular surgery for the interested general surgeon. I don't think all of our general surgery trainees coming out of Chapel Hill are adequate vascular surgeons. Most of them are going into some sort of specialty, including vascular fellowship. Thus everyone finishing a general surgery program is not qualified to do vascular surgery.

DeWeese: What do you see as the future of vascular surgery in the United States? Is it going to end up being done by trained specialists who devote all their time to that specialty, like neurosurgery?

Johnson: I think it will be a long time before all of the vascular surgery in North Carolina is done by certified vascular surgeons. There is just no way they can do it. In North Carolina, there are probably no more than fifteen certified vascular surgeons. Yet noncertified vascular/general surgeons are doing a lot of good vascular surgery in Rocky Mount, Sanford, Fayetteville, and Lumberton. People in North Carolina don't like to leave town. They don't want to come to Chapel Hill; they don't want to go to Duke if they can possibly avoid it.

DeWeese: What do you think about the effect of the current Medicare activities in restricting fees?

Johnson: I have no idea what is going to happen. I went into vascular surgery because I loved doing vascular surgery. I never really thought of making a lot of money. That's not the reason I went into it. There is a tremendous amount of pressure on medical students to go into primary care specialties, pediatrics, medicine, family medicine, and obstetrics. Yet the surgeons keep on coming.

DeWeese: What do you think is going to happen to the superspecialties, cardiac and thoracic, which are now being performed in many towns? Are we going to be regionalized?

Johnson: The cardiac surgeons and even the vascular surgeons who have gone to the community away from training programs are doing well. They are doing a lot of patients with good results and are taking patients away from the centers. They have a very efficient system. Coronary artery bypass grafts and many of the cardiac operations have become pretty commonplace.

DeWeese: As president of the American Venous Forum, what do you think the future of venous surgery holds?

Johnson: The American Venous Forum attempts to attract interest and basic research in venous diseases. I'm impressed with what that organization has done to attract scholarly approaches to the problems of venous disease. Maybe we can improve the treatment of this really devastating group of diseases.

DeWeese: Do you have any thoughts about the future treatment of venous diseases? Are the endovascular techniques that are now being used so extensively for arterial diseases also going to be useful for the treatment of venous disease?

Johnson: I wouldn't think so. However, I never would have thought of taking a gallbladder or an appendix out through a laparoscope. I don't see how it would be used in venous disease, but I am willing to learn. The venous system is, I think, very different because of the low flow and the tendency to thrombose. If we can control the coagulation mechanism better, I think that endovascular instrumentation would have a better chance.

William von Liebig

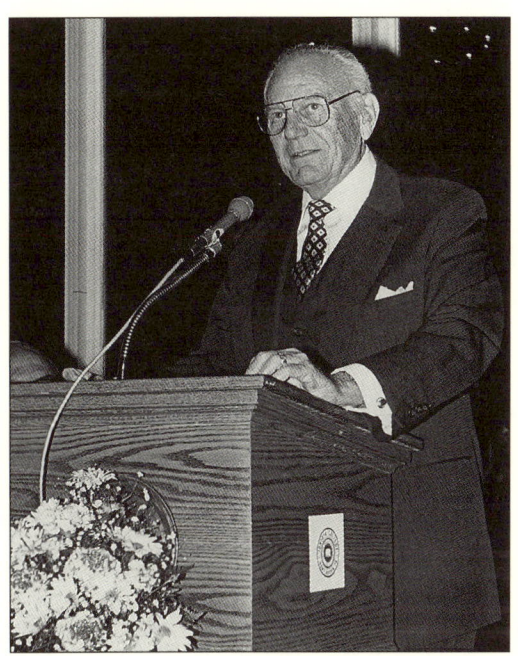

WILLIAM VON LIEBIG is representative of the way in which industry and vascular surgery have grown up in a synergistic fashion. He epitomizes the hard work, determination, resourcefulness, and gambles industry representatives took during the formative years of vascular surgery. The editors include this chapter even though von Liebig is not a physician. He was interviewed December 12, 1988.

Dale: What we really want to do is talk about you as a prosthetic manufacturer, but before that, we want to go back, so tell me first about your parents and where you came from.

von Liebig: My full name is William John von Liebig, and I was born in Huntingdon, Pennsylvania, some seventy years ago, on March 24, 1923. I spent my early years attending Juniata College, where I got my premed degree and had intentions of becoming a surgeon. I won a scholarship to go to Harvard for four years to pursue that career, but during World War II, being in the reserve of the Army Air Corps, I was called up for service and my first alternate won the award. That was in 1943. I spent two and a half years in the service as a bomber pilot, eventually becoming alternate lead of the 8th Air Force in Europe. The operations officer to whom I reported was Lieutenant Colonel Jimmy Stewart with the famous 389th Bomb Group. I flew back to the States with my crew after the war in Europe ended.

Dale: Was Doolittle overall commander?

von Liebig: Yes.

Dale: How many missions did you fly?

von Liebig: Twenty-five.

Dale: And did you have any particular problems with any of them?

von Liebig: Yes, I was shot down on three occasions. The first time we were shot down, we were flying a mission over Magdeburg, a city with a big oil refinery in Germany, and we had an engine knocked out. We were fortunate enough, because this was after the invasion, to be able to cross the lines, and we ended up in a fighter field in Belgium. I was a command pilot of a B-24. We were able to repair our ship and get back to England.

Dale: What did you do?

von Liebig: Working with ground crew, we were able to change the damaged engine and put a new engine in. We were able to get back as a result of that.

The next time was over a target in the Ruhr, where all the major industrialization was. And again we were hit with flak and lost an engine, and again we came down, this time in France. Fortunately, we were able to get back over the lines and we repeated the same.

Dale: You got another engine?

von Liebig: We put it back together and made it back to England. The third occasion was over Berlin. We were able to limp back; at that point it wasn't the engine that was a problem. It was that our ship was pretty badly shot up by flak and fighters, but we were able to get back over the Channel. There was an arrangement in the southern part of England where damaged aircraft could come in on an expensively equipped, long runway and were able to get down safely.

Dale: How long was the runway, do you think?

von Liebig: That runway was over ten thousand feet long.

Dale: Which base were you flying out of?

von Liebig: We were flying out of a base called Hethel, in East Anglia, about eight miles south of Norwich.

Dale: So you got back from the war, you went back to the States, and then they tried to send you to Japan?

von Liebig: I was actually trained in B-29s to go to the Far East. But with the number of points I had acquired during my time in the European Theater of Operations, I was mustered out of the service.

Dale: What did you do next? Tell me about the nurse contingent.

von Liebig: During the course of being mustered out of the service, I had to serve an extra month. They sent me to a base in Sioux Falls, South Dakota, where they really had no assignment, except they did give me a contingent of about fifty nurses whom I had to look after. You know, make sure that they behaved themselves, and bed check every night.

Dale: Were they happy with that?

von Liebig: They were really ecstatic, and I likewise.

Dale: What happened after that?

von Liebig: I came back to my hometown of Huntingdon, Pennsylvania, and went back to Juniata College to brush up and secure my B.S. degree.

Dale: To brush up for what?

von Liebig: For getting back to medicine. As a matter of fact, I planned to continue my matriculation in medical school and get my medical degree. However, I decided during the course of this period that I would go into engineering. This was in 1945.

Dale: What made you change your mind?

von Liebig: A number of my professors indicated that a number of years had gone by, and there would be a long session yet of eight to ten more years before I would be able to get into the final phase of becoming a surgeon. I wasn't getting any younger at that point. Also, my family was involved in textile operations, the Throwing Company in Mifflinburg, Pennsylvania, so there was sort of a family tie-in there.

Dale: What did you make there?

von Liebig: There we produce yarns for all segments of the textile industry: knitting, weaving, braiding, etc. Yarns are made from various fibers, but are mostly synthetic at this point in time.

Dale: How old is Dacron?

von Liebig: Dacron goes back, I would say, to about the mid-1940s.

Dale: Where did Dacron come from?

von Liebig: Dacron came from the DuPont Company. I am not sure who invented it, but it came from DuPont, as did nylon and Teflon.

I finally did graduate with my M.S. degree in textile engineering, having attended the University of Pennsylvania and the Philadelphia College of Textiles and Sciences. I was there for three years and graduated in June 1949. My first position was in New York City with Susquehanna Mills, one of the big three companies in the textile field. They were involved with manufacturing many different textile products.

Dale: What did you do?

von Liebig: That's a good question, Andy. To get my degree we had to spend six months or two summers working in industry instead of writing a thesis. I had spent the six months in the Susquehanna plant at Sunbury, Pennsylvania. When I was hired by the president of the company, Mr. Conza, I asked him what my position would be and what I was expected to do. He said, "Bill, we have a lot of different challenges here; why don't you find what you are comfortable with," which gave me a nice opportunity.

As a result of his giving me this opportunity, I looked around the company and wrote a paper on the performance of the company, which was not really very glorious because they had a lot of problems.

Dale: What did Mr. Conza think about it?

von Liebig: He thought it was a very interesting analysis of the business and was quite surprised to find out what was not happening in the company.

In my early weeks there, I came into an office, and sitting in the corner was an enormous desk with a fellow reading the *New York Times.* I went over and introduced myself and asked him what his position was. He said he was Frank Alexander and that he had been the star salesman for Susquehanna Mills for many, many years. I remembered my father talking about him, because my father and two other relatives had worked for Susquehanna Mills. As a matter of fact, my great-uncle was the treasurer of the company back in the early 1900s in New York City.

So I did have some connections there. Frank Alexander said, "Call me Alex." Alex and I wanted to revitalize the upholstery and drapery division, which had been a part of Susquehanna for many years.

I asked Frank that afternoon if he would be kind enough to introduce me to some of his customers in New York, so we could see what the possibility was of starting the upholstery and drapery division again. Susquehanna consisted of twelve divisions at that time. In 1949 only three divisions were contributing positively toward the bottom line. The other nine were unprofitable. So we decided we would try to make a profitable fourth division.

He introduced me to his best customers, all the big jobbers in New York City, and I found out they were anxious to work with us. So we started up a business in 1949 and 1950, and within a period of one year we were doing over $1 million in upholstery and drapery fabrics from scratch.

Dale: But you were not on your own yet.

von Liebig: Correct. At this time, I was a liaison officer between the New York office and the main factory of Susquehanna in Sunbury, Pennsylvania. Frank and I started this division again, and within two years we were well on our way into a multimillion dollar operation. The president was very proud about this; I reported directly to him. But by 1953 I could see the handwriting on the wall. Susquehanna was going to fail, and I decided I had to start looking around for another position.

Dale: Did they fail?

von Liebig: They failed in March 1954.

Dale: Why was that?

von Liebig: Very poor management. It was very obvious. By December 1953 I had found a new position with the Meadox Weaving Company in New Jersey. The president of the company, Mark Turpan, invited me to come over and be interviewed.

Dale: And how old was that company?

von Liebig: The company was started in 1927. They were in the upholstery fabric business, probably one of the top such companies in the United States. I joined them on January 1, 1954, to turn the company around.

Dale: What was your position?

von Liebig: I was general manager of the company, and had authority to conduct the business totally on my own, reporting only to the owner and president of the company.

Dale: And what did Turpan do? Did he just quit?

von Liebig: He was semiretired. The problem was that he had three sons, each one operating in his own way and not thinking in terms of building the business. An interesting situation occurred. Every Friday afternoon, we would visit the Peoples Trust Company in Hackensack, New Jersey, to borrow enough money to keep the company going.

Dale: How long was your loan?

von Liebig: The loan was ongoing. It was reviewed every Friday afternoon with the executive vice president of Peoples Trust Company, Ken Fisher, who was a friend of mine. The first week after I joined the company, we had our Friday afternoon meeting. During that week I had the opportunity of meeting his three sons and seeing what contribution they were making.

We met in Hackensack Friday afternoon to review the loan. After having reviewed the situation very carefully and having listened to what was going on for one week, I turned in my resignation. I could tell that the company would never be able to survive with the three sons all pulling in opposite directions. A single driving force was necessary to build a successful business.

As a result of this divergence and the fact that I had a close relationship with the executive vice president of the bank, we received the resignations of the three sons that afternoon. I withdrew my resignation and became the vice president of the Meadox Weaving Company.

I began trying to turn the company around and was working at that time to add new products to the line. As a result of my efforts, I was able to establish connections in Detroit. I was successful in producing Meadox automotive fabrics for General Motors, Ford, and Chrysler. We were able to help our manufacturing system right away by producing fabrics for these large consumers.

Dale: But where was your manufacturing unit?

von Liebig: The Meadox Weaving Company was located in Waldwick, New Jersey. We tried to diversify the business, because we were getting a considerable amount of competition from overseas. The Marshall Plan was funding European factories. Fabrics were being imported to the United States and sold at a price less than we could manufacture them.

Dale: Why was that, because of labor cost?

von Liebig: Not just labor, but material cost. Marshall money was funding our allies while we in the United States had to purchase our materials, and our labor was a good deal more expensive, too. Actually, our cost of material was just too expensive.

Dale: How did you feel about that? After all, you had fought and damn near died in Europe.

von Liebig: Well, I could see that this industry was not going to flourish. I am always a believer that fate takes care of things. There seems to be a higher power that guides me in many things I do.

Dale: You mean you are pragmatic.

von Liebig: Certainly so. As time would prove, we were able to be successful by diversifying the operations of the company. Then in the fall of 1954, when the Fontainbleu Hotel opened in Miami Beach, Mark Turpan, the owner of Meadox Weaving Company, happened to be on the beach with an entrepreneur from Chicago and sold the company that afternoon. He called me and said, "You have a new boss, Titus Haffa, from Chicago." Haffa was a Swiss gentleman, I came to know. We became very close, and although he had not finished his eighth-grade education, he was one of the greatest entrepreneureal types I have ever run into.

Dale: Now you're telling me that education doesn't count for very much.

von Liebig: In the case of Titus Haffa, education was not the principal driving force. I am not saying that education is not required.

Dale: What is the important thing that gets a guy to do what he's got to do?

von Liebig: I really think he has within him what he feels he has to do. Generally speaking, a person who is an achiever is driven, Andy.

Dale: What do you mean by driven?

von Liebig: You have an inner feeling that tells you that you should be doing certain things. I feel that I have this, because regardless of whatever successes I have had, I still have a certain drive within me that tells me I must continue to move on and accomplish other things.

Dale: I'm very interested in this. We have some television advertising about "we are driven." What does that mean? Who drives you?

von Liebig: I think it is a force within you. Nobody drives me; of course, my wife has some influence and some of my best friends, but there is something within one. You must know about this yourself, because you are an achiever, one who must accomplish. We who are achievers thrive on what we can accomplish. And if we don't accomplish what we set out to do, we become frustrated.

Dale: Bill, what makes an achiever?

von Liebig: A number of things go into being an achiever. Again, Andy, I think you have to have it within you. You can't learn this. If you are the type to be an achiever, you can become a better achiever by learning, by attending seminars, and by reading up if the talent is within you.

Dale: Do you have children? Are any of them achievers?

von Liebig: Yes.

Dale: How did you trigger that? How does that come about?

von Liebig: I think it comes about naturally. I had three children. Two I have lost. I have a daughter left. My two sons died very shortly after their births.

Dale: I'm sorry.

von Liebig: It's regrettable, because I could have passed the business on to them, and the family name could have lived on.

Dale: Let's go into that, because I have some feeling about that. Would you like to have a child to carry on?

von Liebig: Yes. We are looking into it. We would like to adopt a child, perhaps.

But let's get back to why my daughter is an achiever. Let's say that Barbara is several credits short of her doctorate in psychology, probably at Columbia University in New York City. She has suddenly decided at this stage of her life to counsel young people. She is the only Protestant I know who is top director for the Jewish Youth Council in New York City.

Dale: How do you define a Christian?

von Liebig: A Christian is one who believes in Christ and who believes in the Bible and the teachings of the Bible. Specifically, we are Presbyterians.

Dale: How did you get to be a Presbyterian?

von Liebig: Well, I think this was a carryover from my family. My father came from Wuppertal-Elberfeld in Germany, on the river Wupper. My father, a Lutheran, immigrated to America in 1910 and married my mother, a Presbyterian, from Newark, New Jersey, in 1918. They both attended the German Presbyterian Church. When I was born in 1923, I was baptized in the Presbyterian Church.

We are talking about 1909, when my great-uncle in New York City, the secretary-treasurer of Susquehanna Mills, invited his three nephews from Germany to join him in New York. He would provide transportation from Germany and a job. My father and his younger brother accepted this opportunity, arrived, and were immediately put to work within the company. My father came to New York City, as far as religion is concerned, as a Lutheran. My father spent, I believe, six years with the company in New York City. He reported to the president of the company, and they always lunched at the

Vanderbilt. At lunch one day, they were discussing a difficulty with one of the plants of Susquehanna Mills. At that time they had sixteen different plants throughout the country. My father was saying to the president of the company that perhaps he should be given a chance to straighten out the problems in the plant in Huntingdon, which at that time was the Huntingdon Specialty Company. When they returned from lunch, the president called my father into his office and said, "Bill, thank you. You are going to take a train tomorrow morning to Huntingdon and straighten out the Huntingdon Specialty Company."

So my father did go to Huntingdon, Pennsylvania, and over a period of years did straighten out the problems in the company.

Dale: Now we have to get down to the brass tacks. How did you get into the prosthetic business?

von Liebig: Actually, I sort of followed the footsteps of my father because he, being an entrepreneur, eventually did buy out the assets of the Huntingdon Specialty Company and over a period of years made it the Huntingdon Throwing Mills, which is the family company today. It is located in Mifflinburg, Pennsylvania.

When I graduated from Penn and the Philadelphia College of Textiles and Sciences in 1949, my father reminded me that although the family business was textiles, I was not to be a part of it, because our managerial characteristics are different. He felt that one boss was enough within the company.

Dale: How did you differ from your father?

von Liebig: He really didn't want any competition in the management of the company, because he thought his technique was perfectly great, and he knew that my technique would be different. As a trade-off, he said to me that when I found a business that I would be interested in taking over, he would advance me $25,000 for the purchase of that entity.

Dale: A lot of money at that time.

von Liebig: That was in 1949.

Dale: What is that equivalent to today?

von Liebig: Oh gosh, if we looked at that it would be the equivalent to at least a quarter of a million. I did proceed, as I mentioned earlier, to join Susquehanna Mills and then came into Meadox

Weaving, which was then sold to Titus Haffa. Haffa had an interesting experience in 1954, because his wife had been operated on by a famous surgeon in Chicago, Dr. Ormond Julian. As a result of this successful operation on Mrs. Haffa, Titus decided to give a grant to Dr. Julian to pursue whatever research he was doing.

Haffa had thirty-seven other companies. It was a large conglomerate, and Meadox became number thirty-eight. He had four people reporting to him—his secretary; two controllers, one representing half of his companies and the other representing the other half; and me. Oddly enough, as I did with Susquehanna, I gave him a report on his organization shortly after I had joined, advising him that there were certain improprieties existing. He was concerned and immediately assigned four of his companies for me to manage: the Dormeyer Corporation, the Camfield Company, Paragon Oil, and Webcor.

Dale: You were dealing in oil?

von Liebig: Yes, and Webcor was a high fidelity equipment manufacturer in Chicago. So I had five companies to run, and this gave me a great deal of experience with regard to managing and operating various enterprises. Meadox, at that time, was still a drapery and upholstery manufacturer. Since it did not fit in with the other thirty-seven companies, we decided to sell the company to our competitor, Classic Weaving, in western New York. In the meantime, Dr. Ormond Julian received the grant of money to pursue the research project of his choice. I had a visit from Dr. Julian and the project that he was working on was the development of the first vascular prosthetic graft. He brought with him a friend.

Dale: The year was what?

von Liebig: It was 1954. He brought with him a friend from Columbia University, Dr. Ralph Deterling. The two of them came into my office and discussed the project, which they wanted me to develop for them. And that was really the beginning, as far as I was concerned, of getting into the prosthetic business.

Dale: What was the project?

von Liebig: The project was to develop a tubular structure of a textile fabrication that would be capable of holding blood, being porous, but yet not oozing blood, so that this could be implanted into an animal and would be able to sustain that animal's circulatory system.

My philosophy is that in the years that I have been involved with the health care field, we have never, ever come out with a product, nor have we involved ourselves with the development of a product, that didn't in some way assist you, the surgeon, and benefit the patient to give that patient a better quality of life. We must give Ormond and Ralph a lot of credit for coming up with the concept of developing the first vascular graft.

During this period, I still felt I wanted to go back to medical school to pursue my training to become a surgeon. Julian and Deterling strongly recommended I continue with the research program. They thought I would be more successful in the long run doing what I was doing in developing vascular grafts, than in going back to medical school and pursuing a career as a surgeon.

Ormond and Ralph had done their homework well. They investigated putting in plastic tubes and tried this in animals, which failed. Somehow or other, they came up with the concept that when you pricked this plastic tube with pins it became porous. This allowed the animal to live several days longer, which was innovative. Don't forget that at this time we were still dealing with homografts.

Dale: I remember it.

von Liebig: I was dealing with things like Ivalon Sponge while Dr. Sterling Edwards was busy working out his nylon braided tube with Dr. Tapp from Chemstrand.

Dale: Did you contact Tapp?

von Liebig: I had several conversations with him by telephone. He then said that he had finished the project, so I took it up with Dr. Sterling Edwards. To this day Sterling and I are very close, and we exchange ideas frequently.

We did decide that we would go ahead with our own development. At first we experimented with some fabrics that I procured from Macy's in New York City. This was in late July 1954, as I recall, and I bought several different kinds of fabrics—nylon, Teflon, Dacron, Orlon, and Vinyon.

Dale: Why Macy's?

von Liebig: Because they have a great fabric department where you can buy yard goods. What we were doing was constructing tubes on my wife's sewing machine. Julian and Deterling would then put these into animals and see how they would behave.

Dale: Where was this being done?

von Liebig: This was being done by Ralph Deterling at Columbia Presbyterian Hospital in New York City and by Ormond Julian at Presbyterian St. Luke's in Chicago, in 1954.

Dale: Well, you don't know it, but I was doing it, too. Everybody's had a graft project.

von Liebig: Work continued in our laboratory in New Jersey, but Dacron seemed to be the fiber that responded the best. For me, it was excellent, because at that time DuPont was manufacturing Dacron in various deniers and I was interested in experimenting with these. Teflon was restricted to one denier at that time.

Dale: But DuPont made that too, didn't they?

von Liebig: DuPont made all these fibers. We had one source. Subsequently, many sources, but at that time, one. We began fabricating the first woven polyester graft on our looms in Haledon, New Jersey. It was in the form of a tubular structure in a woven form using 70 denier polyester yarn.

Dale: What about braided?

von Liebig: We did not do braiding. We felt that the braid was not going to be satisfactory, because when you elongate a braid, you narrow the lumen.

Dale: What about knit?

von Liebig: We thought knit was too porous. We did not get into that structure until later. Since we were experts in weaving, that was the natural course to take originally. We pursued that and, in the meantime, Ormond came to us with a number of different sketches of bifurcated grafts. This is the Y-shaped graft that he wanted us to manufacture and in the latter part of 1954 we proceeded to put together on our looms the first bifurcated grafts. The tubular grafts we first made were implanted by Ormond Julian in Chicago, and we also supplied Ralph Deterling with the grafts that he implanted at Columbia Presbyterian in New York.

They worked successfully and, since FDA restrictions had not yet come into play, we began in 1955 to do clinical studies; these proceeded successfully. By that time, we were making the bifurcated grafts, which were used by Julian and Deterling for Leriche's syndrome. A film was made in 1956 of Dr. Julian implanting one of these products at Presbyterian St. Luke's in Chicago.

Dale: Now Bill, entrepreneurs have built America. What about an entrepreneur like you? You can't buy them; you can't breed them. Where do they come from?

von Liebig: You have to seek them out. Along that subject, I mentioned earlier that in 1949 my father promised me he would advance me $25,000 when I found a company I felt comfortable with. I exercised that option in 1961. During the course of events, the complex I was involved with in Chicago, the Titus Haffa conglomerate, started crumbling. I recall that in November 1960 I had a visit from Titus Haffa at the Newark airport. During lunch, he agreed to sell me Meadox Weaving for $25,000. I gave him a $500 check as a deposit, which was about all I had in my bank account. Immediately after we confirmed that arrangement, I called my father and reminded him of his pledge in 1949, and immediately I had $25,000 at my disposal. That is exactly what I bought Meadox Weaving for in December 1960.

Dale: You paid $25,000 for Meadox?

von Liebig: Exactly. That is the entrepreneurial aspect. Recognizing opportunity and pursuing that opportunity because one has an understanding or a feeling that this can develop into something worthwhile.

Dale: How much does education play a part in this?

von Liebig: A great deal, in my life at least. I hold three degrees. My first degree, in premed, gave me an understanding and appreciation for the health care aspect. My second degree, in engineering, ,gave me the background with which to put things together and come up with the answers to problems. My third degree, which I got while I was in New York City with Susquehanna Mills, was taken at NYU. That was my MBA, which is the business aspect of my background. I had the good fortune at that time of studying and working with Peter Drucker, who is considered one of the world's leading industrial consultants.

Dale: How do you motivate the people in your company?

von Liebig: I think the best way to do that, Andy, is by setting a good example and encouraging your employees to be achievers.

Dale: Is it money?

von Liebig: No, you need money to run the operation.

Dale: Where does money come in?

von Liebig: Money comes as a reward to your employees for achievement and is necessary for continued growth of the organization.

Dale: What about for the individual?

von Liebig: It's very important to them to be recognized and rewarded for their accomplishments. We pay one of the highest scales in the nation in the health care field, because we believe, and I believe—it is my credo—that to surround oneself with excellence creates excellence and must be rewarded. We reward not only with money, which is a significant part of it, but also with fringe benefits that cover all health and insurance needs. We take care of their acquiring a home and we also give them participation in ownership of the company. There are a number of things; it is not just money, it's being and owning a part of the operation as a result of their top performance.

Dale: You probably don't want an entrepreneur with you, do you?

von Liebig: Oh yes, I work with entrepreneurs.

Dale: Who do you have with you?

von Liebig: At this time, my successor will be Eleanor Gackstatter, who is presently vice president of administration. I chose her because she knows how to manage. She is intelligent, trustworthy, knowledgeable, and quite capable of understanding people's needs as well as operational needs. In addition, she is a significant contributor to the National Institutes of Health in Washington, D.C.

Dale: You have so much now, it doesn't make any difference about the money. What is the kick you get out of it?

von Liebig: Achieving, Andy.

Dale: Well, there it is. Achieving what?

von Liebig: Goals I set for myself.

Dale: What are your goals now?

von Liebig: Goals within my lifetime are numerous, but I give high priority to developing the ideal implant for vascular surgeons.

Dale: You don't think that will be in our lifetime, do you?

von Liebig: Yes, this will be in the next five to ten years. No question about it, because we have already done it. Problems are numerous, but not insurmountable. With our collaboration with MIT, we have already developed living arterial grafts.

Dale: What are they?

von Liebig: We take a biopsy of the animal's artery and, within a period of approximately a week, we will grow a full-size artery for that animal on a mandrel, with all layers of tissue included, that can be implanted in that animal without rejection. In addition to that, we will be developing living organs, prototypes, which we have already completed in the area of the pancreas and the thyroid. These will be further refined for the human.

Dale: But how can a pancreas be grown?

von Liebig: Through a cellular aggregation technique, by taking a biopsy of the healthy part of the patient's pancreas and putting it into a special kind of cocktail at our laboratories at MIT. This is enriched with many different nutrients, including collagen and a solution that gives rapid growth to these tissues.

For instance, we can develop a patient's skin, an area of, say, one foot square, within a period of one week's time and that skin can then be transplanted onto that patient without rejection.

Dale: Really, that's amazing.

von Liebig: We will be doing augmentation, for instance, for mastectomy patients who have severe mental problems. We will be developing a breast that will equal the original, and it will be tolerated by the patient. This part of the business, Andy, will probably, I would say, within a period of ten years turn out to be a $.5 billion enterprise. When we go public with this, within a period of three to four months it will be a $50 million issue.

Editor's note: On September 29, 1995, William von Liebig sold Meadox Medicals to Boston Scientific for $425 million.

John Madden

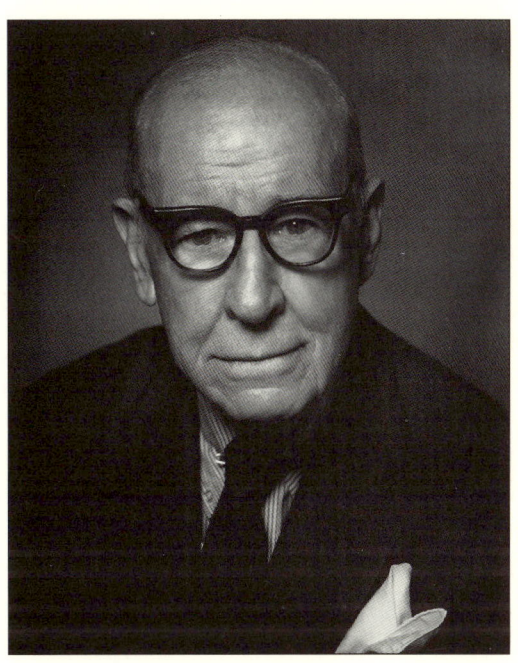

J OHN MADDEN has made innumerable contributions to the
field of surgery, most notably in the field of biliary and pancreatic diseases. He was one of the pioneer vacular surgeons and
should be credited for his early work on the abdominal arotic
aneurysm. Parts of this interview have already appeared in *Contemporary Surgery* 31 (1987): 28–34. Madden was interviewed December
3, 1986.

Dale: John, how did you become a doctor rather than a baseball player?

Madden: My parents were immigrants from Ireland, who later met and were married in Washington, D.C., where my father had a bar and grill restaurant. I was the third of four children—boy, girl, boy, boy. I was born August 15, 1912.

My early heroes were the four members of Connie Mack's $100,000 (pre-inflation) Philadelphia A's infield. They were "Stuffy" McGinnis at first base, Eddie Collins at second base, Frank "Home Run" Baker at the "hot corner" (third base), and Jack Barry at shortstop. In fact, I went to the College of the Holy Cross in Worcester, Massachusetts, because Jack Barry had retired from professional baseball to become the coach at that school, which was the reigning National Intercollegiate Baseball Champion at that time (1930).

At Holy Cross, I was informed that three degrees were available: B.A., B.S. Premed, and Ph.B. In the last (Bachelor of Philosophy), the schedule of classes favored the athletes but did not provide the necessary credits for admission to medical school. Then for the first time, doubt entered my mind. What would happen if I failed to become a professional baseball player? This question was answered by my registration for a B.S. Premed degree.

Dale: Did you have a good baseball career at Holy Cross?

Madden: Actually, I placed second among the twelve candidates who aspired for the second-base position. However, since I had registered for a premed degree, the conflict between baseball practice sessions and laboratory classes ended my "career" in professional baseball!

My family's finances were marginal because of the Depression, but my brother, Joe, who had recently graduated from Georgetown Dental School, provided additional funds that enabled me to attend the George Washington University School of Medicine, from which I graduated in 1937.

Dale: Where was your residency?

Madden: My cousin, Dr. Charlie McLaughlin, urged me to apply to Kings County Hospital in Brooklyn, where he was an attending surgeon. I applied and received a two-year rotating surgical internship from July 1, 1937, through June 30, 1939.

I wished to pursue my graduate surgical training in surgery to qualify as a diplomate of the American Board of Surgery. I then sought the advice of Dr. E. Jefferson Browder, who was the director of neurosurgery at Kings County Hospital and the Long Island College of Medicine, now the Downstate Medical Center. He was the epitome of discipline and awesome intimidation. Levity in the operation room was forbidden, and proper attire was always required. Dr. Browder once stated, half in jest, that he could tell a surgeon "by the way the cuffs of his trousers hung over his shoe tops." He advised that I apply to Lakeside Hospital in Cleveland and recommended me to Dr. Claude Beck, his former classmate at Johns Hopkins.

Dale: Did you have a good experience at Cleveland?

Madden: I enjoyed my time at Lakeside and will always have happy memories of that period. I formed a lasting friendship with many of the residents, particularly with Bill Holden, who would later succeed Dr. Carl Lenhart as the chairman of the Department of Surgery at Western Reserve. However, I had a gnawing, homesick feeling for Kings County Hospital. When I learned that there was an unexpected vacancy on the resident staff, I applied and was fortunate to receive an appointment as a senior assistant resident on the Long Island College Division of Kings County Hospital, under the directorship of Dr. Robert F. Barber.

Dale: Was Dr. Barber a good teacher?

Madden: He was the most unforgettable character I ever met. He often mentioned that he and President Franklin D. Roosevelt were classmates at Harvard in the Class of 1904. He insisted that presentations and writings be in flawless English. During weekly grand rounds, he would be apt to interrupt the speaker with the admonition, "Please use sentences in your presentation." Also, it was always the "operation room" and not the "operating room," because the room does not operate! He subscribed to Michelangelo's dictum: "Details make perfection and perfection is no detail."

Dale: So you finished your residency training just in time for World War II?

Madden: Yes, it ended on June 30, 1942, and on July 4—no holidays in the army during the war!—I was inducted into the Medical Corps of the United States Army in the office of Colonel Frederick Rankin. He suggested that I stop in Philadelphia on the way back to New York and gave me a letter to give to Dr. Stewart Rodman, the secretary of the American Board of Surgery.

While waiting for my orders to active duty, I had the opportunity to visit the various hospitals in New York City as an observer in the operation room. This was due to the largesse of the New York Academy of Medicine, which published a daily bulletin listing the operations being performed.

On one such occasion, I noted that Dr. Allen O. Whipple was listed to perform a pancreatic resection at 8:00 a.m. in the Columbia Presbyterian Hospital. I arrived at 7:45 a.m. and was directed to a glass-enclosed visitors' gallery that looked down on the operation room. The operation started promptly at 8:00 a.m., and I noted that I was the only spectator in the gallery.

Within an hour, Dr. Whipple "broke scrub," leaving the closure of the abdomen to his assistants. When I walked down the steps of the gallery, Dr. Whipple was standing at the bottom. He invited me into an adjoining room, where he reviewed the case history of the patient for me and concluded, "I'm sorry that I could not do anything to help this man."

To have Dr. Whipple, a preeminent surgeon of world renown, spend a half hour discussing a surgical problem with a resident who had just completed his formal residency training program in surgery was an experience that I will always remember.

During this waiting period, I witnessed many surgeons operating, but the one I enjoyed the most was Dr. John Garlock at Mount Sinai Hospital. He was a surgeon whose surgical technique was poetry in motion, and literally bloodless. Not only was he a virtuoso in the operation room, but also as a concert pianist.

My call to active duty was actually delayed until December 1942, at which time I was assigned to the surgical pool at Walter Reed General Hospital in Washington, D.C. Also, I was informed about that time that I had passed Part 1 of the examination of the American Board of Surgery.

Dale: Did you continue to serve at Walter Reed Hospital?

Madden: Yes, in the surgical pool. In April 1943 I received my assignment to the newly opened Bruns General Hospital in Santa Fe, New Mexico. The following month, I took the second part of my examinations for certification by the American Board of Surgery. This second part, that was subsequently to be eliminated, was the performance of a major operation that was observed by a member of the American Board of Surgery. Accordingly, I performed an emergency splenectomy in a corpsman for a delayed rupture of the spleen, which was witnessed by the assigned observer, Major John Koucky. The postoperative course proved satisfactory, and two weeks later, I was informed that I had passed Part 2.

In September I was assigned to overseas duty with the 119th Station Hospital Group. I received a furlough and left Bruns General Hospital with my wife and my first-born child (a girl) for our return to New York. I was also informed by the American Board of Surgery that I was qualified to take my third and final examination. I had a choice, either California or Chicago, and I chose Chicago because it was en route in my travel by car to New York.

In October 1943 I received my certificate as a diplomate of the American Board of Surgery. In December 1943 the 119th Station Hospital landed in Milne Bay, New Guinea, and in February 1944 I was transferred to the Second Field Hospital as chief of surgery. I participated in three landings in the Philippines at Leyte, Mindora. I was later assigned as surgical consultant to the Eighth Army and was returned to the United States in July 1945. I was relieved from active duty in November 1945 as a major in the Medical Corps of the United States Army.

In January 1946 I opened an office in Manhattan for the private practice of surgery and received an appointment to the surgical staff of St. Clare's Hospital concomitant with an appointment to the Long Island College Division of Surgery in Kings County Hospital as an instructor in surgery. Over the ensuing years, I became a faculty member and associate professor of surgery at the Long Island College of Medicine.

Dale: When did you become director of surgery at St. Clare's?

Madden: Following the sudden death of the director of surgery,

Dr. William B. Healy, in 1949, I was offered that position. This produced a dilemma, because of my appointment as a tenured faculty member of the Long Island College of Medicine and my academic responsibilities there. But the challenge of heading a department of surgery at the age of thirty-six was tantalizing. After three days of deliberation, I accepted the position at St. Clare's Hospital and resigned my appointment at the Long Island College of Medicine. Shortly thereafter, I received an appointment as clinical professor of surgery at the New York Medical College.

Dale: What sort of residency program did you develop?

Madden: Our residency training program was approved by the American Board of Surgery in 1950 and continued uninterrupted for the ensuing twenty-five years of my tenure.

In 1952 the National Intern Matching Plan was introduced and caused an immediate change in the composition of our resident staff. Previously, the staff was predominantly graduates of American medical schools, but soon there was a rapid increase in the number of foreign medical graduates. From 1955 through 1975, 90 percent of our residents were foreign medical graduates, and only one failed the examinations for certification by the American Board of Surgery. Interestingly, this resident passed the written examinations, but failed the oral examinations twice. Two others passed Part 1 the first time but elected not to return from the their respective countries for Part 2. A fourth resident never applied for certification by the board.

Dale: Was it unusual for such a hospital to offer research facilities at that time?

Madden: Yes, but Mother Alice, the administrator of St. Clare's Hospital, was an unusual person.

In 1934 she was transferred from St. Francis Hospital in Miami Beach to New York City, to re-open the old St. Elizabeth Hospital; she immediately changed the name to St. Clare's. The hospital is located in West 51st Street, between 9th and 10th Avenues, an area that has the sobriquet "Hell's Kitchen."

In the seventeen years between 1934 and 1951, she transformed St. Clare's Hospital from a capacity of 41 beds to 425 beds. It was comprised of a multifarious group of new buildings that formed an imposing medical center.

Earlier in the expansion of St. Clare's, Mother Alice asked me to meet her in the basement to inspect an area that she thought might be suitable for animal research. This was remodeled at a cost of $25,000. However, not long thereafter, she found a larger area that was transformed at a cost of $40,000.

Next I received a call from Mother Alice to come to her office to see the plans for the new buildings that were being constructed. She then showed me a vacant area that she thought would be suitable for the erection of a four-story research building. I then asked her if she knew how much such a building would cost. She replied, "Doctor, that should not be any concern of yours." Taken aback, I said that I would not know how to begin to construct such a building. Her retort: "Doctor, if I were you, I would be ashamed!" Immediately thereafter, plans were made with the architects and the four-story Institute of Surgical Research came to fruition. This was indeed a memorial to a gracious Franciscan nun, the nonpareil Mother Alice.

Dale: Were the private patients and the staff patients integrated in the teaching program at that time?

Madden: Yes. Each resident would spend an allotted time on both the private surgical and house surgical services. During their third year, residents were assigned full-time to the Institute of Surgical Research for a period of four months. During this stay, experimental protocols were assigned with small and large animal preparations, which proved most instructive. Also they would attend weekly grand rounds and weekly bedside teaching rounds.

In the fourth year, there was an interchange of two months with comparable residents on the gynecologic service that proved most satisfactory. Also in the fourth year, each assistant resident would spend a period of four months as chief surgical resident on the fracture and orthopedic services. At that time, many of the general surgeons had expertise in the treatment of trauma. In fact, the general surgeons so qualified would alternate call for the care of unassigned patients.

In the final year, each of the three chief surgical residents served four months on my private surgical service and concomitantly as the chief surgical resident on the house staff surgical service. When they were on my service, I "opened" and "closed" on every private patient, both for teaching purposes and as a defense in the event of a malpractice suit. Also, should an unexpected intraoperative complication occur, they would see first-hand how it was handled. Since they served during this same period as chief surgical residents on the house staff service, I was better able to discuss with them the various operations they had performed.

During the period from 1949 to 1975, the surgical training was in general surgery, including vascular, head and neck surgical procedures, and the treatment of victims of violent trauma.

An unexpected dividend of their rotation in the dog lab was the fact that each resident was given the option of a sixth year in the Institute of Surgical Research, and 60 percent of the residents exercised this option. It is of interest in this regard that, over a nine-year period, four experimental protocols were presented at the Annual Forum on Fundamental Surgical Problems of the American College of Surgeons.

Dale: Tell me about the early graft replacement of an aneurysm that you did.

Madden: In 1949 we had a patient with an aneurysm of the aorta. It was just six months after Robert Gross had described the use of preserved arterial grafts for long coarctations—so-called adult coarctation of the aorta. I thought that they would serve to replace an aneurysm of the abdominal aorta. I confronted the patient with the diagnosis and suggested we replace it with a preserved graft. He asked, "How many have you done?" I replied, "I haven't done any. I think this will be the first one ever done." He said, "Not on me!" So that was that.

Dale: When did you first repair an abdominal aortic aneurysm?

Madden: It was on June 14, 1952, using a homologous artery graft from the artery bank. William McCann, who had just finished his residency training, did it with me. In fact, we documented it with a film for the American College of Surgeons. The procedure went well, but the patient died of cardiopulmonary complications on the seventh day. The graft was patent.

Dale: I can understand your reluctance to report a procedure that ended with the death of the patient.

Madden: Yes. A few years later, Jim Hardy came to our hospital as a visiting professor. When he learned of it, he remarked, "I'll tell you this—if it had been me, I would have been dictating a paper as I walked out of the operating room!"

Dale: Before we close, tell me about the technique of that early operation.

Madden: We removed the entire aneurysmal sac, which would not be done today. But you asked about the first repairs of aneurysms. The French surgeon Charles Dubost reported the first in Paris in June 1951, using the thoracic portion of the aorta from a nineteen-year-old man who had died in an auto accident. The first American repair was reported by Paul Shafer and Creighton Hardin in 1952, using a frozen homologous aortic graft. My case was the second, and then Ormond Julian's group did the third in Chicago in 1953.

As I said, we showed a film of our case in New York at the meeting of the American College of Surgeons in October 1952. As I was leaving the Empire Room of the Waldorf Hotel, where the movie was shown, a fellow tapped me on the shoulder, saying, "I'm Denton Cooley from Houston, and I'm going to try this when I get back home." Eight months later, in the June 1953 issue of *Surgery, Gynecology and Obstetrics,* he and Mike DeBakey reported eight cases. They had such a large number of cases in Houston and rushed into print as soon as possible, amazingly only six weeks after their eighth case was done.

The explanation for the large number in a short time was that they already had a number of aneurysms under observation, which had been treated by inserting wire in the hope that they would clot and cease to be a problem. They called those patients back and removed their aneurysms and repaired the defect in the aorta with a graft.

John Mannick

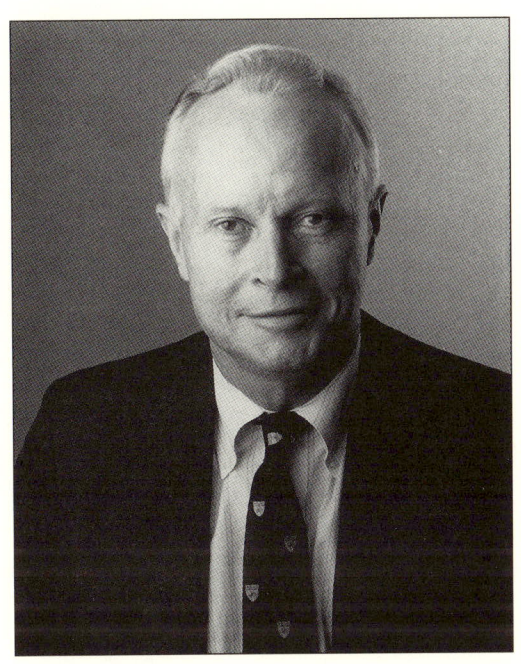

JOHN MANNICK typifies the complete scholar and academic surgeon. After a rugged, rural early life, he pursued an intellectual path and ended up in the academic environment of Boston. He challenges everything and everybody, and has the drive to learn the truth by basic investigation in the laboratory or by well-controlled clinical studies. He was interviewed June 4, 1990.

Johnson: Let's begin with who your parents were, where you were born, and the events of your early life that have influenced you through the years.

Mannick: Well, I was born in Deadwood, South Dakota, on March 24, 1928. I don't remember anything about Deadwood, because when I was just a few weeks old my family moved to the West Coast, where I grew up in a little town called Yakima, Washington. The town was a center for the fruit-growing and farming district, an irrigated valley in the desert east of the mountains. Because the mountains are so high on the West Coast, the area east of them is usually very dry. Yakima was an irrigated desert valley town. My father was a civil engineer who designed irrigation projects, so that's why we were in Yakima.

I went to public high school there. I became interested in medicine in high school, but I wasn't absolutely sure when I applied to college. I always wanted to go to Stanford, because if you were a West Coast kid in those days, that seemed pretty close to heaven down there in Palo Alto. But in the 1940s we had to take the college boards (they're now the SATs) and I guess I did pretty well. Harvard had decided right at the end of the war to embark on a regional distribution program, and they'd never had anybody at Harvard from Yakima, Washington, so they offered to pay my way to Harvard. My parents would've had to pay half for me to go to Stanford. I had been in the navy a few weeks at the end of the war, and when I got home, after about thirty seconds of reflection, my parents had me on a train to Boston. So that's how I got to Harvard. I stayed at Harvard College and Harvard Medical School and got interested in surgery at Harvard Medical School.

Johnson: Did your mother and father influence what you're doing?

Mannick: Because I was an only child, my parents had high hopes for me, and being a doctor was something they liked. They didn't really insist on it, though. They were just interested in my going to the best possible college, and I was often encouraged by them to do as well as possible in school. In high school I was certainly only an indifferent athlete and would have been considered a nerd because I got good grades, and that wasn't very popular at Yakima High School.

I was a National Honor Society member and the class valedictorian. That was a sure way to be an unpopular individual at our high school. It was strictly a grade point average affair, and there were several students who were very close to the same grade point average. I was lucky enough to squeak ahead of a couple of them. They all went to very good colleges, one to Yale and a couple to Stanford. At the end of the war a lot of us had to go into the service briefly, and when we got out, we went off to college.

Johnson: Tell me some of the characteristics of Harvard.

Mannick: Talk about culture shock! That was really something, to come from a small town on the West Coast and suddenly encounter New England. I had never been east of Wisconsin. My mother's family had originally come from Wisconsin. I thought Harvard was the most beat-up old place I had ever seen. Stanford was a pretty place, with Spanish buildings and palm trees, and here was this beat-up old group of buildings that didn't match in a little place with some trees called Harvard Yard in the middle of a dirty town called Cambridge. I couldn't understand how this was possibly a great university. But I got to like the place by the end of the first year, probably because everybody had gotten there because they had done well in school and were interested in intellectual pursuits. So it was like being upgraded; suddenly you were in a place where there was lots of competition and people didn't look down on you if you did well academically. I thought it was a great spot; I still remember that very fondly.

I majored in the humanities, something called the History and Literature of England. History and Literature was the most moss-covered major at Harvard. It was patterned after an Oxford or Cambridge education, in that you were assigned a tutor and in addition to your regular course work you had to read at least one book and write a paper for your tutor every week. It was strictly a volunteer major and you had to pass some scrutiny before they'd let you do it. If you were going to medical school in those days, a lot of the university advisors suggested that you devote your undergraduate time as much as possible to something other than science. These days that would be considered pretty ridiculous; in those days it was pretty popular. I took the premedical requirements on the side.

I had decided to go into medicine by my freshman year. I'm not at all sure what influenced me to make that decision. Looking back on it, I'd gotten this interest in high school. I can't really tell you that there was a doctor in town who was a hero of mine. It just seemed like an interesting thing to do. No one in the family had ever been a doctor. In high school it seemed like something they'd let a nerd do. I had the usual childhood illnesses, and was impressed by the doctors who took care of me. At first I thought I wanted to go into psychiatry. Freud was very big as an intellectual conversation subject right after the war. All over the country, Freudian psychology got to be a very big subject of interest; it seemed to be a nice marriage of medicine and the humanities that I was majoring in. I figured the thing to do was go to medical school and make use of this background in the humanities and be a psychiatrist.

Johnson: So Freud even trickled down to the undergraduate schools at Harvard?

Mannick: Absolutely. Freudian interpretation of nearly everybody was rife on the campuses in those days. All the famous authors were quickly being reinterpreted by Freudian principles. There were all kinds of pseudo-analyses of famous men being written in those days and people loved to throw what we now call "intellectual claptrap" into every discussion of a poet or an author or a statesman. So it was just rife; it seemed as if we had hit the mother lode. This was the explanation for human behavior, and if we just understood more thoroughly what motivated people, we wouldn't really have any trouble in the world.

Johnson: Who at Harvard had a strong influence on your future life?

Mannick: I was impressed with a number of teachers. I suppose the one who really was the intellectual leader of the humanities in those days at Harvard was a man named F. O. Matthiessen, who was an interesting character. He was the head of the Department of History and Literature. He'd grown up in California but somehow got himself to Yale. He became a scholar, but in the midst of his undergraduate years he had run off and joined the Royal Flying Corps in World War I and had actually flown SE-5s in combat and come back to Yale. Later he was hired by Harvard. He was a great intellectual in the humanities doing the things that were very popular then, such as writing intellectual criticism, particularly criticism of poetry, analyzing poetry with what was a kind of offshoot of the Freudian principles. He became interested in the metaphysical poetry of the seventeenth century, probably led there by T. S. Eliot and Ezra Pound. He used those poets as models for some of his work. T. S. Eliot was the hero of the day, and Matthiessen was the great interpreter of poets with what was called the New Criticism. A lot of the New Criticism, however, came from the South, where Cleanth Brooks held forth and the *Sewanee Journal* was one of the real intellectual touchstones of that era.

Johnson: Do you still like poetry?

Mannick: To tell you the truth, I probably do, but if you ask me if I have read any lately, the answer is no. I probably have totally buried that side of my life in my professional years.

Johnson: What about the rest of Harvard?

Mannick: I had a wonderful time. I was fortunate enough to be in the first class that started at Harvard College after the war, and had some very mature roommates who had been in the war a long time, had a large number of discharge points, and got out early enough to get into college in late 1945. It was a great group to be going to school with. They were very interested in educating themselves and had clear goals in mind; they were mature. They partied hard, but they also certainly studied hard. They brought us kids along a lot just by their influence. So it was a great time going to school. I did a little rowing because I was the right size for the 150-pound crew, but I stopped that after my sophomore year. I was in some plays; I was editor of a yearbook; I did a lot of stuff that was fun; and I really had an awfully good time.

I applied to Harvard Medical School and got in. Somehow or other it seemed that by then I'd gotten the Harvard bug. I started Harvard Medical School in 1949, and I must say I thought it was a big disappointment compared to Harvard College. As opposed to being an intellectually stimulating atmosphere, I thought Harvard

Medical School was intellectually stultifying. Everything was by rote. You weren't asked to think conceptually at all. I thought it was terrible. I still regard it as a very unpleasant couple of years.

There was a series of lectures that you were supposed to parrot back on your exams. Some of them were poorly presented, a lot of laboratory work seemingly bearing little relation to any human disease. I think I only had a minimal scientific background. The pedagogy was poor. There were some exceptions; the pharmacology department was very stimulating. They had marvelous lectures and made things interesting and related them to the world of human disease.

I thought it would be okay once I got to the clinical years and I could really try my wings in psychiatry. I had my first rotation in psychiatry and found out that it was absolutely, totally different from what I had anticipated, and I began more and more to believe that in its Freudian form, which was practiced in those days, it didn't seem to be helping people much at all. So I was very disillusioned.

After that, I was on internal medicine. I really thought that was an incredibly difficult way to go through your life. Endless rounds and discussions of the problems, nobody ever arriving at a conclusion to anything, and they drove me nuts. By the end of the third year, I sat down and tried to decide if there was any discipline that I thought I liked in that whole third year. And the only thing I could think of that I liked was dog surgery. So I thought, I've gone three-quarters of the way through medical school and the only thing I like is dog surgery; maybe I ought to look at surgery as a career a little more carefully. I took quite a few surgical electives as well as the required courses the fourth year. By the middle of the fourth year, it was very clear that I seemed to fit all right into surgical services, whereas I didn't into the medical services. So I scurried around and applied for a whole lot of surgical internships.

Johnson: You had been an intellectual all your life until this point, and then all of a sudden your whole career is going to be changed by a technical aspect.

Mannick: Exactly. Strange, isn't it? I had sense enough to realize that your life's work should be something you enjoy doing. The only thing I'd actually enjoyed very much was operating. The time on the surgical wards was not bad, either. I took a lot of electives the fourth year and that confirmed it. I went into surgery, and I have never regretted it.

Johnson: Were there any heroes?

Mannick: Lots of them. We were influenced as students in surgery a lot by Franny Moore's lectures; he was an extraordinarily charismatic lecturer. We were influenced by Bert Dunphy, another great lecturer who was still at Harvard in those days. Dave Hume at Brigham was another charismatic individual. I didn't know him terribly well as an undergraduate in medical school, although he was the faculty advisor to the club to which I belonged. That dates us, because they had clubs in medical school in those days. That would not be politically correct any longer, I'm sure. The club I belonged to was called the Lancet Club; it was a pretty wild outfit. I knew Dave Hume a little bit that way. Down at the Mass General, I think we were clearly stimulated as students by people like Claude Welch and Richard Sweet. The latter didn't pay much attention to students, but he was very good with house officers. Claude Welch was good with students, and Marsh Bartlett was very good with students. We had people, like George Nardy, on the junior staff who were very nice to us as students, and John Raker, who later left to go down to Philadelphia. We had some heroes all right. They were nice people, took us under their wing, taught us a lot, made us feel comfortable.

Johnson: How did your analytical mind go from here?

Mannick: I tried to sign up for what seemed like the best surgical program to me at the time. I was quite surprised to get into Mass General, to tell you the truth, because my medical school record was not bad in the clinical years, but it had been pretty spotty in the basic science years. Mass General was a pretty competitive place; it was certainly my first choice. The Brigham, where I've spent an awful lot of my lifetime, was not a top choice in spite of Franny Moore, because it was a small hospital and there was very little operating. The residents spent a long time before they got to do much in the way of surgery, whereas at Mass General the tradition was to start operating in the intern year, and everybody on the house staff did a lot of surgery. It seemed to me that if you're going to be a surgeon, you probably ought to go where the operating is.

With regard to my future interest in vascular surgery, I had a strange beginning in my internship. The chief of surgery at Mass General, Dr. Edward D. "Pete" Churchill, had a stroke right before our intern group started in 1953. He was always a very distant figure after that—never operated again that I can remember. A few house officers later got to know him well, but I never did. The person who was chief of surgery when I started my internship in 1953 was Mike DeBakey. He had dropped his work with his new Department of Surgery at Baylor and moved into the MGH for three to four months to take over for Dr. Churchill. He really worshiped the man; he had gotten to know him in the war. Mike DeBakey found Dr. Churchill worth dropping his own practice to come to the MGH and replace him for a while. I also found myself on a service headed by Stan Crawford as chief resident. With Stanley Crawford as chief resident and Mike DeBakey as chief, I suppose if I hadn't developed some sort of interest in vascular surgery, I would have had to have been unconscious. Mike, in fact, was the guy who did the first aneurysm replacement at Mass General. It wasn't Bob Linton, as one might have thought, but Mike DeBakey, in early 1953. So vascular surgery at Mass General essentially began the year of my internship. It was the new thing.

In 1954, right after my internship, I went into the air force during the Korean War for a couple of years. This was just before the hostilities were over. I didn't go anywhere near Korea.

Mass General in those days had a policy that they were going to try to finish everybody they started. Dr. DeBakey had come for a few months when Churchill had a stroke; then Churchill came back and served as the surgeon in chief during my training program. The training was quite good. We wouldn't recognize it as being socially acceptable any longer, in that you helped the private surgeons on one side of the hospital and then you operated on the patients who could not afford the private surgeons on the other side of the hospital; the private surgeons never helped you. These days, we help our residents do cases, but it was totally foreign in those days of our training. We operated independently.

Johnson: Were there any heroes on the faculty?

Mannick: I was working my tail off as an intern and never came into contact with Dr. DeBakey, but Stan Crawford was probably my first hero. He was so extraordinarily able, both technically and in deciding which patient needed what done to them. He was a role model you could certainly put your trust in. I developed some other heroes on the senior staff in time. Richard Sweet was an extraordinarily gifted operator, and so was Bob Linton. I was very fortunate to have been assigned twice to Linton's service during my residency. Usually you didn't get assigned twice to that service, but I was, for reasons that I don't think were anything other than accidental. I got to spend eight months of my residency with him, and I got to know him well. I operated with him on a lot of vascular cases and learned his technique of putting vein grafts in the leg. He was one of the few who hadn't abandoned vein grafts by the time I finished my residency in 1960.

Johnson: Who were some of your colleagues?

Mannick: It was a varying group. One was called in for military service during the Korean War, and I hadn't had enough time in the navy to avoid that. People kept getting called out of residency and coming back, so you didn't have a class that you went through with. The only one I started out with who was in vascular surgery was Ed Salzman. Another guy I came to know was George Zuidema; we were in the same intern group. I ended up finishing with Gerry Austen. Those were probably the ones who are now known nationally. Ahead of us in the residency were people like Hermes Grillo and Jack Burke.

In the middle of my training, I became interested in the new field of transplantation, which was not yet a clinical field. I think I now understand a lot better than I did then how impolitic I was about it. Paul Russell, who had then taken over as the boss of the house staff at Mass General, had been in the laboratory of Peter Medawar, who went on to win the Nobel Prize in 1960 for his work in transplantation. So Russell was a guru in that field; I went to him to ask if I could go work at Cooperstown, New York, with a young man named Don Thomas, who was doing bone marrow transplants in dogs. It was very clear that you could not, with the techniques available then, transplant organs in mice, which were the animals Medawar and other basic scientists used. But you could transplant organs in dogs. So I wanted to go up there where these guys could make chimeric dogs with bone marrow grafts, and sew organs in them. Russell didn't think much of that. He thought I ought to go work in England, and he had arranged a job for me in the radiation laboratory in East Grinstead. I still don't know where East Grinstead is, but instead I chose to go up and work with Don Thomas in 1958. Understandably, that was not a decision which was well received at Mass General.

It was a very exciting year, because when I got there they were unable to do bone marrow transplants between dogs and keep the donor alive. They killed the donor to get enough marrow cells. My job as a surgeon was to figure out how to get enough bone marrow out of a dog and keep him alive. We figured that by opening the bones in an anesthetized dog and draining the marrow out and sewing the legs up again, you could keep the donor alive, and then you had an organ donor available. We managed to pull off a kidney transplant in a chimeric dog that year.

This was totally eclipsed in the minds of the public by a fellow named Joe Murray, who performed the first nonidentical transplant in a human that same year. Thus, the dog transplant at Cooperstown lost a little bit of its luster since they occurred at the same time.

Don Thomas is a hematologist and an extraordinarily gifted investigator. This wasn't so clear to my mentors at the MGH at the time, but Thomas had had Ph.D.-level training in biochemistry at MIT as well as an internal medicine residency at the Brigham. He was a very clinically-oriented investigator, as opposed to strictly a laboratory doctor. He was interested in bone marrow transplantation to cure leukemia. He was interested in all applications of bone marrow transplantation. I've since thought with some amusement about all that. When I got back to the MGH, no one ever asked me what I had done that year.

Johnson: Did you ever work for Joe Murray?

Mannick: I never did. I used his technique of how to transplant a kidney in a dog when I got to Cooperstown in 1958. He had done a

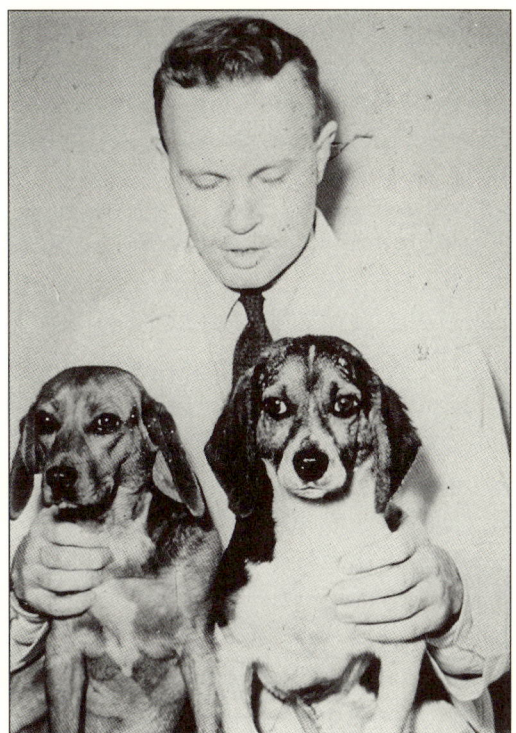

Sam and Sally received the first vascularized organ graft in a chimeric animal at Cooperstown, N.Y. Sam had a lethal dose of radiation and a bone marrow transplant from Sally, then had a bilateral nephrectomy and received a kidney from Sally.

lot of autotransplants in dogs, polishing up for the first identical twin transplants he did the year I went into the service in the Korean days. He was putting the kidney in the pelvis and implanting the ureter in the bladder. He'd worked that all out in dogs back in the early 1950s. I knew who he was because I had been present as Don Thomas's research fellow in the discussions that led to that first nonidentical twin transplant. Joe had called Don to talk about what they might do for immunosuppression. This was before the days of any immunosuppressive drugs. And so it was decided on sublethal radiation, which they gave this poor individual. Whether that was necessary, we'll never know, but it worked.

I was fortunate to have had my research time with a future Nobel laureate, no thanks to my ingenuity, and to have had a chance to work eight months with Bob Linton. When I got out of the residency, I was definitely not in good odor with the management at the MGH. The only job I was offered was by David Hume, whom I had known slightly as a medical student. Since Hume was something of an iconoclast himself, I think he sort of took to me. He offered me a job in Richmond.

Dave was a marvelous guy who was a great inspiration in the sense that he had more ideas per twenty minutes than anybody I've ever seen. Some of them were brilliant and some of them were awful, but he just kept having them. It was stimulating to work around him. He was an absolutely disorganized individual. For example, he refused to ever answer any mail. When I first went to work for him, I walked into his office and his big horseshoe desk was piled so high on all sides of the horseshoe with unanswered letters that I couldn't see whether he was there or not. I don't think he ever did answer any mail when I was there. I suppose he's a good example of the fact that good department chairmen can come in all sizes and shapes. He was quite a good chairman, because he was good at picking people and he was good with ideas. But he was a mess as far as administration was concerned.

With him was a young man named Dick Egdahl, to whom my career owes an awful lot. He made sure that I got into the right societies, that I got abstracts sent to the right meetings, and that I learned how to be an academic surgeon.

Our job was to mount an academic effort in a hospital that was used to being a practitioner's hospital. We were not very popular with the staff or the citizenry of Richmond. Naturally, Dave, with his "spit-in-your-eye" attitude, didn't exactly make himself loved. When I left my residency, the first and last conversation I think I ever had with my boss, Dr. Churchill, was when he decided that he should do something for me, and he wrote me a letter of recommendation to Dr. Carrington Williams, Sr. I carried this letter with me when I reported to work a couple of days later to Dave Hume, after I found out there was someone behind that desk. I said, "By the way, Dr. Hume, I have a letter from Dr. Churchill, who was my chief, to Dr. Carrington Williams on your staff. Where would I find him?"

He said, "Well, I don't think I'd deliver that letter just yet. Last night at the Richmond Academy of Medicine, Dr. Williams suggested that I be publicly horsewhipped." I think that there was that feeling about Dave when he first started down there. He, of course, later became a local hero.

Johnson: Was that before or after his death?

Mannick: Before his death. I think he became an international superstar, and Richmond really kind of took him to her bosom after that, but the early days were rough going.

Johnson: What did you do at Richmond?

Mannick: We did general surgery, some vascular surgery, a lot of endocrine surgery, worked in the lab on transplantation, and actually began to do human kidney transplants during my tour down there. About midway through that four-year stint down there, Dave Hume decided that Dick Egdahl and I ought to split up some of the clinical assignments. He decided that one of us should focus on being a pancreatic and liver surgeon, the other one should focus on being a vascular surgeon, and we both ought to be interested in transplantation. We actually flipped a coin, and Dick was the pancreatic surgeon and I was the vascular surgeon. We had all been doing everything until then. So I was put in a vascular niche largely by accident, though I had done more vascular than anybody else on the staff other than Hume himself, because of my time with Linton. Hume was quite interested in the fact that Linton had been doing vein grafts in legs, and so I started doing Linton-style vein grafts. Hume sniffed around and thought that was pretty interesting. He started doing vein grafts. Then we carried the vein grafts down to the tibial vessels and thought we were the first, but we discovered that Andy Dale was probably the first. There was a fellow named dePalma in Argentina, who reported that he had put vein grafts in there, but the pictures suggested that was just to the distal popliteal artery.

I think Dave and I put the first vein graft into an anterior tibial artery. Andy hadn't thought of doing that. We did one of those in 1962 and reported it in 1963. We did vein grafts more and more frequently; the coin was certainly fortunate for me.

Johnson: Did you actually flip a coin?

Mannick: We did. Dick Egdahl and I flipped a coin. It was a quarter, as a matter of fact.

Johnson: You should have saved the quarter.

Mannick: It did not seem a very important event at the time.

Johnson: How long did you stay at Richmond?

Mannick: Four years. I went up to Boston University with Dick Egdahl, who had been my real guide and mentor, who was organized enough to have gotten me into the societies, made sure I was taken care of.

Dave and I parted under amiable circumstances. He hired Mel Williams immediately as my replacement, which wasn't a bad bargain. And Dick Egdahl and I went up to Boston University, where I started doing vascular surgery pretty much full time.

Johnson: Who had been doing vascular surgery at Boston University before you came?

Mannick: Dr. Smithwick had done some, but when he retired from the chairmanship, he just plain retired. A chap named Charles Robertson did some vascular surgery, but they were doing very little arterial reconstructive surgery at the time. It was pretty fallow ground to start cultivating. I had an open field to try to run as far and as fast as I could with vascular surgery. The the university hospital wasn't a very big hospital; it was about the size of the Peter Bent Brigham. We were associated with Boston City Hospital and took over its management some years later, but we did our surgery largely at the university hospital.

Because of our Richmond experience, Dick decided it would be a good idea if we didn't try to compete with general surgeons, and we tried to focus on some specific clinical areas. My assignment was transplantation and vascular, and his was going to be endocrine and pancreatic cancer.

Johnson: How long did you stay at Boston University?

Mannick: I spent twelve years of my life there and matured clinically and as an investigator. I started out as an associate professor in 1964 and in 1966 was promoted to full professor. When Dick Egdahl became the vice president for medical affairs at Boston University in 1973, they made me chief of surgery. I moved up the ladder largely, I think, through Egdahl's influence. I did research in transplantation;

ran the transplant unit, which was strictly for kidney transplants; and also did vascular surgery.

Johnson: Why did you leave Boston University?

Mannick: It became clear to me that Boston University was simply not well enough financed to compete successfully with Harvard in the same town. It was very difficult to recruit top individuals, to get recognition for what you did, to influence already formed public attitudes, or to obtain financial resources to allow you to realistically compete. I concluded that before I was too old to get another chairmanship I ought to try to get one somewhere else. I had been approached by UCLA, where Bill Longmire was retiring. This was another accidental event. The more I think about what I've told you this afternoon, it seems like almost everything that's happened to me was accidental.

I was offered the job finally at UCLA. My wife and I were in my office at Boston University waiting for a taxi to take us to the airport to go out and look for houses in Los Angeles when I got a call from Gene Braunwald, who was head of the search committee for the Brigham job. He asked me to be chief of surgery at Brigham. As you might imagine, Ginny and I flew out to Los Angeles in a total quandary; we didn't know what to do. I had talked to the Brigham search committee eight or nine months earlier and never heard anything more from them, and I thought that that was a dead issue. I hadn't even considered it and was all set to move to Los Angeles. But the more we thought about things, it seemed somehow that we ought to stick with the old university that we had started out with, and so we chose to remain at Harvard.

Johnson: You hadn't accepted the job at UCLA?

Mannick: No, we were going to go out and sign the contract and buy a house and work out the details of the final settlement to take the job. I took two weeks off to try to decide what to do. We went on vacation to think about it for a while and to come to some conclusion. At the end of the two weeks, we decided to take the Brigham.

Johnson: Tell me about the early days at the Brigham.

Mannick: I got there in 1976. The main problem at the Brigham was that it was too small, and I would not have taken the job had they not already had a hole in the ground for a new hospital. We had to struggle with that small hospital for the first four years I was there, and then in 1980 we moved into a bigger hospital, 720 beds. It became far easier to develop a Department of Surgery in a hospital of adequate size.

Johnson: What were some of the highlights of your time at the Brigham?

Mannick: Well, goodness, George, I don't know. My time at the Brigham is still ongoing. I guess what I've enjoyed more than I thought I would is trying to bring on people in the department and watch them flourish. It is very satisfying. I've been fortunate to have some very good people come our way both through the program and recruited from elsewhere.

Johnson: Tell us about Ginny. She obviously influenced your life.

Mannick: Oh, very much so. Ginny and I were college classmates. She was at Radcliffe and I was at Harvard. I knew who she was because we both took organic chemistry from Louis Fieser, who was a great teacher. He had exam every few weeks called an hour exam. It was possible to get a 100, but he also had an extra-credit question at the end of the exam. If you got all of the exam correct, and you answered the extra-credit question, you could get a 105. I never got any better than about 98. There was this damned strawberry-blonde girl in the class who kept getting a 105 or 104 on her exams, so I knew who she was in those days. She was dating somebody else, as I was in our undergraduate years. We finally began dating when I was in medical school and she was in graduate school getting a Ph.D. at Harvard Medical School in the Division of Medical Sciences. She got a Ph.D. in biochemistry, which she certainly seemed to have talent in, from my undergraduate experience of her exam scores. So we started dating, and then we got married after my third year in medical school. A wife like Virginia who is academically-oriented herself has made it very easy to have an academic career. I was very fortunate.

Johnson: That's a great story, John. What do you see in the future of vascular surgery?

Mannick: Well, I've never been able to predict anything in my life, certainly not my own career, but I would say that we have had some quite significant advances in the field over the last decade. Two seem very clear to me. First, with better technical skills, we can put in vein grafts in the legs and get limb salvage in the 85 percent range at five years. It is really quite astonishing. We were just not doing that a decade ago. That's been a signal advance. Another thing that's been a very big advance is keeping people from dying of heart attacks after vascular surgery. Aneurysm patients are now surviving our ministrations in amazing percentages in most big institutions, whereas when I moved up from Richmond, aneurysm repair mortality was in the neighborhood of 10 percent to 15 percent. I think those trends are going to continue.

Johnson: And the interventional radiologists?

Mannick: Interventional radiology has helped us a lot. I do not think it's going to replace vascular surgery. They treat entirely different spectrums of disease than we do; I see nothing in their armamentarium at the moment that suggests that they're going to start being able to duplicate what we can do about distal arterial reconstruction, for example.

Johnson: You are in a position to monitor the relationship between general surgeons and vascular surgeons. What are some of your thoughts?

Mannick: Well, there certainly are a group of general surgical chairmen who are very unhappy with their lot. They are not able to articulate, at least to my satisfaction, precisely what it is they're unhappy about; perhaps they feel they're not getting sufficient acclaim, or something. I feel that vascular surgeons for the most part are general surgeons. I won't argue with the board, who tell us that vascular surgery is a part of general surgery. I think it is. I think it is a very specialized part, just like I think hand surgery is. Most of us cannot do hand surgery very well if we only do it occasionally. I think vascular is a similar kind of thing. But then, you know that in big academic centers, general surgeons are not doing general surgery at all. They are specializing in an area of general surgery, and some areas haven't yet gained recognition, so they're low in morale at the moment. They do a lot of superb, new, high-tech surgery, and they don't get any certificate; maybe that's what's bothering them. The vascular surgeons have gotten some recognition, and I think that gripes the GI surgeon, who has also carried the field to new heights technically. Maybe that is behind some of this unhappiness.

Johnson: John, I've always marveled at your ability to be a vascular surgeon and yet have interests in areas that have very little relation to vascular surgery. How have you done this? Is that a paradox?

Mannick: You have to remember that I started out as a vascular surgeon and a transplant surgeon. I gave up transplantation when I became a department chairman after a couple of years, simply because I couldn't administer a department, be a vascular surgeon, and be a transplant surgeon. One of the three had to go, and what went was the transplant surgery. Now, that left me in the schizophrenic position of doing research in immunology and doing vascular surgery clinically. In recent years, I have tried to turn the immunological research towards something that is generally applicable to surgery, studying what happens immunologically to people who've been injured, since surgeons not only care for injured people, they also produce injury. All surgeons probably ought to have some interest in the abnormalities produced from injuring patients, and I've focused on immunological research. So it may not be quite so schizophrenic as it first sounds. I admit that it might fit a lot better, in terms of people's view of what I do, if my research were in endothelial cell biology rather than immunology. But you know those two fields are now approaching one another very quickly.

John Ochsner

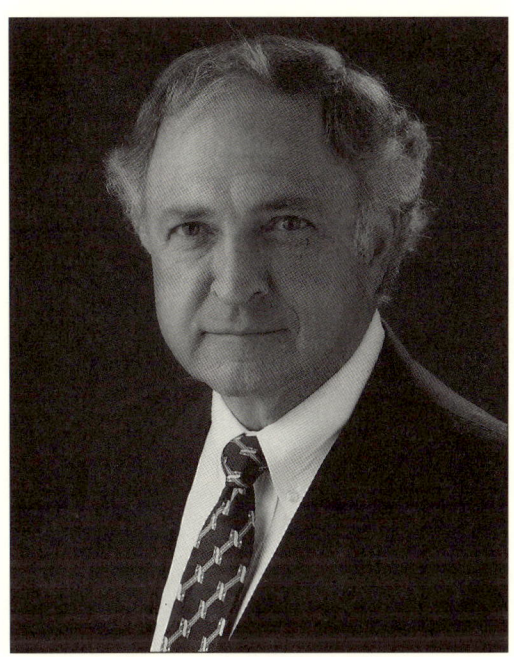

JOHN OCHSNER was raised among the early leaders in vascular
surgery: his father was Alton Ochsner, he was a guest as a youngster in the home of Rudolph Matas, and his babysitter, Mike
Debakey. He was also later trained by DeBakey, as well as by
Denton Cooley. With his intelligence, ability, leadership, enthusiasm, and wit, he has accomplished much in the development of vascular surgery. He has held leadership positions in societies, boards,
and committees for both vascular surgery and cardiac surgery, and

his diverse achievements have been well recognized. His community of New Orleans once honored him by naming him the Rex of Mardi Gras. Despite all of these achievements, Ochsner remains a warm, friendly, down-to-earth person.

He was interviewed October 10, 1993.

DeWeese: When were you born, and what schools did you attend in your youth?

Ochsner: I was born February 10, 1927. I attended the public school system in New Orleans, the Audubon School, through grammar school and then attended and graduated from a prep high school, Darlington School, in Rome, Georgia. At that time, it was Darlington School for Boys, the same school from which Andy Dale, Bill Scott, Ben Wilcox, and Lew Flint graduated.

DeWeese: Why did you go into surgery?

Ochsner: I went into surgery because I assumed it was the only thing to do. I had two brothers and all of us went into medicine. We grew up with a very dominating father and assumed that what he did we should do also, and I don't think there was any question in the minds of any of us that we would not go into medicine.

DeWeese: Where did you go for surgical training?

Ochsner: I began my surgical training with an internship at the University of Michigan at Ann Arbor and did one year of surgical residency. This was in 1954, and at that time I was drafted into the Korean War as a physician. There were many of the older residents coming back from the Korean War, and Dr. Coller, who was chief at the University of Michigan, was very compliant to the needs to these men and accepted all of them back into surgical training. Hence, with time, there was a plethora of surgical residents, and they were allotted a very small amount of time on the wards and spent the majority of their training in the surgical clinics. Although there were many who could obtain adequate training in that mode, I was convinced I could not, so prior to leaving Michigan for the service, I called Dr. DeBakey, who was professor pro tem at Harvard in Mass-

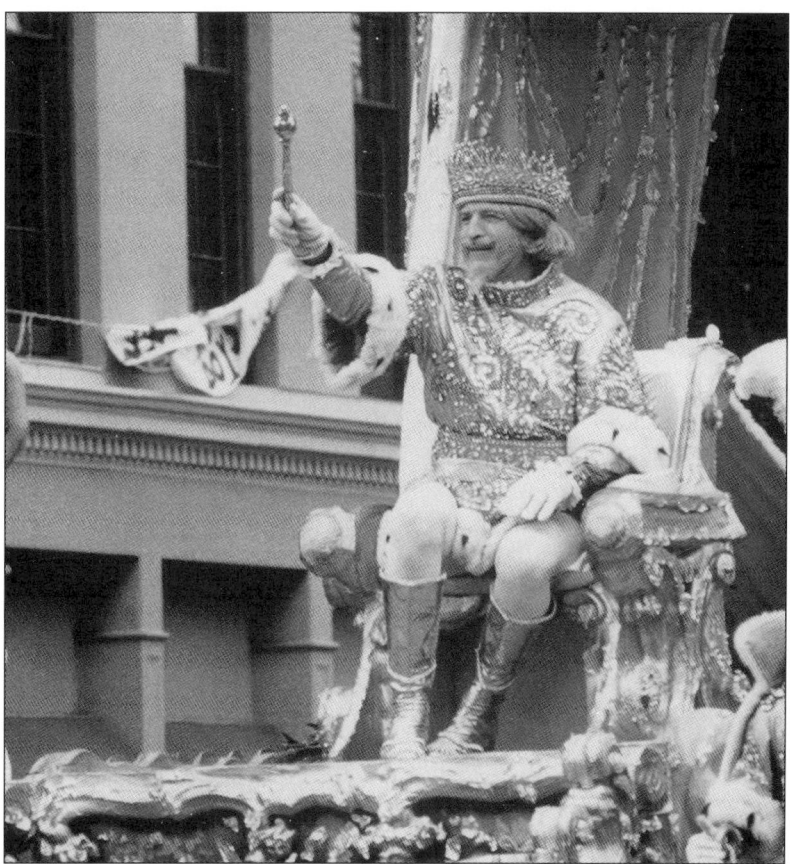

John, Rex of the Mardi Gras, 1990.

achusetts General Hospital, and asked him if I could enroll in his program at Baylor Medical School in Houston; he said that of course I could. Hence, at the completion of my service, I went to the Baylor-affiliated hospital system in Houston to complete my surgical training, first in general surgery and second in thoracic-cardiovascular. At that time, the major teaching hospital at Baylor was Jefferson Davis, which was a city-county hospital and the precursor to the present Ben Taub Hospital. Almost exclusively, our surgical training was urgent or emergency care, as this was the trauma center for the area and housed all the care for the indigent. We had a huge operative experience, which was mainly unsupervised except from senior residents.

My thoracic training really consisted of a single year. At that time this was the usual course: to receive thoracic boards after being in a program during general surgical residency in which there was a considerable amount of thoracic training as well.

DeWeese: Who were your teachers?

Ochsner: My teachers were many. At Michigan, Dr. Coller was the chief, although Buxton and Berry were very instrumental in my training, as they were the young staff men who were most active in the training of residents. At Baylor, Dr. DeBakey was chief, although George Jordan and Stanley Crawford were very active in the training of the residents. When I finished general surgery, I asked Dr. DeBakey if I could spend a year with Denton Cooley, who was just gearing up to do open-heart surgery. He said yes, if I would then come with him on the staff. So I was fortunate to be Denton's assistant in the early days of heart surgery when things were just beginning, and we were probably busier than anyone in the world.

DeWeese: When did you get married?

Ochsner: I got married in between the time I left Michigan and went into the service. I married Mary Lou Hannon from Shaker Heights, Ohio, whom I met at Michigan when we were both in a wedding.

DeWeese: What was your military experience?

Ochsner: My military experience is interesting in that I enlisted as a seventeen-year-old in the naval reserve in World War II, serving in the merchant marine as a purser pharmacist, after training in Sheeps Head Bay, New York, for a short period of nine months. I served for two years, and although I was exempt from draft in the Korean War because of my previous World War II experience, I was drafted as a doctor under the new draft act and served in Hokrado, Japan, for two years. We were stationed right across from the Russian border at a time when there was a lot of tension, but, of course, no major conflicts. Thus, unfortunately, I ended up serving in two wars under two different draft acts.

DeWeese: What was your relationship to Dr. DeBakey?

Ochsner: My relationship with Dr. DeBakey was very unique in that I knew him as "Mike" as a child when he was a resident and young staff man with my father. He actually was our babysitter on many occasions. In fact, when he and his first wife, Diana, married, they spent their honeymoon at our house while my mother and father were overseas on a visiting professorship. When I went to Houston in 1956 to begin my residency, John Overstreet and Oscar Creech, who were former residents of my father and serving on the staff of Baylor at that time, took me out to lunch and gave me some of the best advice I have ever received in my life. They told me to forget Dr. DeBakey as "Mike" and remember that henceforth he was "Dr. DeBakey," never to make an excuse, and never to talk back. Therefore, during my entire surgical training, my answers to Dr. DeBakey were invariably "Yes, sir" or "No, sir," and nothing else. In fact, I can remember vividly that one time during the middle of my residency, Dr. DeBakey grabbed me by the shoulders and said, "John, can't you ever say anything but 'Yes, sir' or 'No, sir'?" and I said, "No, sir." He never again questioned my answers.

I remained on the staff at Baylor for one year before returning to New Orleans at the Ochsner Clinic. It was a very difficult decision for both Mary Lou and me to make, whether to stay in Houston or return to New Orleans. Obviously, I was in Houston at the time Houston was the hottest spot in the world for cardiovascular surgical care, and yet I had such a desire to return to the Ochsner Clinic and help build it, particularly in thoracic-cardiovascular surgery. Thus, I left, although Dr. DeBakey had given me a tremendous offer to remain on the staff. I have remained very devoted to Dr. DeBakey and am grateful for all that he did for me in guiding me through my training. I am also grateful and devoted to Denton Cooley, who has become a close personal friend, for the opportunity he gave me to be with him during those early formative years of cardiac surgery.

DeWeese: What is the history of the Ochsner Clinic?

Ochsner: The history of the Ochsner Clinic is somewhat unique, in that it was started by five professors of surgery in different surgical specialties at Tulane University in the hope of forming a university practice. However, Tulane would not support this role and would not build a hospital or a clinic for these endeavors. Hence, these five men raised money and put up their own capital to form a clinic that they named after my father, who was more or less the leader of the group. That was in 1942, and the clinic has grown to be the largest medical practice group in the South, now having over five hundred doctors and an equal number of residents. At the present time, the Ochsner Clinic is somewhat in the forefront of the change in medical practice, in that we began an HMO some eight years ago and our administrators saw the value of spreading out with multiple satellites and other hospitals, so as to give us a broad base. Only time will tell whether these extraordinary, bold ventures will prove to be positive.

DeWeese: What is the future of cardiac and vascular surgery?

Ochsner: I believe that both cardiac and vascular surgery will continue to flourish, although most of the advances will be in basic science as it relates to surgical practice, rather than in the clinical and surgical techniques, as it was during my era. I was lucky enough to come along during an era in which one could do research and clinical experimentation without interruption from other bodies. If during a surgical procedure we felt the need for the use of any foreign material or untried operations, there was no question as to our direction, and approval was accepted by all. The same was true in performing any experimental research. It was not uncommon during an afternoon when one did not have any clinical commitments to call up the animal lab and ask for an animal of a certain size to do any sort of experiment one desired without going through any review boards and red tape. As you know today, before one can do any sort of experimental work, it takes practically three months to get the paperwork done for approval.

I do think that many of the operations we as cardiac and vascular surgeons are doing will continue in the future. However, many will be done by interventionists, be they cardiologists, radiologists, cardiac surgeons, or vascular surgeons. The emphasis to perform procedures without major incisions and in such a way to decrease hospital stays will be paramount.

Of some distress to me is the fact that it appears that medicine in the immediate future is going to be price- or cost-driven, and not so much quality-driven. There will be quality control, but that will not be of the strength that cost control will mandate. I believe some of this will change with time when it is realized that severe cost restraint is not necessarily the ideal way in medicine.

Malcolm Perry

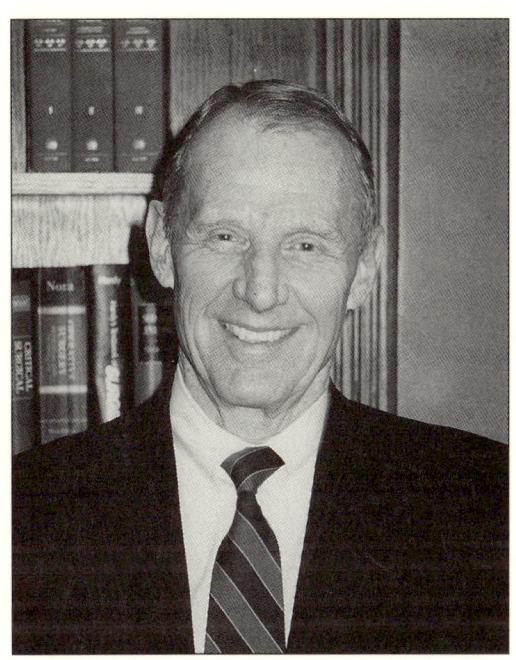

A TEXAN, Perry made the full circle around the United States
and returned to Texas. His contributions to vascular surgery
stand out, beginning with his extensive experience with vascular trauma at Southwestern in Dallas with Tom Shires. His leadership role in vascular surgery has touched everyone, and his criteria
for potential vascular trauma have stood the test of many years. Former president of the Society for Vascular Surgery, he is a true southern gentleman and also an avid airplane pilot. He was interviewed
June 3, 1990.

Johnson: Where were you born, who were your parents, and what did they do?

Perry: I was born in Allen, Texas, a town of four hundred, on a Saturday, September 3, in 1929. I was delivered by my grandfather, on the screened-in porch at his home. My father died when I was four, and I was subsequently reared by my grandparents. My grandfather was a country doctor who practiced medicine in Collin County, Texas, for fifty years. So I grew up with all the heroes that you might expect, and it's almost inevitable that I'd end up going in to medicine just because of Granddad.

Granddad was a country doctor. He drove four or five thousand miles a month, I suppose. I thought for a while I might be a doctor, but then I wanted to be an aeronautical engineer. I actually was interested in flying. Granddad used to talk to Sam Rayburn, the former Speaker of the House from Bonham, Texas. My grandfather always said you should never discuss religion and politics with anybody, because you'll always have a furor. Granddad never talked about what party he was in or how he was going to vote. A lot of the people thought he was pretty important. I can remember that when I was in junior high school, Mr. Rayburn would come by and sit in the waiting room of the office and wait for Granddad to come back in from calls to talk to him. I guess he figured that since Granddad delivered so many kids and had so many patients in that county that he might be influential in that regard, even though he never talked about it. So Granddad called Mr. Rayburn and secured me a preliminary appointment to Annapolis. I was going to go into the navy in aeronautical engineering and be a pilot. At the time I was vacillating between that and medicine.

In Allen, Texas, we played six-man football, and I played on the basketball, football, and baseball teams; I also ran track. I decided to transfer to Plano High School, which was five miles away, because they played eleven-man football, and I wanted to get a chance to go to college on a scholarship. In addition, they had chemistry, physics, and advanced mathematics at Plano, which weren't available at my little country school. I subsequently ended up going not to Annapolis but to the University of Texas. I played football and basketball, but I sat on the bench for the most part. I broke my shoulder playing football, and I'm almost over the disappointment, some forty years later, of not quite being good enough. I got in at the end of the game for a minute or two, when it was safely away. Good enough to get a uniform, but not good enough to play.

Johnson: Where did you go to medical school?

Perry: University of Texas–Southwestern. It was the Southwestern Medical Foundation, and I was at medical school after I got out of the University of Texas as an undergraduate. Southwestern had just been taken over by the University of Texas. It was an independent medical school, private, and in 1951 it became part of the University of Texas system. Galveston was the first branch of the University of Texas. Later, of course, a branch in Houston was added. Southwestern at that time was comprised of quonset huts out behind the hospital. It didn't have a medical school as such. There were ninety students admitted that year.

Johnson: What are some of the ways in which your grandfather influenced you? What can you remember about him?

Perry: I had two older sisters, and there was a cataclysm along about the time I was in grade school: one of my sisters went to live with an aunt and the other with my mother. I stayed with my grandparents. I was nine or ten when all this happened. It was a big emotional thing about moving, but I stayed with my grandfather. I used to go with him in the car and stand up and hold onto the dashboard. And many's the time I went with him and fell asleep in the back of the car when he was delivering a baby or whatever he was doing. I'm told—of course, I don't remember this—that when people would ask me who I was, I said I was Doctor Perry. My grandfather was a remarkable person. You know, he did everything; he even delivered babies in the home. I remember him setting fractures by touch with basswood splits. Then they'd send them to the nearest town, which was McKinney, because they had an x-ray machine.

My grandfather didn't believe in local anesthesia for things like eye lacerations. He just sewed them up. He did everything, things that would just terrify you to think about now, with no antibiotics, no blood, no fluid—only ether, chloroform, morphine, phenobarb, novocaine, all those things. Yes, he was a remarkable person. He delivered a baby three days before his final and fatal coronary at age seventy-six.

Johnson: Where were you when he died?

Perry: I was there. I laid out between college and medical school and worked with Procter and Gamble. I needed some money to go to school, so I worked in field advertising for them. I was in Louisiana working for P & G when he got really sick, so I came back to Dallas. He was at the Dallas Medical and Surgical Clinic on Live Oak, where Dr. J. Warner Duckett practiced. Granddad used to send all his cases to those surgeons. Dr. Duckett is another guy of some name. He did the first patent ductus operation west of the Mississippi. He came from Johns Hopkins. His son is professor of pediatrics at Pennsylvania, really an outstanding pediatric urologist. At any rate, I got back there and was at his bed when he died. My grandmother had already had a fatal heart attack and died in the stands when we were playing in the state quarterfinals in high school. She hadn't missed a game. Granddad lived to see me accepted to medical school. He died in the March before my freshman year in medical school. He was very proud of me. When you asked what influence Granddad had, I think he influenced everything.

Johnson: What happened to your mother?

Perry: My mother died this last year at eighty-six. I don't remember much about living with her, because after I was four I lived with my grandparents. One of my sisters lived in Los Angeles; she committed suicide about six or seven years ago. My other sister, who is two years older than I, lives in Kilgore, Texas. She's had a coronary bypass; she had her first coronary at age thirty-eight. She was a smoker, overweight, and all that. My father died of some strange thing. Granddad said the post didn't show anything. He was twenty-seven and he was a heavy smoker, but Granddad thought it was probably some electrical event.

Johnson: What did your father do?

Perry: He was a licensed funeral director. When he was seventeen, he ran off and joined the navy instead of going on to school like his sisters did. He was the eldest of four. He then got married, so Granddad told him he could do whatever he wanted to do. His younger sisters—the twins and my other aunt—all went to college and became teachers. Dad was apparently a very personable guy, but a grasshopper. He was always here and there and yonder.

Johnson: What happened when you got into medical school? What motivated you to be a physician? How did you become a vascular surgeon?

Perry: I guess you'd really have to blame Tom Shires for that. I got into medical school with a lot of kids I'd gone to school with at the University of Texas; they were real scholars. My first two years at Texas, my grades weren't grand. I was trying to play football and basketball and take a lot of the courses in the summer. I worked at one of the local swimming pools, taught swimming and diving, and worked as a lifeguard. I hardly took lab courses, because I was trying to carry only about fourteen hours in the fall so I could play ball. I was really having a hard time. During the last two years, I guess, I have to thank Jack Grey, the basketball coach, for medical school. I got a uniform as a sophomore, but he called me and said, "What are you going do with your career? You're premed. Frankly, you're not good enough to make the team unless you can be out here every day. You're missing two days a week going to laboratory. If you were my son I'd advise you to concentrate on medicine rather than athletics."

So I did not try to play the following year, and I was accepted to Southwestern. It turned out I was accepted at three schools: the University of Texas–Galveston, Tulane, and Southwestern. Southwestern was close—it was there in Dallas—and it was relatively less expensive than the others. And I had to go somewhere I could afford. Jeannine and I were married one week before I started medical school. Our honeymoon consisted of a trip from Wichita Falls to Mineral Wells. She went to work, and I went to school in the fall. During school, I actually started to do internal medicine. Don Seldin, who was chief of the program in medicine, invited me when I was a third-year student to come and work in his laboratory. And so I worked as a student research fellow in the Department of Medicine for a year. Dr. Seldin wanted me to go to Columbia in New York to intern and then come back to Southwestern as a resident in internal medicine. I was broke and had borrowed a lot of money, and I was a little unsettled about internal medicine. I told Jeannine, "I'm going to go ahead and volunteer for the air force to try to pay some of our debts. I'm not sure I'm ready to do internal medicine." I did an air force internship at Letterman Army Hospital. The air force had no hospitals, so they sent us to the army. I went to flight surgeon training and stayed in the service three years. During that time, I decided I really wasn't suited for internal medicine. I needed to be more actively involved in what was happening.

Johnson: But you did learn how to fly?

Perry: Well, at that time flight surgeons received some preliminary training, and I also joined the air club.

I then wrote Ben Wilson, who was chief of surgery. He'd been Carl Moyer's protégé. Moyer brought Dr. Wilson with him when he came from Michigan. I told him I'd decided that I really didn't want to go into internal medicine and that I thought I was more suited for surgery. He accepted me in the residency. I found out when I got there that they paid fifty dollars a month, and you worked every day and every other night. It was a pyramid. Twelve started and four survived. But you didn't ask any of those questions. I figured we'd survive. When I got out of the service, I came back as a first-year resident. I remember when I saw Dr. Seldin ten days later, he stopped in the hall and said, "You've been back three weeks and you haven't been to see me. And I'm pretty mad about it." And he grinned, like he always did, "But I forgive you." You know Seldin; what a character. He just retired after thirty-five years, and his successor is Dan Foster, one of my classmates. But Dr. Seldin and Dr. Wilson were responsible for my attitude towards medicine. Near the end of my residency, I was looking for a place to go into practice. I went down to Baytown and various places in Texas. Dr. Schulze of San Angelo said he was worried because my surgical training was so limited. He said, "You know, Charlie Mayo did cataracts and everything. You seem to be so limited in what you're able to do in general surgery. You don't do cataracts. You don't do ENT. You just do general surgery." And I said, "Yeah, that's what we do now." But Dr. Schulze was worried about my making a living in San Angelo, since I'd had such a limited training. During that time Tom Shires was trying to recruit the faculty. He'd just become chairman.

Johnson: What year was this?

Perry: It was 1961. He was appointed chairman that year, and he recruited Bob McClelland, Charlie Baxter, and me to stay on the faculty. And he said, "You know, you like to teach. You have a gift for it. The residents and the students like you. You need to do something; perhaps you'd be interested in vascular?" And I said to him, "But I don't do heart." As you remember, in 1961 and 1962 the heart patients all died. You'd go in there and do a lot of good work and you never could get them off the pump. My personality's such that I get depressed when everybody's dying, so I don't do that. Tom talked to John Howard, Charles Hufnagel, and Wiley Barker. Wiley was interested in such training, but Longmire said, "No, it would disrupt the residency."

Johnson: Was Jesse Thompson a vascular surgeon at this time?

Perry: Yes, he and Dale Austin were the guys who helped me. Jesse was the chief of our vascular service, *ex officio,* but he and Dale and Leroy Kleinsasser looked after us. They were our vascular consultants, and they came over all the time. I'd worked with Jesse some; he'd covered me and I really enjoyed it. Jesse said, "Well, I'll tell you what. My classmate from Harvard, Jack Wylie, might be interested in having Mac come out there for a year, unofficially." So I went to the SVS meeting that year in Chicago, and Jesse introduced me to Wylie. We sat down and talked about all this and what I wanted to do.

Jack told me, "There's no money for it." I had a little house with a four and a quarter GI loan. I had to sell my house to get enough money to travel because there wasn't any money for the fellowship, and the residency wasn't going to pay for it. Dr. Goldman was willing for me to come as long as it didn't disrupt the residency. So I drove my Volkswagen to San Francisco. John Tapley came out in a T-33 and picked me up at Hamilton Air Force Base. I left my car there with a colonel and found us a place to stay. A month later I drove out with my family.

Unofficially, the residents greeted me with undisguised hostility. It turned out that Bob Siegel and Dee McGonigle were on the service, and we all became good friends when they found out I wasn't there to steal their cases. I was there to learn how they operated, and it turned out to be quite a change in my whole life. We were able to get together $5,000 to pay for some stuff that needed to be done in the lab. We were looking at ischemia of the kidney and later published the data. I returned to Dallas at the end of August 1963 as an assistant professor of surgery after my year with Wylie.

Johnson: What were some of the highlights of your year with Wylie?

Perry: You know Jack: tough and demanding. I remember that Wylie was always determined to do things properly the first time. I will always thank him for that and for the concept of durability. He said, "Many of the operations you do can be technically satisfactory, but if they're not durable and you have to re-operate two or three weeks from now, you're not doing the patient a favor." He said expeditious surgery is not what you want to do; you want to do something that is complete and durable. He was determined.

I remember that one day we were doing a popliteal aneurysm using an iliac autograft. We'd take the external iliac and replace it with Dacron and use the segment of external iliac for repair of a popliteal aneurysm or for repair of an infected carotid. In this particular case, we'd taken the external iliac and replaced the popliteal with it. And we used completion arteriography. The suture line didn't look exactly right; it was open but it didn't look right. We re-did that thing three times, each time with an on-the-table arteriogram. We finally made it satisfactory. It was a really long afternoon, because it was the second or third case we'd done that day. And so we got done and I finally said, "This gets pretty tedious, doesn't it?" And Jack turned to me and said, "Would you like to do hernias all day, every day?" And I said, "No." He said, "That's why we do this." It did not have to be done again.

And so perseverance and determination were important parts of vascular surgery. There wasn't a format. It wasn't "take things out," it was "fix it." You had to persevere, whatever it took to get it right, however long it took. And so I learned something about attention to detail that I think is extremely important for all vascular surgeons. Because, as you and I both know, in vascular surgery, if

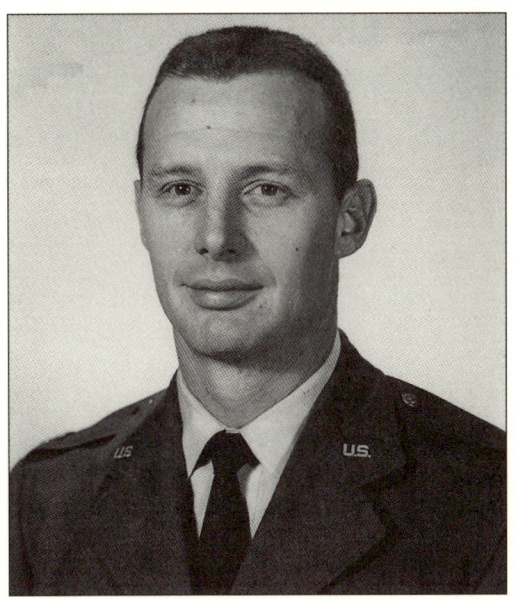

Malcolm in the Air Force, 1955.

you're there at the right time, for the right reason, and if you're a good physiologic surgeon, then the results are going to be directly related to how skillful you are. So we hope to have all three of those things lined up. I think Wylie exemplified that, as Jesse did, too, when I was a resident. You want to be there at the right time and for the right reason, but you've got to do it right when you get there and be sure it is right. Jack was his own strictest critic. He was very critical of himself, as well as of what we did. He made sure at the operating table and at the conferences that we did it right. He wouldn't accept anything less. I think that was a very important lesson.

Every Wednesday afternoon, we had our critique conference. Jack presided and many of the people in town came, as well as some of the former residents. Bud Murray would come back down from Napa and Shel Levin would come from across the Bay; it was really quite a spirited place. Blaisdell was the chief at the VA at the time. He and Wylie didn't always agree and we had some really spirited sessions. I knew very little about the way they did things, but that didn't exempt me from being asked a lot of questions. In the clinic earlier that day, we'd see all the patients ourselves, he and I. John Najarian was chief of the lab. He had just returned from Scripps. He and Bill Silen were both assistant professors that year, which was fortunate for me because I was around them and they were terrific. John was running the research lab. I usually spent two days a week in the lab and then three days a week operating with Wylie. That was kind of the way things were set up; there was no such thing as a fellowship. It finally sorted itself out as the year went on and other residents rotated on the service. I'd do one of everything with the resident if Jack wasn't there. And, after a while, I became kind of a junior staff surgeon. Initially, Wylie and I would do the cases, and then as the year wore on and the residents got better and he gained more confidence in me, I'd help them do things. I first assisted Jack or the resident, in that case the junior staff. Ron Stoney was a third-year resident at the time, as was Wes Moore. And, of course, we became friends. They are outstanding people. By the time the year was out I think we were all pretty good friends. I was not a paid employee and as such I wasn't really staff, nor was I a resident. We had to walk a little carefully. But Jack used to say, "You can get any-thing you want if you know how to ask for it."

If you ask for it right, people will be willing to help you. Gener-ally, that's true. It changed my life, of course. The time at UC helped me meet many people who've become good friends. I learned a great deal from it. But it changed my whole approach. I had to go back to Dallas, but I was offered a job to stay at UC and it was one of the most difficult decisions I've ever made. That was the second time I had lived in San Francisco. I used to tell Jack, "I think I'll go down to Polk Street and open an office." That's where his private office was at that time, on Union Square. And he used to tell me, "You don't have enough gray hair to compete down there." Although I really wanted to stay when they offered me a job, I had an obligation to Tom and Jesse to return to Dallas and bring back the things that I'd learned to Southwestern. Tom and I had agreed, so I went back to Dallas. The next year they got another fellow, Freddy, and I've forgotten who the next one was. Anyway, the fel-lowship was established that year, and a couple of years later became formal. Ehrenfield came four or five years later.

Johnson: But you were the first fellow?

Perry: You really couldn't call it a fellowship. I was the first one in Jack's program. Jesse took Mark Kartchner two years later. It was Jesse and Tom's idea more than Jack's.

Johnson: What year were you in San Francisco?

Perry: It was 1962—I came back to Dallas in August 1963. I love San Francisco. I'd go back tomorrow.

Johnson: And so then you went back to Dallas?

Perry: I stayed on the faculty as an assistant professor. The whole department consisted of Tom Shires as chairman, Bob McClelland, Charlie Baxter, and me. We didn't have a cardiac surgeon. Bob Walker was head of oral surgery; Kemp Clark, of neurosurgery; and Charlie Gregory, a marvelous man, was chief of orthopedics. Charlie died prematurely at age fifty-seven. He was a great guy; like Jesse, he was a Rhodes scholar and a real intellectual. And then Paul Peters came on as an assistant professor. Tom brought him from Indiana. We were a pretty small group. We used the City-County Hospital, and the VA Hospital was fourteen miles away.

Johnson: When you went back, did Jesse still come to Parkland?

Perry: Yes. Jesse was so much help to me. He and Kemp Clark particularly looked after me. I guess that's one of the reasons Jesse and I are such good friends now. I don't know what I would've done without him. In the following year, we invited Jack to come. Jesse and I acted as cohosts and had a marvelous time.

Johnson: Was there a vascular program at Parkland?

Perry: There were some vascular surgeons there, but we did not have a program as such. Each of the trauma services carried an appendage, as a specialty; Trauma 3 carried vascular. That was my service. Our elective cases were vascular. We didn't have enough cases at the outset at City-County Hospital that were elective for an active service, although we got pretty busy in a few years. My interest was in vascular trauma. I also covered vascular surgery in the VA.

Johnson: Did you ever work with Jesse?

Perry: We had some conferences together and that sort of thing. But I didn't work with him.

Johnson: During this period, you became known as the expert in vascular trauma throughout the world, even though there was a lot of vascular trauma at other hospitals in the United States. To what do you attribute the fact that you became so knowledgeable in the management of vascular trauma—the "Perry" indications for angiography, and so forth?

Perry: I wish I could take credit for that, George, but you and I know that I learned some of that from you and others. All through the years, you and I were on programs together and shared many thoughts. I can't take credit for all of that. That's an amalgam of what you and I and all the rest did. We did a lot of trauma surgery because we had a lot of it, and thus had a lot of vascular trauma. I didn't have much elective surgery, and so I was able to concentrate on trauma.

Tom had done a lot of surgery and knew how to do it. I could always sit down with Tom and talk to him. He has good surgical judgment, and it didn't make any difference whether he did vascular or not. I accumulated a lot of cases early on. Tom would just say, "We're going do this, we'll have these services, and we'll do it that way." I pretty well had a free hand to do what I wanted. Tom, like all good CEOs, said it was my service, as long as it ran alright. If I needed help, I would talk to him; otherwise he'd leave me alone. The things I'd learned from Jesse, from Wiley, and from Tom about the management of patients, I applied to vascular trauma. You may not always be right, but at least you get some semblance of order in what you do.

Johnson: You and Dr. Seldin worked together during this period?

Perry: Yes, you know I'm a great admirer of Don Seldin's and said for years that if he and Tom could have ever gotten together, they could have ruled the world. They are two of the smartest people I've ever known. Both of them are walking around with 150–160 IQs. Don Seldin was absolutely one of the most stimulating people I've ever known. He is still a power to be reckoned with. A true renaissance man. For example, he could tell you who was an all-pro guard with the Cleveland Browns in 1960.

Johnson: You certainly made an impact on vascular surgery at Parkland. Tell me about the move to Seattle.

Perry: Seattle, and on to New York. It was difficult. I didn't go with them initially. At Parkland, it was the age-old battle between the basic science/internist and the surgeon regarding the teaching of surgery. Tom foresaw that there was no way to teach and train residents and attract good faculty if you only had the City-County Hospital. You need a private service and other types of patients; you don't need everybody with an incurable breast cancer. It's an educational problem. A university hospital needs a "gold coast ward" where you can have private patients. We all had private patients, but they usually wouldn't come to Parkland more than once; then I'd have to take them to Presbyterian or St. Paul. He recognized that we were going to have to commit ourselves clinically. Our cardiology friends can put in one person with a myocardial infarct and train three residents, two fellows, and two staff people with that one patient for three weeks. You and I can't do that. We've got to have a number of different types of patients. We have to have volume. The internists do not require that many patients. They can use one patient for teaching purposes. They wanted it to be a basic science research institute. Tom is dedicated to basic research, but also believes that you ought to have a first-class clinical program.

That led to his departure. He took the job in Seattle. Jim Carrico, Pete Canizaro, Bill Curreri, Bob Jones, and David Heimbach all went with him. I didn't go because I'd visited with Gene Strandness and David, and it didn't look to me like there was anything there for me to do. And I didn't want to move. I told Tom, "There's no place for me there."

Dean Odegaard, who had made all the arrangements with Tom, had a heart attack after everybody moved. They brought John Hoagness back from Washington, and he became the new boss. He appointed Tom Grayston, an internist, as his executive officer. Hoagness unilaterally abrogated about 90 percent of the agreements that Odegaard had made with Tom. Tom didn't stay more than one year as a result.

In May, Tom called me and said, "Gene's renting an office over in Bellevue, and it appears that he's going to go into practice. I need you; will you come and help?" I sold my house and we moved to Seattle.

Johnson: You stayed in Seattle, although Tom stayed only a year and then went to New York. Pete Canizaro and Bill Curreri and all of them went to New York with him, but you stayed.

Perry: Pete and Bill and Joel went with him. I said, "Tom, I really don't want go to New York." His answer to that was, "Find me a better place, and I'll go with you." Three years later he talked me into going. I had stayed in Seattle four and a half years by then. As a matter of fact, and I'm surprised to hear myself say this, I really miss New York City. I miss New York Hospital and a lot of the friends I made there.

Johnson: What happened when you stayed in Seattle? How was it there without Tom?

Perry: Well, initially it was really hard, because there was some animosity between various people when I arrived. John Schilling followed Tom as chairman at Tom's recommendation. John did a good job. He had a little help from Carrico and me, and we tried to work some of the things out. We finally got it done.

Some of the bad feelings were the result of a lack of communication more than anything else. I had no personal problem with anybody myself. As things sorted themselves out, of course, people said that Gene Strandness and I would feud, but actually we didn't. Our problem was the fact that when I arrived there were already a bunch of legal problems; but I was not part of them. After Tom left, the administration changed, and it all went away. Gene and I parted as friends. I don't think he and I had a problem other than the circumstances into which we were thrown. It was a shame it had to happen.

Johnson: Was there a fellow?

Perry: No. We didn't have enough cases for a fellow at the outset. Everybody rotated on the services, and there were fellows from time to time who worked in Gene's lab. But there wasn't much volume. When I got to the University Hospital, I did very little surgery. I looked at the previous ten years of operating records to see how much vascular surgery was being done, and there was not much. Most of the vascular surgery was at the VA and a little at the public health hospital.

Johnson: And then you moved to New York?

Perry: And ran into a lot of your old friends, some of whom were glad to see us, and some of whom were not. They had eight guys there doing "pick-up" vascular surgery, but no one who really did it regularly.

Johnson: How long were you in New York?

Perry: Ten years, from 1978 to 1988.

Johnson: How would you characterize the New York era?

Perry: The first two years were a real struggle. I was watching everybody else operate, and I didn't have any cases. You rearrange your diplomas or whatever you have on the wall, your pictures, string your paper clips together, or something. I like to operate, and you can spend only so much time in the office and the lab. I was busy trying to get a grant renewal, so I had some work to do in the lab. I was covering at Jamaica Hospital in Queens, as well.

Johnson: What stimulated the move to Vanderbilt?

Perry: I actually wasn't looking for a job at all. One of the problems at New York was that I was never going to have a vascular program of my own. We had eight or nine chief residents. With that many, there was no way we were going to have enough volume to have a separate program.

Another problem was financial. As you are well aware, when you try to do the academic business and you're away from home, the bills are still there and you're not making anything. At Cornell, you had to support yourself with your practice. The last four years I was there, I was losing money. I never got in the position where I could make any incentive money. Once you covered your expenses and your guaranteed salary, you got to keep half of what you made over that. I never got there because my expenses were going up every year. Liability was up to $78,000, rent was $31 a square foot, the secretary's salary was $37,000, etc. I suddenly realized that all those years of working for $15,000 or $20,000 a year as an assistant professor didn't put much in my retirement fund. I was nearing sixty. I wasn't going to have a vascular fellowship. I couldn't get rid of a couple of problems I had there at the hospital; they were going to be there forever. There was no way to hire a couple of young scientists whom I really needed. It was either give up some of the academic business and concentrate on building my private practice, or not be able to survive financially. The last year I was there, I put $450,000 in the kitty and broke even. So I moved mainly for those reasons.

One, for a fellowship; two, for an opportunity to do a little building; and three, for financial reasons.

Andy and John Ochsner and Jesse Thompson talked to John Sawyers at Vanderbilt and suggested that he might talk to me. I was not looking for a place. Frank Moody had asked me to come to the University of Texas at Houston. I went down there and looked at it. Frank and I are old friends. He wanted me to come down there and be chief of vascular and vice chairman. I really wasn't ready to move at that time. I think Jesse, John, and Andrew all knew that I was struggling. When John Sawyers said, "If you come, we'll make you the first recipient of the H. William Scott Chair of Surgery," it was impressive. An endowed chair sounded pretty good. I hated to leave. I'd been with Tom twenty-five years, and I miss him terribly.

Johnson: Tell me about how you met your wife.

Perry: Blind date. Jeannine's roommate was dating my roommate when we were at the University of Texas. I went out with her as a favor to Herky Vaughn, my roommate. She went out with me as a favor to Pat Owens, who was her roommate in the Tri-Delta house. Jeannine didn't want to go out with me for two reasons. First, I was a Kappa Sigma, and they were noted for boisterousness. Second, I was one of the athletes, and she didn't usually date them. I had a great time, and I said, "What are you doing every night next week?" and she said, "Nothing." She says I startled her; she actually had a couple of dates that she had to break.

Johnson: Well, you've been in the national scene over the years, an association with Jack Wylie, Jesse Thompson, Tom Shires. From your perspective, what has happened to vascular surgery during the years that you've been associated with it? How could you sum it up?

Perry: I don't know if I agree with all of it. I got crossways with Wylie for a couple of years. At the time, Tom was chairman of the American Board of Surgery. Jack had the mistaken impression that I influenced Tom in regard to resisting the concept of vascular surgery as a separate specialty. Nothing could be farther from the truth. I think we were at Monterey when Jack got after me and was a little unhappy about my not having set up a program in Dallas. Later it all went away, and we were okay.

I thought vascular surgery should remain part of general surgery.

And my idea at the time, which Jack didn't like, was that we should put the onus on the program director for the quality control. I didn't think we needed a separate board or a separate examination process; I wasn't even sure we needed a separate certificate. My feeling was that vascular was part of general surgery and it should stay part of general surgery. Both for training reasons and for educational reasons, I saw nothing wrong with people like Jesse doing general surgery. It didn't bother me like it did Jack. I thought that, rather than having all these separate things, we should require the program director to ensure proper quality control and make this an educational effort.

Now we've done all that, and we've alienated a number of people. I don't know whether we've improved it or not. It is better educationally, but I'm not convinced that the board examination per se sorts these people out. It gives them a certificate, but I don't know what that means. The focus on specialization has been good as far as some of the training is concerned, but I'm not sure it's been good overall for vascular surgery or for general surgery. I think it's the people who are training the guys that make the difference. I don't know that the boards make that much difference. We're all concerned about the "endovascular group." Well, I find it boring as hell. We have a laser program at our place. We just finished the FDA phase-one study on the tunable dye laser for plaque ablation. It doesn't make any difference what laser medium you use, it's the delivery system that's the key, as you and I know. I viewed the hot tip and balloon dilation as a way station. We've done that, and it doesn't work. Little durability, as Wylie would say. At UC that year, we did fifty long fem-pop TEAs with distal vein patches. Every one worked. Two years later, 30 percent were working. Everything works for two years, and after that you find out whether it's really durable or not. So I figured all this stuff wasn't bad. The hot tip laser is sitting on the shelf like you'd expect. What's going to happen, now that all the cardiologists and radiologists are doing it, is worrisome.

We need a better way to go at it. We need to understand the physiology and the biochemical changes. What we've done is to do the clinical cases without the research, and it's coming home to roost.

Balloon dilation and hot tips and all that stuff are a way station. That does not take care of the disease process. The emphasis has been on the wrong place. Vascular surgery has been on a sandbar for ten years. Technically, we've done about what we can do, and just like we were talking about this morning, we are recycling everything. I'd like them to take some of it back to the lab and not talk about it again for about five years. Then perhaps we'll know what we're really doing. The basic physiology of the endothelial cell is where the work is going to be. And we need to do that before we start any clinical trials.

Mark Ravitch

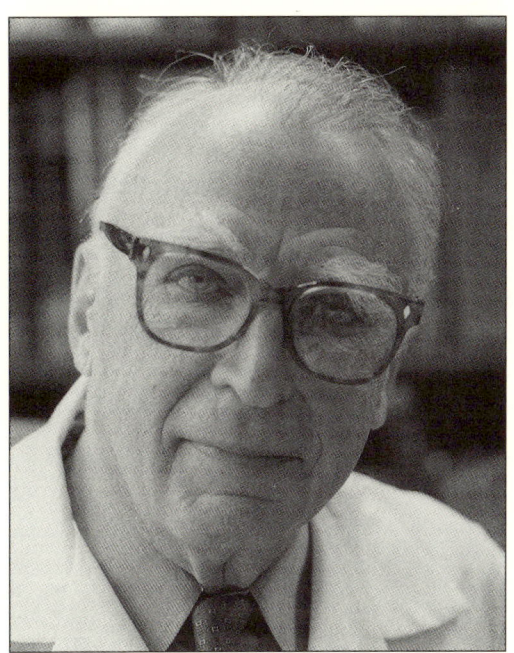

MARK RAVITCH represented the true meaning of being
one of "Alfred Blalock's boys." He was a friend of everyone, in his gruff, opinionated fashion. His untimely death
in March 1989 left a void in the field of surgery. The editors have
included his interview as an example of the time when surgery was
king and the chief was a dictator. He was interviewed January 19,
1987.

Dale: Mark, tell me about your parents and where you came from.

Ravitch: My parents were both Russian immigrants. My father actually escaped from the police because he was a social democrat. He and my mother were both practicing dentists. She practiced all of her life, until she was over eighty, as a matter of fact.

Dale: What year did they emigrate?

Ravitch: About 1908. He came first and she followed him. They were married in New York. She came with the intention of marrying. I was born in 1910.

Dale: What was your early education?

Ravitch: I was educated in the schools of New York City at a time when the teachers were dedicated and devoted and wonderful. I can remember the names of grade school and high school teachers. One got a superb education in those days. I got a Regents scholarship to Columbia, but instead I went out to the University of Oklahoma. I had an uncle and an aunt who were both on the faculty, he in mathematics and she in modern languages, French and German.

Dale: Were they named Ravitch?

Ravitch: No, my aunt's name was Ravitch, but my uncle's name was Court. He was quite a distinguished mathematician. He wrote a lot of books, popular books and college texts, and, I think, did very well with them. I established residency in Norman, Oklahoma, and as a resident of Norman, I could go to school for, as I remember, twenty-five dollars a semester. That was a bargain, and I got away from New York and learned what America was really like.

I got my degree in 1934 and I applied to a lot of medical schools.

Dale: What other interests did you have in college? Were you a writer then?

Ravitch: I wrote book reviews for the Oklahoma City daily newspaper.

Dale: Did you take a premed course?

Ravitch: No, I did not, but I knew I was going into medical school, or at least I hoped I was.

Dale: What made you want to do that?

Ravitch: I'd always known since I was a kid that I wanted to go into medicine. I've said elsewhere that I remember talking to my mother once, saying I was going to be a dentist, like her, and she said, "Don't do that. It's kind of boring." I suppose she planted the seed in my mind, but she was too smart to let me realize it. I always knew I wanted to at least study medicine, and I wrote my father from college and said, "I want to go to medical school, but don't get me wrong. I don't really want to be a doctor. There are just a lot of things I want to know about the human body."

Dale: Which school did you want to go to?

Ravitch: Well, I wanted to go to Harvard. I'd taken organic chemistry in summer school, and I was absolutely smitten by Harvard Medical School, then a very new marble building, and the medical museum. I remember there were displays of a crowbar that went through a man's head, and so on. So I was bitterly disappointed to be turned down by them. I was accepted by Rush in Chicago; that was before the University of Chicago Medical School was founded. I was turned down by Yale, Andy, and that made me mad, because I realized even then in my innocent youth that the Yale medical school was not the school that a great university should have. Never has been. I was a zoology major, actually a graduate student, and my professor of zoology, Aute Richards, said he wanted me to go to Hopkins. I'd never heard of Hopkins, never been in Maryland, but I had been tractable in the face of authority, so I did what he told me and they accepted me, so I went there.

Dale: I accept those words with a smile, Mark. Go ahead.

Ravitch: I went there and it was extraordinarily good fortune.

Dale: Had Dr. Blalock already arrived when you went?

Ravitch: Oh, no, no. I came there in 1930, and he didn't get there until 1941.

Dale: So who was there? Lewis?

Ravitch: Well, Dean Lewis was professor, a forbiddingly authoritative figure. He was a great figure in American medicine; he was or became president of the AMA; he edited the *Archives of Surgery,* which was a great journal in those days. He was their first editor, I believe. He edited a great big twelve-volume system of surgery. An encyclopedic mind. He impressed us all at clinics by calling for a

German text or journals and reading them off, translating them effortlessly. Lewis was omniscient. He remembered the literature, French and German, and read it, and expected us to know it; he told us to read German or French articles. With a grin he would say, "I know it says in the requirements of the medical school that you must have a reading knowledge of French and German, so I know you do!" He knew it might be very difficult for some of us. But he insisted on it. He had an absolutely incredible recollection. Six months after he'd asked you to look up something, he would come back and say, "Where is that boy from wherever, Kansas City, or Little Rock?" Then he would ask, "What did you find?" It was terrifying and people used to be afraid that he might call on them. Some students, therefore, never went to his great Friday noon conferences, for fear that he might call on them. But on the other hand, those of us who wanted an internship in surgery sat down in the front row, to dare him to call on us and to test us mentally and project ourselves to him.

Dale: Perhaps that's where Barney Brooks got his style. Sounds a little like him.

Ravitch: Barney Brooks had left Hopkins in Dr. Halsted's days. I just think they were of another generation.

I had gotten my internship in surgery, but then, without telling Dr. Lewis, I had gotten an internship in pediatrics at Hopkins. He said to me in the corridor one day, "I hear you're going to intern in pediatrics." I said, "Yes sir, but I want to come back into surgery the next year." And he said, "Are you going to be a surgical pediatrician or pediatric surgeon? Haw! Haw!" And I guess we had that conversation two or three times, but in the end he let me come back, so I went to work in the laboratory.

Dale: What were you working on in the laboratory?

Ravitch: Well, I worked on the Brown Pierce rabbit carcinoma and on tetanus, and had my own project on adrenal hemorrhage. I probably am the only man in the world who ever spent a year in a research laboratory and didn't have a paper to show for it. Dr. Firor had one to show for it, but I never did. His was a clinical paper on adrenal hemorrhage and I got it together for him, but I decided then that I was not going to spend my life in cancer research because it

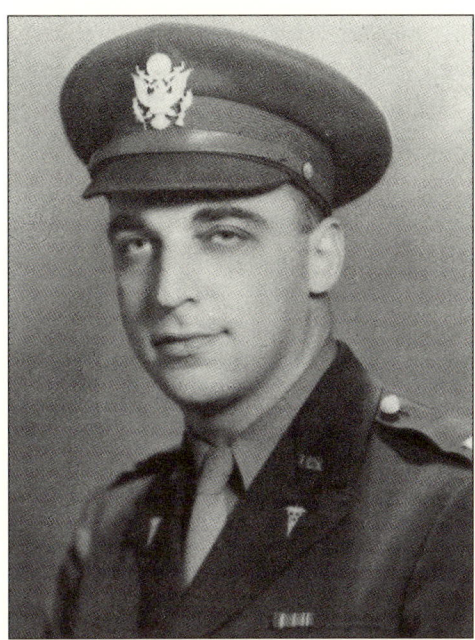

Mark with the Army Medical Corp in England.

would be so easy to go down a blind alley and spend your life in that blind alley. I didn't have any confidence in myself to stick to the mainstream.

Dale: What about Dean Lewis and Dr. Firor?

Ravitch: Well, Firor was the acting chairman and, of course, he and Bill Reinhoff were the two in-house competitors for the chairmanship.

Everybody else was an assistant resident, and I was on the house. I had an extraordinarily good relationship with Dr. Firor, who was the most brilliant teacher for the medical students and the role model we all aspired to; he was a superb surgeon, a very good investigator, and just a fine human being. He then and for years afterwards was, in a sense, my sponsor or protector. He did a lot of things to strengthen the department. We had never had a departmental conference or meeting before, and he set up conferences and meetings and so forth. Things were very different in those days. House officers never went to national meetings or any other meetings except the local meetings.

Dale: They just worked?

Ravitch: They just worked. I had nine years in a white suit and I was allowed to go to the AMA meeting once, but I had a paper to present on blood banking. I was allowed that morning to go to Cleveland and to come back that night. Period. We'd go to all of the hospital meetings, to the meetings of the state medical society and the Baltimore Medical Society, but we never went to any other. The professors, Dr. Lewis and Dr. Firor, would tell us about the meetings they had been to and the places they traveled to.

Dale: And that was, no doubt, stimulating?

Ravitch: It was as stimulating as it could be. As a matter of fact, when Lewis came back from Australia, he talked to us about a man named Hipsley who introduced the treatment of intussusception by saline enemas. That stimulated me, and it has been a lifelong interest ever since.

Dale: So finally Blalock came along?

Ravitch: Blalock came in 1941. I was the fourth man in line for the residency, and I had been there eight years. I had been in a white suit for seven years, but Aldus Jonas, Jim Mason, and Bill Watson were all ahead of me. Blalock came in to interview everybody. He smoked incessantly then and thereafter, and I don't think his interview with me took more than about three puffs of the cigarette. He said, "I'd be glad to have you stay on for next year." I said, "Will I then be in a position to compete for the residency?" He said, "It will be wide open," so I said yes. I think, in the first place, he had an evaluation of the house staff by Firor, and I would guess my evaluation was satisfactory. In addition, by the greatest good fortune, I had been assigned, by the administration of the hospital, the responsibility for creating a blood bank, and I was ready. I had just written a paper that appeared as the lead article in *JAMA,* and that was made to order, for Blalock was interested in shock and blood replacement. He told me that he would like to work together, and that was typical of his gentlemanly style. He didn't say, I want you to work for me or with me, he said he would like to work with me in that field.

Dale: Had his book on shock and related subjects come out by then?

Ravitch: Yes, within a year or two before that. That was the only book he ever wrote and I believe he wrote it as part of his plan to become a department chairman. He told me once that he didn't have much interest in writing books. He said he was more interested in original work and creative thinking and producing new knowledge. For once I was diplomatic and didn't point out to him that Osler and MacCullum and Kelly and Howell and all the other greats at Hopkins had not done badly with their books. I didn't say that, but we came back to the residents' suite after the interviews. To Aldus Jonas, he said, "Well, you've been here such a long time, I know you want to go back to your father in Omaha. You can take the first four months of the year as the resident." Then he said to Jim Mason and Bill Watson, who also had fathers who were prominent surgeons, "You two can split the rest of the year." He told me and Ken Pickerel that we could compete. He told two residents, who were then on Dr. Dandy's brain team, which was part of the rotation in surgery, that he knew they wanted to be neurosurgeons, so they were out.

He told me once after I had become the resident, and I guess at a time when he was probably displeased with me, "You know, I didn't have to keep all you boys."

And so we assembled that night in the residents' suite and a letter to Dr. Blalock was drafted that said, This is outrageous and unjustified; we haven't been treated fairly.

Dale: All the guys signed it?

Ravitch: Well, at that point, I said, "You know I can't really say that for myself," and Pickerel wasn't saying anything, because we were both given the opportunity to compete. So the letter was changed a little and we signed it and that was taken down to Dr. Blalock's room. Mary Blalock subsequently said she had never seen him so absolutely infuriated as he was upon the receipt of that letter. You know him; you can imagine what the reception was. This was a man who knew his own mind, he knew his priorities, he knew his authority, and he didn't brook insurrection. Well, he came back the next morning and saw us all, one by one, and if I said it took two or three puffs of his cigarette the first time, he didn't even have time to puff once this time. One cigarette covered the whole series of conferences with each of us, and what he said, in essence, was, take it or leave it. Everybody, of course, took it and, in point of fact, it worked out exceedingly well. The war came on and Jonas and Watson were in the Hopkins unit. Jonas wouldn't have completed his year, Watson wouldn't have gotten any of his year, and Mason wouldn't have gotten much more than he got because he was in the second auxiliary surgical group, so it worked out very well. Dr. Dandy then created, or was urged by Dr. Blalock to do so, his own training program, and Tennesack became his first neurosurgical resident, independent of his general surgical training program. They, of course, have become distinguished neurosurgeons.

Dale: What happened to you during the war?

Ravitch: Well, I served for twelve months as the resident. It was a marvelous time and a very difficult time. The house staff was decimated, because so many of the junior house staff went off to the war. The visiting staff was decimated, and since it was known that these were abbreviated programs for the three men proceeding me, very little passed down to me except appendices, hernias, and hemorrhoids, so I'd never done a cholecystectomy until my ninth year in a white suit.

The result was that I did operations for the first time as operator, assisted by assistant residents like Herb Sloan, who had never even seen the operations done before. He, of course, was magnificent as my mainstay and has since become a distinguished thoracic surgeon. We worked very hard and I remember telling the house staff that a lot of peripheral people on the faculty and visiting staff would be "glad to help out," that is, to get their hands on the house cases and if I ever heard of one of them complaining to Dr. Blalock that they were tired, that would be the last thing they ever said in this institution. The chief resident could pretty well say that and mean it. In those days you had great authority. It was very hard for months, certainly many, many nights. The only sleep I got was on a litter in the operating room, between cases. At the end of that time, Dr. Blalock said that he'd like for me to stay on the full-time staff, and I accepted with alacrity.

Within a week or two, I just felt miserable. All of my friends were overseas. I felt very strongly about the cause for which we were fighting and I was perhaps made more miserable by the fact that I knew I would do more good for my country, for the hospital, and for medicine if I stayed behind than if I went into the army. Nevertheless, I talked to some of the people I respected on the faculty, came back to Dr. Blalock, and said, "I've just got to go." Although he knew as well as I did that in many ways it was the wrong decision, and he certainly needed my support, he didn't say a word to dissuade me. I went to Washington, to the Surgeon General's office, and had an immediate offer to go somewhere in the South with Crenshaw Briggs, who had been resident when I was an intern. It would have been lovely, but I said that I didn't join the army to stay in the States and that I had to go overseas. I went eventually with the Fifty-sixth General Hospital, which was a pick-up unit. The chief of medicine was Dan Rutledge from Hopkins, and the chief of surgery was Bill Moore from Cornell. We were picking up our officers mostly from those two institutions when we were suddenly alerted to go overseas. This was the day my wife came down to join me.

Dale: Where did you go overseas?

Ravitch: We went to England, France, and Belgium. There was a general hospital in England, near Bristol, that was a great break for me, medically speaking. We expected an epidemic of flu and our commanding officer went to the director of the Bristol Royal Infirmary (BRI) and said, "We can't take these flu people when they come, but when the time comes if you want to evacuate your convalescent patients to us from your general operations, we'll be happy to handle them." Well, as so often happens, there was no flu epidemic and the next thing I knew the colonel said to me, "They called me from the BRI and wanted to know if we'll take their elective male waiting list in surgery." I said that could be arranged, because we were delighted. We hadn't really evaluated our nurses, our technicians, our procedures, or even some of our officers. For some months I constantly had about thirty beds filled with elective male patients, most of them with hernias. And that became a consuming interest of my lifetime.

Dale: How long were you in service?

Ravitch: I was overseas two years and on active duty almost three.

Dale: When were you married? Let's talk about that.

Ravitch: We were married when I was a second-year medical student, which for medical students was not illegal but uncommon. At that particular time, it was extremely prejudicial to becoming a surgical house officer, so we kept it quiet, and Dean Lewis actually didn't know about it until the year I was an intern in pediatrics, which was four years after we got married.

Dale: Well, that was pretty quiet. Mark, as we conclude, tell me about your relation with Hank Bahnson, who was a classmate of mine at Davidson. When did you first run into Hank?

Ravitch: I think I met Hank in the dining room, when he was applying for an internship. I don't have a clear recollection of that. I do have a clear recollection that I ran into Denton Cooley that same way, and then I went off to the war before they came. When I came back, Hank was in the navy. His beautiful wife, Louise, was still in Baltimore and Hank came back and went through the residency while I was on the full-time staff. For most of that next ten years after I returned from the army, I was really Dr. Blalock's lieutenant in charge of the house staff. There were Bill Scott and Rollo Hanlon and I.

Hank was an absolutely incredible person and performer then and ever since. I remember his extraordinary daring at amputating aneurysms with big Kelly clamps and ordinary surgical sutures, including one huge abdominal aneurysm that I think in retrospect must have been so big that it involved some of the vital branches, but I don't remember that anything was reported. I think it may have been presented at the American Surgical Association. That patient got an abdominal infection and I had to take care of that while Hank was on vacation or off somewhere. Hank was just a golden boy. Dr. Blalock loved him. He was just an assistant resident assigned to the heart team.

At first there wasn't any heart team. There was just the resident, Bill Longmire, and me. I went back in a white suit for about three months because there wasn't anybody ready to be the resident and Bill Longmire had it as long as he could take it. I was glad to do it, because military surgery was pretty coarse and I knew I needed a refresher course. So I went back on the heart team. Dr. Blalock didn't think I was helping him as well as Longmire did. He would say to me, in his usual whiny voice, "You know, Bill Longmire didn't do that," or "Bill Longmire was able to do this for me." You know from your Vanderbilt days what a whiner he was in the operating room, saying, "Won't somebody please help me?" The other great remark he would make was "If you can't help me, don't hinder me." After my military experience and coming back essentially with an appointment on the faculty, I was back in a white suit at a resident's salary, which was not much. I perhaps was not as cowed by him as I had been as a resident, although in general, I don't cow very easily.

If my relationship with Dr. Blalock was different in any sense from that with the other marvelous people that he had trained, it was that I always spoke my piece and it wasn't always diplomatic. There were others, like Hank Bahnson, who, if they were in disagreement, simply would say nothing. But there were many who took another stance. He knew that he would always get an independent opinion from me, whether he liked it or not.

Anyway, he said, "There are too many of these patients coming in and you don't have time for them. We've got to have somebody just assigned to cardiac surgery." My recollection is that Denton Cooley was the first person who was assigned. He was a brilliant man, as he is now, although I don't recall at that time saying, "Why, this is the hottest technical surgeon to come down the pike." They were all very good, and he was very good with them, but he too had his own independence in a variety of ways.

Norman Rich

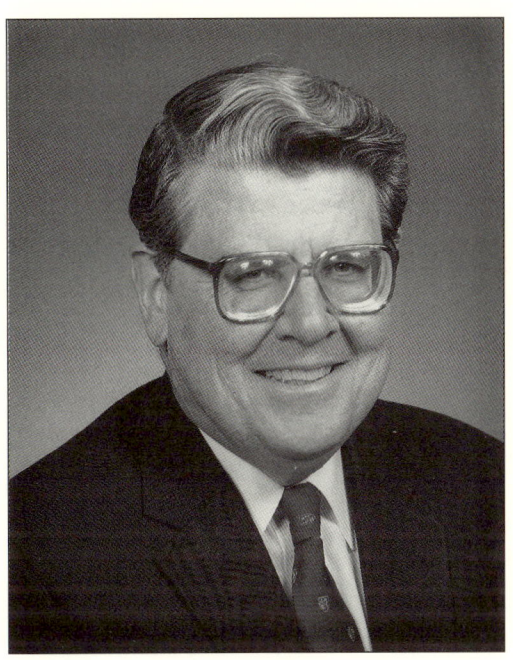

NORMAN M. RICH has taken his place in vascular surgery as one sensitive to international relations in medical fields, a stance that grew out of his experiences in the armed forces. The creation of a military vascular registry and his campaigns for recognition of military medicine in the surgery arena have given him the respect of his colleagues. He was interviewed September 12, 1990.

Johnson: Norm, tell me about your beginnings, your heritage.

Rich: I was born on January 13, 1934, in the southeastern mountains of Arizona, in the town of Ray. Ray was settled in 1882 and lasted until 1965. My father was from Jerome, Arizona, another mining camp, and my mother was from Gilbert, Arizona, a small farming town outside Phoenix. My parents were both schoolteachers. Ray was in the middle of nowhere, at the end of a fifteen-mile dirt road.

The town was made up of workers from Kennicott Copper Company, but an adjacent town had about 5,000 Mexicans, while in another small town there were about 125 Spaniards. All of this was on the fringe of the San Carlos Apache Indian Reservation; thus, these cultural differences and activities were an inspiration for my current international interests.

The surgeon for Kennicott Copper Company was Otto Utzinger, an undergraduate from Stanford and a Johns Hopkins Medical School graduate. He trained under John M. T. Finney at Union Memorial in Baltimore. He was offered a position by the Mayo brothers in Rochester, but while driving to the Mayo Clinic he stopped for a vacation in Arizona and decided that's where he really wanted to live. He was among the first to receive his certification by the American Board of Surgery in 1937. He traveled all over the state as a medical consultant and became president of the Arizona Medical Association in 1943.

Dr. Utzinger was my first idol; I always wanted to be a surgeon like "Doctor." He encouraged me to do what his middle son had done—go to the University of Arizona, then transfer as an undergraduate to Stanford and compete for the medical school—which is what I did. There was no one in my family who had been even close to medicine, so it was the influence of this head surgeon for Kennicott Copper Company that convinced me to become a physician.

"Doctor" retired from the Kennicott Copper Company in 1953 and moved to Scottsdale, worked for the Samuel Gompers Crippled Children's Hospital for many years as a consultant, and died in 1976 at age eighty-seven.

I went to the University of Arizona because I was given a scholarship. I couldn't afford to go to Stanford right off the bat. I worked very hard. I took the examination that was required to transfer and was fortunate enough to be one of ten transfer students that Stanford allowed in that year. Culturally, it was a phenomenal change for me, because my first twenty years were in a very small environment in Arizona. The University of Arizona only had four thousand students, and I knew about half of the students on campus. To transfer to a school like Stanford, even though it was still relatively small, was a whole different situation.

Through Dr. Utzinger, I made contacts with Dr. Emile Holman, Dr. Victor Richards, Dr. Carleton Mathewson, and people on the Stanford staff. Dr. Utzinger's second son, Bill, was in the training program at Stanford, and I was trying to emulate what had made him successful.

I arrived at Stanford in the fall of 1953. Bill Utzinger was the chief resident, and he wanted me to come into the operating room at the old Stanford-Lane Hospital. Bill had explained to me that the new chairman of the Department of Surgery, Dr. Victor Richards, would be helping him do a big case. This was before I knew Dr. Emile Holman. An elderly gentleman came in, got a lift, started peering over Dr. Richards's shoulder, and kept saying to him something like "Damn it, Vic, I thought I taught you better than that." All I could do was think to myself, Who is this old guy making remarks like that to the chairman? I found out later that Dr. Holman was the epitome of the educator. We all benefited from his incessant drive to teach.

Dr. Holman, Bill Utzinger, and Bill Blaisdell had a great influence on my becoming a vascular surgeon. When I became a third-year medical student, Bill Blaisdell was the Stanford chief resident at the San Francisco City-County Hospital, as they called it in those days. I'd already met Bill when I was a second-year medical student, and he was a resident on the Stanford service, so I had known him since about 1957. I came under the influence of Bill Blaisdell twenty-four hours a day.

In those days, Stanford had its hospital on the corner of Clay and Webster. There were two hospitals there, the old Stanford Hospital and the Lane Hospital in San Francisco. Stanford ran a "Red Service," as it was called, and Cal ran a "Blue and Gold Service" at San Francisco City-County Hospital, which was the trauma hospital. Stanford and Cal shared everything. I met Ron Stoney and Bob Lim in the emergency rooms on the Cal service. This was 1955 to 1959. In 1959 Stanford pulled out of San Francisco, and we went back down to Stanford in Palo Alto. They sold the Lane Hospital, which was torn down, and the Presbyterian Medical Center stands there now.

I used to wait tables in the faculty dining hall, and I could hear it coming. Stanford was one of the first schools, in about 1958, where the other departments, out of jealousy or whatever, literally ganged up and destroyed the Department of Surgery. Surgeons at Stanford had essentially run the medical school from the beginning. The previous leader and dean, Yank Chandler, had been very supportive of Dr. Holman as chairman of surgery from 1926 to 1953. There was a host of very strong people in surgery during that period. About the time that I was getting ready to move into my surgical education, the Department of Surgery was literally destroyed. Essentially everybody, including Dr. Richards, stayed in San Francisco when the medical school moved back to Palo Alto—"Back down to the farm," they said. I was in the first class as a senior to go back to the Stanford undergraduate campus in Palo Alto. Everything was in turmoil, and people like Dr. Carleton Mathewson, who was rapidly becoming one of my real idols, and Dr. Roy Cohn said, "Why don't you get your army service over with, because it's mandatory, and you're going to be drafted if you don't. Come back, we'll have the program straightened out, and you can complete your surgical training here at Stanford." So I volunteered to go on active duty as an intern.

I graduated from Stanford in 1960. I will always remember the associate dean—I won't mention his name, because he had a lot of names attached to him—who called me in to point out that no one from Stanford had ever volunteered to go on active duty. I'm sure that was an overexaggeration, and I'm sure he wasn't threatening me. However, he did tell me in no uncertain terms that it didn't look good for the image that Stanford was trying to create for training academicians to have anybody volunteer for the military. It was a very solid message and gave me a lot of heartburn, but again, people like Dr. Mathewson just laughed and said, "Don't pay any attention to him." I ended up with a military internship at Tripler. I was at Tripler during the regular internship year and stayed another four months at Scofield Barracks. In those days, the residency didn't start until September, so I had about sixteen months in Hawaii.

The way I ended up staying in the military wasn't by design. They offered me the opportunity to go back to Letterman in San Francisco to complete my surgical training, and I knew that if I went back, I would be under the tutelage of people like Carleton Mathewson, who had helped set up the program at the end of World War II, along with General Heaton and others. I jumped at the opportunity to go back to the type of outstanding education that I had known before, at San Francisco and Stanford; Letterman was part of it.

Johnson: What did you do while in Hawaii waiting to go to Letterman?

Rich: In the summer of 1961 I had three or four months out in the "jungle," as they called it, running around Hawaii with the Sixty-fifth Engineers. There was a man at Tripler named Werner F. Bowers, who was a University of Minnesota product of Dr. Owen Wangensteen's program, a real surgical educator who decided to stay in the military after World War II. He had the rank of full professor, but he liked being a colonel and had stayed on. He was one of the people at Tripler who was very academically and surgically oriented. He stressed to me that I should first be the best general surgeon that I could, and then I could do whatever I wanted to, be it vascular or whatever. During that internship year, one of the people who influenced me greatly was Carl W. Hughes, who had been in Korea and had a great deal of interest in the vascular arena.

I came back to San Francisco in September of 1961 to start the four years of general surgery training at Letterman. San Francisco General was much like the program I had known before at Stanford. Even though Stanford was out of the circle, many of the former Stanford professors, like Victor Richards, Carleton Mathewson, and Don King, had joined the University of California at San Francisco clinical staff. Bill Blaisdell came back in 1963 from Baylor to the VA Hospital and then back to the County. We had them as consultants at Letterman. Many of the University of California people were very

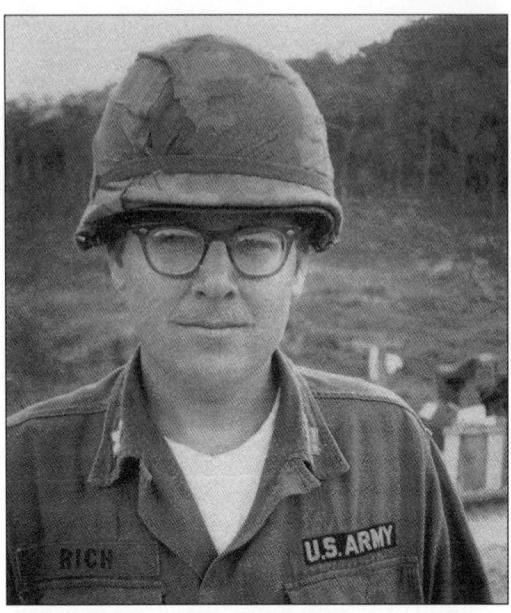

Captain Norman M. Rich, An Khe, Republic of Vietnam

dedicated to the Letterman program. Dr. J. Englebert Dunphy came about that time, and the Cal residents used to remark with envy that we saw Dr. Dunphy more than they did; he was very committed to the military. He recalled his World War II service, as did Dr. Mathewson. They came to Letterman once a week for two to five hours. They would scrub quite frequently. Bill Silen was still at UCSF at that time, and he used to come over and scrub with us on the pancreatic cases. There were a number of senior people, like Dr. Paul Samson in cardiothoracic and Dr. Frank Gerbode, who had been at Stanford, who helped get the pump team started. I was becoming more obligated to the army all this time. By going to Tripler and taking an army internship, I owed the army four years.

At Letterman I continued to be influenced by people like Bill Utzinger, Bill Blaisdell, and Carl Hughes, who was my chief. They fanned the flames of my interest in vascular surgery. I had a lot of time with Dr. Gerbode, even though he was a cardiothoracic surgeon. Of course, Dr. Holman was always available. One of the things that I really appreciated from Dr. Holman was what he called "high tea" on Sunday afternoon, to which I was fortunate enough to be invited several times. He patterned it after his experience at Oxford in 1915. He would have a handful of people over, and it would usually be a student or a resident and a couple of senior people, sort of a no-holds-barred discussion where, for three or four hours, six or eight people would sit around and have tea and crumpets and talk about anything they wanted to talk about. Of course, it was a thrill to me to be in the presence of someone who had contributed so much.

When I finished Letterman, I was assigned to Fort Dix. My plan was to pay back my four years and get out of the military. Before I could even get my household goods packed, the Bay of Tonkin occurred, and President Johnson proclaimed that we were going to commit more troops to Southeast Asia. For about three or four months, I was quite in limbo. I was attached to the Second Surgical Hospital, which had not been out of its container since World War II, when it was deactivated in the Philippines. It happened to be in some warehouse at Fort Bragg. I was sent there along with a number of other people. A few months later, we were flown to the docks in San Diego and placed onboard a World War II troop ship called the *Simon Bolivar Buckner III*.

It was an interesting cruise through the Pacific. *Simon Bolivar Buckner III*, as I rapidly found out, was what they call a "one-sacker." There was no stabilizer on it, so it bounced all over the place. We had a significant storm for a couple of days, and literally everybody was down. We were finally thrown out on the beach near a city called Quinyon, a coastal city in the middle part of the Republic of South Vietnam. We were sent into the central highlands to support the First Air Cavalry Division, which was the first enclave, as they called it in those days, to be put into Vietnam. Our hospital, which had been put on ships in North Carolina, took two and a half months to go through the Panama Canal and catch up with us in Vietnam.

I was a captain through almost the entire time in Vietnam. Because I was regular army, I was made the chief of surgery even though I'd just finished my training. This was a small surgical hos-pital; we only had eighty-six personnel. My commanding officer was a lieutenant colonel who had served in Korea. We rapidly discovered that it was very valuable to have somebody who had been there before. He had been trained in cardiothoracic as well as general surgery. He let me be the chief of surgery, and only interfered when I needed support. I had an orthopedist, who was fully trained and somewhat senior to me, who was very kind and more than willing to let me be the chief of surgery. We had a handful of partially trained surgeons, but that was about it.

Johnson: Were there a lot of surgical hospitals in Vietnam?

Rich: No, not at that point. We were about the fifth hospital to go into Vietnam, and the first one to go into the less protected area. We were out in the middle of the jungle. By the time I left, the numbers had gone up to twelve or fifteen. We had about twenty-nine at one time, if you count the navy hospital ship and supporting activities. We were technically a mobile hospital, but we didn't move. We were given orders a couple of times to move, and interestingly enough, at one time, it would have been into Cambodia, but that was rescinded. Because of the experience and the ingenuity of my commanding officer, by the time we received our hospital equipment we had built some quonset huts on cement slabs and were able to become more fixed. The entire time I was there, the officers slept in tents in the mud, so it was fairly primitive.

We were located in An Khe, in the central highlands of the Republic of South Vietnam, near the mountain city of Pleiku. It was Montagnard country. These were the more primitive mountain people who were never really part of the Vietnamese culture, and they weren't Chinese. They were their own people, their own ethnic background. They have been fighting with the Chinese and the Vietnamese for three thousand years, so they were part of the fighting force.

Johnson: How did the vascular registry begin?

Rich: Two things precipitated the vascular registry. One was Carl Hughes showing me a big piece of cardboard on which he had written down a number of cases he had worked on in Korea and that he had tried to follow. That interested me. When we were together at Letterman, we talked more about it, and then Carleton Mathewson, who became my very favorite professor, had stressed the importance of documenting experience. Going over by ship, there was an incentive to have a project, and by the time we arrived, I was all set to develop a registry. I was able to document 750 consecutive cases of my own. I tried to determine the wounding agent, the type of injury, and the follow-up. Out of those 750 cases, to the best of my recollection, there were about twenty-nine patients with arterial injuries that we repaired. I cannot remember how many venous cases were included, but it was not a huge number. My idea was to pull as many of the individual experiences together as I could. Before I left the United States, Colonel Hughes had come back to Walter Reed to be the chief of surgery. The Surgeon General, General Heaton, wanted him to develop a vascular registry. Colonel Hughes told me this was my opportunity to tell General Heaton what I wanted to do next. I told him, "I'd like to come back from Vietnam and work with you." General Heaton assigned me to Walter Reed. That in itself is an interesting little story, because when I was sinking in the mud in Vietnam, I got a letter from an army medical service corps colonel, who said, "Congratulations, you have been given the first fellowship in vascular surgery at Walter Reed." Well, they didn't have a program, and nobody knew what a fellowship was. The reason for doing this was for me to sign on the bottom line and owe them another year. And I can always remember writing back to Carl Hughes and a few other people and telling them I was not anxious about signing up for another year. The answer I got was, "You've been in so long, what difference does one more year make?" That's what set me up to come back to Walter Reed and to work on the vascular registry. By the time I got back, people like Tom Whalen and Carl Hughes, who both became general officers quite soon after I got back, were most anxious to help me because they were both interested in vascular surgery. Hundreds of people contributed to the development of the vascular registry from 1966 through 1971.

Johnson: What were the mechanics of the registry?

Rich: There was a surgical consultant in Vietnam from the beginning, from 1965 through 1973, each serving for one year. Since I knew all of them, they were kind enough to distribute the Vascular Injury Report Form. Through General Whalen's assistance, the Department of Defense was kind enough to allow me to do this through the "big system." We even had the Veterans Administration helping us. If we missed vascular injuries in Vietnam, we picked them up through surveys in the Philippines, in Japan, or through the hospitals in the United States. It is important to emphasize that Vietnam was unique. It was almost like Dr. Halsted's clinical laboratory. We controlled the air power, we had fairly stable hospitals, and most of the injuries were spread out over an eight-year period. We had the luxury of being able to not only gather this information but to get the follow-up and make sure of our documentation. Out of approximately 600 surgeons who served in Vietnam, I think I personally met and got to know about 375 of them. I have reams and reams of material that augmented what the original charts said. Collectively, we identified roughly 90 percent of the wartime vascular injuries.

Johnson: How about the follow-up of these patients?

Rich: When I came back to Walter Reed, everybody we trained went immediately to Vietnam. I had all my trainees and friends helping, which was a phenomenally supportive network. Through the American College of Surgeons exhibits and through presentations, the word got around, and I received hundreds of unsolicited follow-ups from people in the VA system and from individuals who wanted to help.

Johnson: How many vascular injuries are in the registry?

Rich: It's never been absolutely completed, so I can't give you an absolute answer. We have nearly 7,500 patients included in the registry, and if we added up all of the arterial and venous, it would be in the range of 10,000. I hope to someday have the final documentation. The reason that I have not pushed for completion yet is that, after an interim report of one thousand acute arterial injuries, I realized how much labor was involved. I kept hoping that the computer would help. We've been through about six different systems. We started out with the Jonker Multiple Punch Card System for the data. We got caught in some of the mainframe computer headaches, and when the microcomputers came along, we didn't have the funding support. One of the reasons I'm still in the federal system is that I would like to complete this very important job.

Johnson: Do you feel that you can trace them even further?

Rich: Yes. One of the things that I was able to do was to get the veterans claims numbers for maybe 85 percent of the people. They will receive checks from the federal government for the rest of their lives, so it's very easy to trace them, because they want to get their checks.

Johnson: What do you think is the most significant thing that came out of the vascular registry?

Rich: Korea had really demonstrated that vascular repair could be successful, even under less than ideal circumstances. Probably one thing we added is the fact that we had some six hundred surgeons who did these cases. In Korea there were maybe only six or eight surgeons specially trained in vascular surgery. Literally all surgical training programs in the United States were represented, and they almost universally did a good job in vascular repair. That was a good demonstration that our surgical training programs provided that type of training. As for specifics, we had more arteriovenous fistulas and false aneurysms than we anticipated, 558 cases to be exact. Just the sheer number was interesting. All the surgeons in Vietnam were looking for vascular repairs to do, yet 7 percent of the patients presented at a later time with unrecognized injuries. Venous repair is probably one area where we added some important emphasis to surgery, particularly the importance of lower extremity venous repair. It's interesting because Dr. Frank Spencer, who had been in Korea and had even written on the subject, wasn't convinced that it was that important. When he was helping me with the book, he kept saying he wasn't convinced that the repair of lower extremity venous injuries was that important. We have numbers and continue to have the follow-up that I feel will stand the test of time and be very important for the future.

Johnson: How did you get interested in venous disease?

Rich: One of the most frustrating cases I had at four o'clock in the morning was repairing a popliteal artery only to have to amputate the patient's lower extremity forty-eight hours later because of what was obviously acute venous hypertension. I came from Stanford, where we had 756 hours of anatomy. I recalled that the anatomy of that area was such that most of the venous return had been interrupted in this case. When I got back, I told Carl Hughes that I was very perplexed with this case. He smiled and said, "Well, we had the same problem in Korea." One of the first retrospective reviews we did in the vascular registry was of 125 patients who had popliteal arterial injury ending in amputation. We determined collectively that 19 out of 125 had required amputation because of acute venous hypertension. It wasn't just my own personal experience; it was a combined experience of a number of people with anecdotal cases.

M. L. Montgomery, as far back as 1932, had worked on the physiology of acute venous interruption. Bob Hobson, Creighton Wright, Ken Swan, and a number of other people helped us work with it at the Walter Reed Army Institute of Research. We were able to put a more physiologic basis into some of the clinical observations. We then went back to the clinical setting and followed up more of the patients from Vietnam and began to realize that chronic venous hypertension was a major problem, at least in the lower extremity. However, it was much like the patient with a postphlebitic syndrome in which the sequelae may not show up for fifteen or twenty years. Some of these former casualties have actually become personal friends. They have benefited from the use of graded support hosiery. It controls the edema fairly well, and I think it probably has limited some of the sequelae that might have developed.

Johnson: We left you at Walter Reed, and you had agreed to come back for a one-year vascular fellowship, which meant two years. Why did you stay on?

Rich: The day I arrived at Walter Reed, they received notice of the death of Gary Wratten, who was one of General Heaton's favored former residents. He had been one of the junior staff at Walter Reed who went over shortly before I came back. He had been killed with the Forty-fifth Surgical Hospital. It was a very difficult time. The person who was going to work with me in vascular surgery was a former resident named Bob Benson, who was also one of General Heaton's favorites. He was shipped off to Vietnam a couple of months after I arrived. I was supposedly going to be a fellow under him, Joe Baugh, and ultimately Carl Hughes and Tom Whalen, the four of them. But Bob Benson was sent to Vietnam, so for all intents and purposes, I became the chief of the service and the chief of the program. By September, which was nine months into my fellowship, I had my first fellow. He outranked me and had three years of additional surgical experience, so that made for very interesting times. I had the support of Joe Baugh, Carl Hughes, and Tom Whalen. One thing led to another; I became busier and busier, and as we all know, when you're busy and work hard, you don't think about other things too much, so I stayed and stayed. I didn't take some of the bonuses they offered, because I was still planning to get out. Dr. Chase at Stanford, who was the chairman of the Department of Surgery then, was someone I really respected. Dr. Chase and I met on a number of occasions, and I was all set to go back to Stanford, but he got in a disagreement with Norman Shumway. As the dean of Stanford said at that time, he had to make a decision, and he opted to support Shumway, who was going to support Stanford more financially than Bob Chase. So Bob Chase either was fired or resigned his position. That sort of destroyed my dream to go back to Stanford. This was circa 1972. In 1975 Steve Wangensteen, who was going to Arizona, knew that he could pull my heartstrings and offered me the opportunity to be the co-chairman with him, to "share in the glory," as he said. I told him that I was getting smart enough to know that it wasn't glory that we were going to share. The thing that kept me from even seriously considering that opportunity was an emergent laminectomy with a number of long-term complications that ended my flexibility. With the years running on, I decided I might as well stay and retire. I was offered the position of chairman of the Department of Surgery at the Uniformed Services University of the Health Sciences in early 1977. Much against my better judgment and the better judgment of all my friends and consultants, after four months of negotiating with the Army Surgeon General and the dean, I decided to do it, but with the proclamation that I would not remain beyond my retirement of twenty years in 1980. I really planned to leave at that point and would have gone if John Collins at Stanford or Art Baue at Yale could have worked out something. Both of those individuals were in tenuous situations, and I was offered the opportunity to stay at the Uniformed Services in a retired capacity. At that time, the investment in time and effort had been great enough that I made the decision to stay and see if I could continue to contribute. I would say, in reflecting, I haven't been sorry for the decisions I've made.

Charles Rob

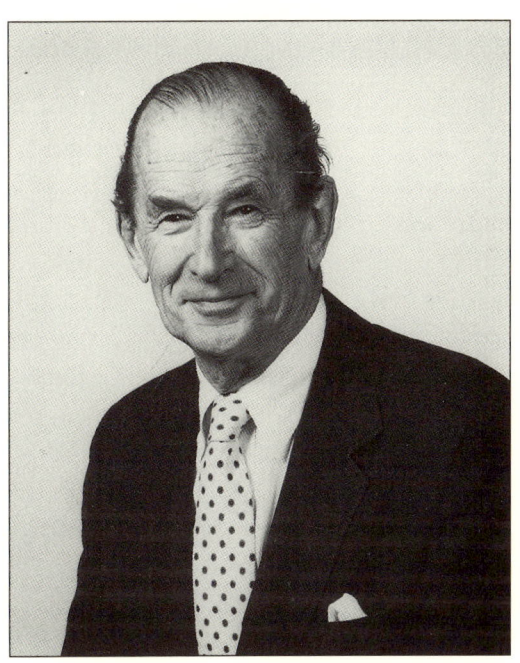

CHARLES ROB'S career began when he became chairman of a large department of surgery in London, after which he transferred to the University of Rochester in September 1960 and developed an outstanding clinical program to complement active research activities. At once he proved to be a splendid leader and administrator, a skillful operator and clinician, a stimulating teacher, and a charming person. His impressive books and articles are surpassed only by his extemporaneous remarks at countless surgical meetings, in which his opinions are highlighted by subtle wit, pleasant anecdotes, and articulate summations. After his official retirement in 1978, Rob worked for five years as a professor and strong supporter of Walter Pories's department of surgery at East Carolina University in Greenville, North Carolina. More recently, Norman Rich lured Charles and Mary Rob to a more urban residence in Washington, D.C., where Rob serves as professor of surgery in the Uniformed Services University of the Health Sciences Medical School. He was interviewed December 8, 1988.

Dale: What was your background and how did it lead you to enter the medical field?

Rob: My father was a physician and surgeon, a graduate of Cambridge Medical School, so I was brought up in a medical household. He had done three years of surgical training, and at the time that was considerable. Then he married and did not pursue further training. My mother, Maud Smith, was a clergyman's daughter. She was interested in medicine but did nothing formal in the field. But she was an excellent doctor's wife. Many of my relatives were farmers, so I learned about animal biology, illnesses, accidents, and breeding while I was young. I was born in 1913, on May 4.

Dale: What triggered your interest in surgery?

Rob: I also went to Cambridge and early on was attracted to surgery, partly because I was helping my father in his practice from high school years on.

My primary surgical training was at St. Thomas' Hospital in London. There was also a bit at McGill University in Montreal.

Dale: How long were you in Canada?

Rob: I went there just before World War II for a year. I was cut short by about three months at the onset of World War II.

Dale: Who were your teachers, the people you respected?

Rob: I was fortunate in two ways. One teacher, whose name was Maybury, was a surgeon at St. Thomas' Hospital. He had been the assistant and associate of Sir George Makins, who wrote a book on gunshot wounds of blood vessels during World War I. As a result of my contact with Maybury, although he didn't do vascular surgery in the modern sense, I learned about bypass grafting and other modern procedures. To my knowledge, he was aware as early as the middle 1930s that atherosclerosis was a segmental disease. Of course, that was not generally recognized at that time, so I was fortunate in that before World War II, I was aware that people with intermittent claudication had a lesion potentially treatable by surgery. At that time few people in the medical profession knew that. During World War II, I was fortunate, too, in working at a Field Surgical Unit, and I also worked for a year or so at the British Vascular Diseases Center in Italy. We mostly had aneurysms and arterial-venous fistulas, ligature of arteries, and things like that. We did a few arterial repairs, but not on acute patients.

Dale: Who were the senior surgeons in that unit?

Rob: Mason Brown, who subsequently went to Edinburgh. But it was controlled by a British Committee on Vascular Disease which was formed at the beginning of World War II. Maybury was a member of that committee.

Dale: Did you do any vascular anastomoses there?

Rob: Yes, we did a few, but not for acute problems. We put in a few vein grafts for aneurysms or AV fistulas. We did have the capability to do angiography.

Dale: What contrast material?

Rob: The same as we used for intravenous pyelograms; frankly, I forget what it was called.

Dale: So you placed some vein grafts, then. Which vein was used?

Rob: We used the saphenous vein. I think we did three or four out of a total of several hundred patients. In other words, it was not a subject that you talked about or heard about, but you knew about it.

Dale: Did you know about Pringle's cases in 1914?

Rob: Yes, I knew about Pringle's cases; also I knew that in World War I and even before that, the Germans, particularly on the Eastern Front, had done a good bit of vascular surgery; by that I mean approximately fifty cases of aneurysm repair. Maybury told me that before World War I there had been a Balkan War; the Red Cross had organized a hospital and Maybury did a rotation through it in

1912–1913. He was associated with a surgeon—his name was Sub-botich, from Belgrad—who did a number of chronic arterial repairs before World War I.

Dale: What other early vascular surgeons did you know?

Rob: I knew people like Lexer. I met Pringle, I met Makins, and I met Carrel, but I didn't know them. On the other hand, I knew René Leriche; I visited his home once. He was a real pioneer in the field. He developed the idea of arterial spasm and its relief by removing a segment of blood vessel. Subsequent studies have shown this to be incorrect, but he was a dynamic personality who stimulated his colleagues. So he was a great force in French surgery, but during World War II things were difficult for him. He had a problem during the war but it is difficult to be critical of that if you were in a country which was occupied. He worked with the people concerned—the occupiers—and this I think caused a certain amount of dislike, particularly after the war, but he lived that down. He was very much the great man of French surgery.

Dale: Had you finished your training completely by the time of World War II?

Rob: I was the chief resident at St. Thomas' Hospital in 1940 and 1941, so I joined the British army at the end of 1941 having completed my residency. I went to North Africa and then to Italy and stayed there until after the war. That was not a bad thing for me, because there was continuous surgery.

Dale: Did you run into the Vanderbilt unit that was stationed at Naples?

Rob: Yes, I met them, and also Mike DeBakey was there for a time. Also Simeone and a lot of other fellows. The Vanderbilt unit was in a large hospital on a hill in back of Naples. The British had a hospital, the Ninety-second General, below them on the same hill. I worked there and I visited and met a large number of Americans in the Naples area. There was a good conference organized during World War II on the surgery of war. It was organized by the British with the Americans as guests.

Dale: What rank did you come out with?

Rob: I made lieutenant colonel. In World War II, if you had your boards or the equivalent before you went in you couldn't miss.

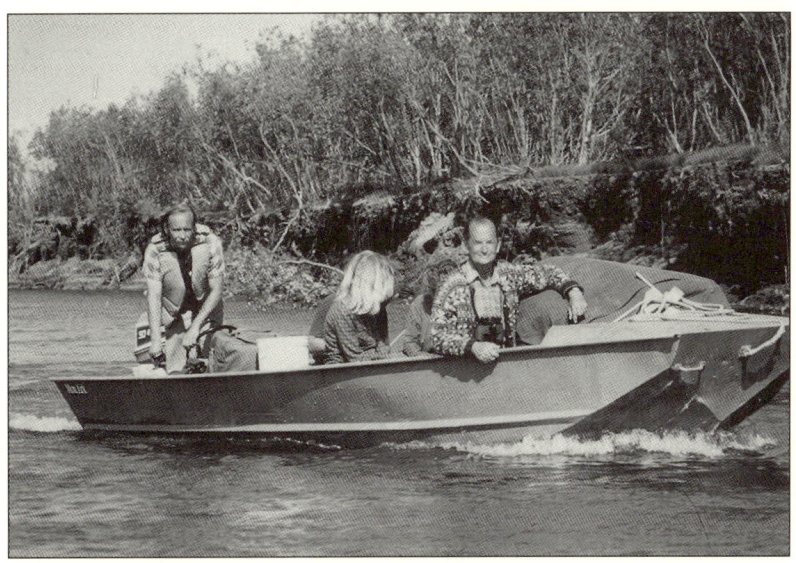

Charles and Mary with their children on the Neatak River, 1982.

Dale: Did you stay in the reserves?

Rob: Yes, but that was not a major activity. I returned to St. Thomas' as attending surgeon. In 1950 I moved to St. Mary's Hospital as professor of surgery.

Dale: How did you get started in vascular surgery? Was it in the laboratory?

Rob: At St. Thomas' Hospital I became interested in vascular surgery. We worked in the laboratory; there was a good dog lab there. I worked away, continuing this idea that had really been put in my mind by Maybury and other people, regarding the direct surgery of atherosclerosis before World War II, so when I came back from service it seemed the natural thing to do. It was the world's most common disease; why not see if you could treat it?

Dale: Do you recall your first vascular case?

Rob: You mean an arterial reconstruction. We did a few in Italy in 1944–1945; then were doing them in 1950. We did vein grafts in thromboendarterectomies.

Dale: Were you aware of Jean Kunlin of France, who first reported a successful femoral-popliteal vein graft?

Rob: Yes, he reported the first long femoral-popliteal bypass. I did know Kunlin, who was an assistant to René Leriche in France. He spoke excellent English. Kunlin, however, had a problem similar to that of Leriche in that he was not fully accepted in Paris. He never had privileges at a major hospital.

Dale: There has been a bit of discussion regarding priority for the first successful carotid artery reconstruction. I have thought that the Carrea team of Buenos Aires and the DeBakey group of Houston first did it in 1951 and 1953 respectively, but their reports did not appear until after your report in 1954.

Rob: The first thromboendarterectomy was done and reported by Elliot Hurwitt in New York in 1953. It was not a success. I was aware that he had done a carotid reconstruction before we did ours and published it. In the first paper that I wrote on the subject, his previous operation is mentioned. It was done on a complete occlusion and he didn't get a good result.

Dale: What about your first patient?

Rob: Well, it was an elective case. Before we did the operation we knew that a complete carotid thrombosis was not a good candidate. I had heard that from Elliot Hurwitt, so from the very first we looked for carotid stenosis rather than complete occlusion and we found one and it was a success. I consider that we were one of the first to deliberately operate for carotid stenosis and, of course, once we had done one successfully they came fast. We probably did twenty-five within the next three months and one hundred during the year after that.

Dale: Did you use the open technique?

Rob: Yes. I never liked the semiclosed method, although I have used it for the external iliac artery. We used general anesthesia with hypothermic cooling to protect the brain while the artery was temporarily clamped.

Dale: How did you cool her?

Rob: In a bathtub with ice. Felix Eastcott did the operation, but I found the patient and set it up for him. She had a localized arteriosclerotic plaque in the carotid artery. It was easy to resect the artery and anastomose the ends after removing the diseased segment. The second case, done a week later, had a true thromboendarterectomy.

Our first patient did well. She was sixty-eight in 1953 when we operated upon her, and she lived about twenty years afterward.

Dale: What sort of angiography did you use to find the plaque?

Rob: We did a direct needle puncture of the carotid artery. Inserting a catheter came a bit after that. When I was practicing in London in the early 1950s a nurse was sent to me from the Belgian Congo. She had renovascular hypertension, which had been demonstrated by an excellent arteriogram of the renal arteries done by a Swedish radiologist in the Belgian Congo. I think it is a true statement that a catheter arteriogram was done in the Belgian Congo before it was done on the North American continent.

Dale: Tell me something about Felix Eastcott. Have you known him a long time?

Rob: When I first went to St. Mary's Hospital in 1950, Eastcott was just finishing his surgical training. We arranged for him to go for a year in Boston because Francis Moore and others had set up an exchange system of residents between our two institutions. Eastcott was the first man to take this exchange. When he returned, he became my close associate and we were thus associated for ten or more years in which he was an active member of the surgical team and helped me in the development of vascular surgery.

Dale: In the States, our experimental laboratories were important to the development of vascular surgery and its experts. I have heard that such was difficult in England.

Rob: It was and it wasn't. It wasn't too bad if you knew how to play the game. In other words, if you obtained a license, it wasn't difficult to be able to do anything you needed. There was no problem about the ordinary simple vascular procedures—that is, doing long-term or short-term vascular experiments on dogs. The long-term ones were a bit tougher. The short-term ones were no problem if the animal was put to sleep and didn't wake up from the anesthetic. If the animal woke up from the anesthetic, you had to submit to an inspection, but if the animals weren't clearly suffering there was not a great problem.

Dale: What about the monetary support?

Rob: We were lucky in two things. We had a fairly good financial situation ourselves, generating income from patient care, and we also had a fair amount of grant support from commercial sources. I happened to know the director of the Wellcombe foundation very well; believe it or not, he had the same name as you—Dale—and Henry Dale won the Nobel Prize. When I was at Cambridge as a student he was active there, so I knew him from those days. He was quite a help in making funds available for anybody doing reasonable research at the time.

Dale: When did you first become aware of the development of synthetic grafts which Arthur Voorhees published in 1952?

Rob: It essentially came in to us in England about the same time it was done in New York. I have always said in jest that a new idea took about three weeks to cross the Atlantic and about three years to cross the street. In other words, the further it comes, the quicker it is accepted. New ideas did cross the Atlantic quickly at that time, so we were aware of Voorhees's work actually before the paper was published.

Dale: Did the development of vascular surgery depend on the laboratory in England, as it did in our country, or did it depend on the operating rooms?

Rob: It depended much more on the operating rooms than it did in the States, because laboratories were not widely available. We had one, but not everyone did. The difference between the surgical program that I ran in England and the program I subsequently ran in Rochester, New York, as regarded the laboratory, was that in England you could not use it to train or teach. In other words, it was not possible to learn the suturing of blood vessels on animals the way you can in the States; we only used the laboratory to do experiments.

Dale: How do you view this philosophically? Is it good or bad?

Rob: Well, I think it's bad. I believe that the animal lab is useful for learning certain things. One of them is vascular anastomosis.

Dale: It seems that way to me, also. Almost without argument, it seems that a person should make his learning error on an animal rather than a human. Did you know the dos Santos family, father and son, who respectively pioneered aortography and thromboendarterectomy?

Rob: The father, Reynaldo dos Santos, in 1929 did aortography in

Portugal. He was before my time. His son, João Cid dos Santos, was the one I knew. He was a charming person, a fine man. He spoke several languages and was totally fluent in English; French; Portugese, of course; and Spanish.

Dale: Toward the end of his life, when I knew him, he considered himself cursed by politics.

Rob: Until a few years ago, Portugal had a dictator. João Cid dos Santos opposed him. In fact, he ran for parliament once on an opposition ticket. I don't know whether or not he was elected, but he felt strongly about political matters.

I think the Portuguese dictatorship wasn't as repressive as some others, and obviously that dictator, whose name I can't remember, was not as repressive, because dos Santos did move around rather well even though he was an opponent.

Dale: Did you know any of the Italians?

Rob: There were a number of Italian surgeons whom I did know during the war. A gentleman called Bastionelli was practicing in Rome. He was an old man in his late eighties when we got there and he still had an active practice. But the most interesting event in Italian surgery at that time was the operation of the internal mammary artery ligation for angina pectoris. At the time, it probably was about as effective as anything. It became widely practiced and it was supposed to improve the collateral circulation in the way the diagram showed, but I felt the whole thing was a phony.

Dale: What about the Germans? Did they lose it all with World War II?

Rob: There was a closer relationship between England and Germany before World War II than many people realize. The welfare systems of the two countries were integrated even before the First World War and remained intact until the Nazis destroyed the relationship. I have a lot of German friends, including Linder, who is now professor and chairman at Heidelberg. He was a student in England, where I knew him before World War II. The Germans developed a formal system where the professor was always right. Sometimes he became hostile toward anyone who might be a competitor. They have subsequently recovered well, and there are many excellent departments of surgery in Germany.

Dale: What explains the rapid rise of the French "school"?

Rob: There were a lot of excellent people, including Leriche. There were many other French surgeons whose names are hard to remember now. Leriche stood out because he had a number of good pupils, including Fontaine, dos Santos, Kunlin, and Hubinot. Charles Dubost, who first resected an abdominal aortic aneurysm, was not a direct pupil of Leriche, but he is a very great surgeon.

Dale: I think you told me one time that Jacques Oudot crashed in an automobile accident.

Rob: Yes. He was what you might call a colorful figure. He was the first to replace the aorta, and he did it for a lesion which was really an aortic occlusion. He went as the doctor on a French expedition to climb Annapurna in the Himalayas. Subsequently he crashed his Maserati into a wall. He was a colorful figure, you know, driving fast cars, climbing high mountains, all that sort of thing.

Dale: Does it seem to me only that British developments in vascular surgery were dormant through this period of French progress, until you and Eastcott and other people came along?

Rob: In Britain, thoracic surgery was developing well at that time and the beginnings of cardiac surgery were coming along. Vascular surgery really didn't get moving until after World War II and then it went quickly, but in the immediate postwar period of 1945–1948 it was the French who were pushing on.

Dale: In our country who were the surgeons who put it across?

Rob: The direct surgery of atherosclerosis was started by a number of people. One was Ormond Julian's group in Chicago. Around 1952 they published an excellent paper titled "Direct Surgery of Atherosclerosis," by which time they had done a number of vein grafts, as well as thromboendarterectomies. Jack Wylie at that time in 1952 was in the U.S. Army in Europe. When he came back, he started strongly in San Francisco. The DeBakey group of Houston really didn't get moving well until the Dacron prosthesis came along. They were working with homografts, but their real volume work came with the Dacron prosthesis, which they popularized. They have excellent, high-quality work, such as the first resection of the entire aortic arch.

Dale: How about Robert Linton, of Boston?

Rob: Bob Linton was a great man, too. He has one thing in common with me: We were both born in England. He used to come over when we worked in London and watch me a lot. I remember well, about 1951 or 1952, doing a popliteal thromboendarterectomy with him watching, and he said it would never work, but, fortunately, it did work. He was a man whose earlier vascular practice included wiring aneurysms and performing sympathectomies; then from homografts he moved very rapidly to femoral popliteal bypass, grafting with veins, and aortic reconstructions.

Dale: Why did he never advance in academic status at the Massachusetts General Hospital and Harvard beyond an assistant clinical professor? Was there some story there?

Rob: Well, he did head the vascular unit and so was essentially from the end of World War II onwards the man in charge of peripheral vascular surgery at the Massachusetts General. I believe their chief, Dr. Churchill, was a great man, but he was not very farsighted in the development of cardiovascular surgery. As you probably know, the Massachusetts General Hospital was one of the last large hospitals to get going with cardiac surgery. I don't know for a fact, but I always felt that Churchill was not particularly interested in what Linton was doing. Linton was an active practitioner of surgery, and he had a big practice, and it may have been that his practice was so large that he was a source of jealousy for some.

Dale: What do you think about the development of the "vascular guidelines" and examinations?

Rob: We do need to define who can do vascular surgery. Unfortunately, we have conflicting interest groups. There are the general surgeons, the cardiothoracic surgeons, and the peripheral vascular ones. Clearly, it really doesn't matter much which interest group is right, as long as the citizens of North America are operated on by people who are skillful and properly trained.

Dale: So, then, it may be just a matter of politics.

Rob: I myself broke into vascular surgery by simply declaring one day that I was a specialist. There was no board; I just sort of said, I am a vascular surgeon. But now that we've set techniques and established practices, some formal training should be required just to protect the public.

Dale: Does Rochester have a vascular training program now?

Rob: We have a vascular service there, but that has been set up very recently. When I was chairman we always had sufficient volumes with Jim DeWeese and myself, so that every man who went through his chief residency had more than the minimum requirements set by the various committees. What essentially happened in Rochester was that every man was trained in vascular surgery. What we had was my service, which was probably about 70 percent vascular, and Jim DeWeese's service, which was probably 30 percent peripheral vascular, plus a few other men doing it.

H. William Scott

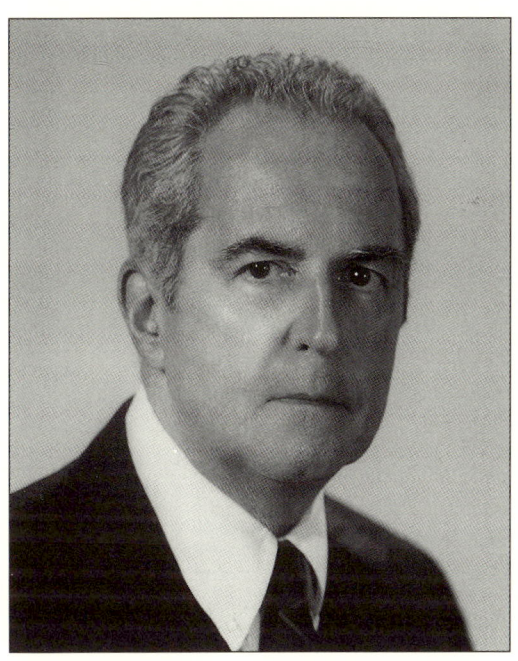

BILL SCOTT has represented for years the epitome of the academic surgeon. He went to Vanderbilt University at an early age and rebuilt a dying service into a dynamic program that soon began to attract the best young doctors from all parts of our country. His service was tough, he himself demanding, but his fairness, high ideals, and superb capabilities as a teacher created a much-sought residency program in surgery. Bill Scott's reputation spread internationally. He was invited for numerous visiting professorships and for lectures all over the world. His peers in the many surgical organizations to which he belonged eventually elected him as president of most.

A few men are fine public speakers, most with detailed preparations. It is unusual to find a man who on a moment's notice can organize his encyclopedic knowledge and extemporaneously deliver a well-organized discourse on any subject of surgical science. H. William Scott can deliver a prepared lecture with brilliance, discuss your subject with organized knowledge, or charm an audience with humorous anecdotes. He was interviewed on December 8, 1986.

Dale: Bill, how and where did you begin your life?

Scott: I was born August 22, 1916, and I grew up in Graham, North Carolina. My father, Henry William Scott, was a manufacturer, having been in the cotton mill business with his father for quite a number of years. My mother was Clara Turner Scott. She grew up in Raleigh but was working as a secretary in Graham, where my father was a widower, having lost his first wife to cancer. He and my mother married in 1914. I was their first child; I have a sister who is two years younger. We grew up in Graham, where I attended a private school for the first six grades. I started in the public school in the seventh grade, but I was two years too advanced, since I was only ten years old. Every day at recess I had a fight during the first year in the public school.

Dale: Why was that?

Scott: Because I was automatically a "sissy," coming from the group of people who ran mills instead of those who worked in them. Everybody wanted to fight me. Most of the time they won.

Dale: That wasn't much fun.

Scott: No, but it was a good experience. I learned to protect myself.

Dale: How did you happen to go to the Darlington School in Rome, Georgia?

Scott: I spent five years in the high school at Graham but didn't apply myself to learning very much. I was interested in athletics and girls and playing my trumpet, so I didn't distinguish myself. My family didn't think that I was a candidate for college, so they decided I'd better have a year at Darlington and learn how to study. That did make a big difference, because that's exactly what I learned to do.

Dale: So you had one year there?

Scott: Yes—1932 to 1933. Let me tell one story about my first interview with Mr. Wright, at that time the head of the English department. Since I was a high-school graduate, he interviewed me to see whether I could qualify for something that he had cooked up called "Flying Squadron English." He started off by saying, "Now, Mr. Scott, what literature did you study last year?" I said, "Mr. Wright, I remember it was a red book, Greenlaw and Stratton, Book IV, and we used that all year." He said, "Yes, but was it American literature or English literature?" I replied, "Mr. Wright, I am not sure that I can answer that question." He exclaimed, "Scott, don't tell me that you don't remember whether you read William Cullen Bryant, Sidney Lanier, and James Whitcomb Riley—or did you study Shakespeare, Keats, Shelley? Don't you remember which you had? It's been only three months since you were in the class!"

I had to say, "Mr. Wright, I just can't tell you." That's the most embarrassing question anybody ever asked me. And to this day, I don't remember which it was!

Dale: Did your year at Darlington help you?

Scott: Yes. I really got tremendous good from Darlington because I learned to study. That, plus being away from home, working hard both in athletics and in my school work where the learning process first came to me, did me a hell of a lot of good.

Dale: What athletics were you particularly interested in?

Scott: Oh, baseball, football, basketball—everything.

Dale: What about the trumpet?

Scott: Well, I had played the trumpet in a pick-up dance band in Graham before I went to Darlington. When I went there, we got organized as a group that played jazz and popular music.

Dale: Did you organize it?

Scott: No. I joined with a guy named Ward who was a very good piano player. He was the driving force in getting us together, and we had a nice little band. We played on the radio in Rome—the "Darlington Hour"—once a week. I can still remember the announcer saying, "This is Station WROM, the voice of Three Rivers and the Echo of Seven Hills, where the Oostenalah and the Etowah come together to form the Coosa." That was the standard announcement of the station.

Dale: That was certainly a formidable announcement. After all that, you went on to college at the University of North Carolina. Did you study much there?

Scott: I started as a freshman repeating everything I had had the year before at Darlington—even the same books during the fall quarter—but I did a lousy job. I had been on the honor roll the whole year at Darlington, but as a freshman my first quarter grades included a B, two C's and a D—I remember them very well. My father took a look at those, and he laid the law down clearly: "I had an obligation to see to it that you went through high school. I have no obligation to see that you go through college. That is a privilege; it is not your right. As a businessman, I expect a return on any investment and on my investment in you. The only return I expect is good grades. If you don't make good grades, I must assume that my investment is a poor one, and I will apply it somewhere else." He made the matter very clear to me!

He went on, "Now, you can go back to Carolina, and you can go all the way through if you want to, paying your own way by your own work without my help. If you make good grades, I will continue to help. If you don't make good grades, I will withdraw it and it will be entirely up to you."

Dale: Now let me jump ahead many years, because a few years ago you were honored as a "Distinguished Alumnus" at Carolina. Is that correct?

Scott: Yes. I was named a Distinguished Alumnus.

Dale: What were your extracurricular activities there? Did you once tell me that you learned to play cards there?

Scott: We did play bridge and poker at the fraternity house. It got to be so bad that we had a lot of friends and some non-friends dropping in on the weekends to learn when the game was going to start. We finally took stock and did a little legislation to eliminate the gambling that had been going on in our fraternity house.

Dale: How did you become interested in going to medical school?

Scott: Well, I developed that interest in high school. I liked my family doctor very much and was impressed by his ability and his knowledge. There were some incidents that showed me what a doctor could do to help people. I remember one that happened in high school. When I was a freshman, I was watching a high school football game. The hero of our Graham High School team was a tall guy named "Tadpole" Davis, who played center. Tadpole had a chronic problem with his shoulder, so that it dislocated quite easily. During this particular game, which we were all watching from the sidelines, he threw his shoulder out, which naturally was very painful. A cousin of mine, Dr. Mel Thompson, who was the team physician, proceeded to reduce Tadpole's dislocated shoulder. It was an impressive thing to me because not only did he do it very skillfully—flipped it back in—but Tadpole fainted as he did it, which was also very impressive. I thought, "Well, he's the only person in that crowd who knew what to do for that dislocated shoulder." That got me interested in it, and I just stuck with it and thought that medicine was what I wanted to get into.

Dale: You graduated at Chapel Hill and went on to Harvard Medical School?

Scott: Yes. I was a rather naive and perhaps a cocky guy. Since I had graduated as a Phi Beta Kappa, I thought that I had some things that many other people didn't, but I learned quickly that I was just a small person in that particular group. Among the hundred or so in my class, there were seventy-five Phi Beta Kappas. There were also several guys with Ph.D.s—one who had been an instructor in histology for two years in a veterinary school before he came to medical school. That was impressive competition, I must say.

Dale: So you found that you were in the fast lane?

Scott: Without question. I was in the fast lane.

Dale: How did you become interested in surgery?

Scott: The thing that interested me more than anything else in the first year of medical school was the anatomy of the nervous system. That summer I stayed to take the brain modeling course, which they offered during the summer months. I worked under a wonderful man, a neuroanatomist and neurologist named David Rioch, who ran the brain modeling course. We learned the three-dimensional concept of the flow of the various nerve tracts and how the brain and cord worked. That major interest led me to read a good deal about neurophysiology, so I became very interested in becoming a neurologist. Through the first two years of medical school I was fairly sure that I wanted to do something concerned with the central nervous system. I joined the neurologic discussions held by the Department of Neurology, sat in on their seminars, and went to all their rounds as a third-year clinical student.

One day it suddenly occurred to me that once you make the diagnosis and locate the lesion within the patient's brain or cord, what do you do about it? The answer was that a neurologist didn't do anything about it. He tried to obtain an autopsy to see if the diagnosis was correct.

Dale: So it chiefly became an intellectual diagnostic exercise?

Scott: Yes. The people who could do something about the lesions were the neurosurgeons. So I made the jump from neurology to deciding to become a neurosurgeon. I went into my internship and residency thinking that that's what I wanted to do.

Dale: Where did you intern?

Scott: I interned at Boston Children's and Peter Bent Brigham.

Dale: Two different years or one year?

Scott: There was a combined internship between Peter Bent Brigham Hospital and Children's Hospital that was superb. It lasted twenty-eight months. They started a new intern every two months; I was lucky because I got my first choice of hospitals and starting date. I wanted to be the last man in our intern group who started so I could first spend ten full months in pathology. So that's the way we started, but then there was a little something called World War II that came along and changed it all.

Dale: What happened?

Scott: I started off at Children's Hospital in pathology on July 1, 1941. They had a wonderful group of people, including Tom Weller and Fred Robbins, who later joined with Dr. John Enders to work on viral diseases and ended up as Nobel Prize laureates.

Dale: All three were selected for the Prize?

Scott: They were junior partners with Dr. Enders in all his work.

Dr. Enders was offered the Nobel Prize. He wouldn't accept it unless his coworkers Robbins and Weller were also named. So it was a great privilege for them to work with him.

Dale: Who were the surgical chiefs at Children's and Brigham?

Scott: Dr. William E. Ladd at Children's was the professor of pediatric surgery. His junior right-hand man at that time was Dr. Robert E. Gross. At the Brigham, Elliott Cutler was professor of surgery. He was known among medical students as a man who was fond of saying to a new class of students, "There's plenty of room up here at the top." He had a very great sense of self-confidence.

Dale: Did you like him?

Scott: Oh, he was a delightful, likable person. I didn't see much of him as a student because he didn't appear before our class often. As an intern at Brigham I scrubbed with him only three or four times before he left with the army. So I didn't see very much of Dr. Cutler during the time I was a Brigham intern.

As I said, I started in the pathology laboratory, but as my colleagues went to war, the surgical staff pulled me out of the lab, and I began as a surgical intern at the Brigham in November 1941. It wasn't long until Elliott Cutler and the Brigham unit left to go overseas.

Dale: Was it a good intern experience?

Scott: I had a wonderful experience in the basic Prussian-type philosophy that had been handed down since Cushing's day. You did not go to sleep at night until all your work was completed. And it was a tough disciplinary system that stayed with me for a long time. It didn't make for an easy life. And you didn't get much sleep.

Dale: What happened during the war?

Scott: I stayed on in Boston throughout the whole wartime period. I had a duodenal ulcer, and I had planned to go into service after my internship. All of us were told that we were never going to become surgeons, that we were going to be pulled into the service after an internship and then used essentially as a corpsman during the war. No one knew how long the war was going to last, but we figured that when we came back, there wouldn't be any jobs available. We'd be too old to go back into training, so we were going to end up as general practitioners with a one-year internship.

My roommate and I went down to volunteer for the navy. I was commissioned as a lieutenant j.g. About a month after I thought I was all set, I was called down to the Boston Navy Yard and the commandant exclaimed, "Scott, what the hell is this about a duodenal ulcer?" I hadn't told them, so I replied, "I guess I do have one." He replied, "Do you think that the navy is going to accept damaged goods?" I said, "I don't know. It doesn't bother me." He said, "Well, we'll see about that." So I had a navy GI series, which confirmed the fact that I had a duodenal ulcer. They kicked me out of the navy.

Dale: Later, in 1954, you finally had an operation for the ulcer. What sort of operation was it?

Scott: I had a vagotomy and antrectomy by Dr. Leonard Edwards and Dr. Rollin Daniel, and I've never had any further trouble.

Dale: So you continued your surgical training?

Scott: I stayed on through the surgical residency at Boston Children's, 1942 through 1944. After that, Dr. Frank Ingraham offered me the opportunity to spend a year with him as resident in neurosurgery. Dr. Ingraham was one of Cushing's former residents and at that time was the neurosurgeon in chief at the Brigham and Children's. I spent a perfectly delightful year with him. But after about two months I learned that I did not want to go into neurosurgery. I went down to Johns Hopkins in Baltimore to apply to Dr. Blalock for a general surgical residency continuation there. He kindly accepted me.

Dale: How long were you at Hopkins as a resident?

Scott: I was a resident there from January 1946 through May 1947, and the chief resident for the last six months.

Dale: So you had a rather lengthy training for that time, six years in all. Did it seem long at the time?

Scott: No, it didn't. The time passed rapidly. As I look back, it probably was the most delightful period of my life.

Dale: What was Dr. Blalock working on at that time?

Scott: When I went down to visit him in March 1945, he had just done blue baby operation number three in his series. He knew that I had worked with Bob Gross and that we had operated on many children with patent ductus arteriosus. He asked me to listen to one child's murmur to learn if I thought it sounded like a ductus murmur. Quite frankly, I thought it was a very weak and unimpressive murmur. You can be sure I didn't tell Dr. Blalock that. The child looked pretty blue to me, too, but Dr. Blalock was very proud of him and thought he was greatly improved, and I could only agree with him, since he was ready to go home at that point. Dr. Blalock was just beginning to do those cases. By the fall of 1945 when I went to Baltimore, his series was up to about fifty, and so he was really beginning a production line program of operating on blue babies.

Dale: Was that because Helen Taussig was finding them and bringing them in?

Scott: That was certainly a large part of it.

Dale: What was the inside story on Vivien Thomas, the laboratory technician, and the development of the operation to relieve blue babies?

Scott: Vivien was one of God's noble gentlemen. He was one of the most delightful people that I have ever known. He started off at Vanderbilt with Dr. Blalock and had worked with him from about 1933. When Dr. Blalock moved to Hopkins, he went also. The professor would produce an experimental plan and then Vivien would run up the numbers. He was one of the best surgical technicians the world has ever produced. Vivien would always do things in a sitting position. He'd be comfortable. He'd work things out so that he'd have two hands free, and he would use rubber bands and things of that type as retractors while performing experimental surgery on animals. He was clever as could be and operated without any assistance whatsoever.

Dale: How was the operation developed?

Scott: The whole thing started at Vanderbilt, where they were attempting to produce pulmonary hypertension by anastomosing a systemic artery to the pulmonary artery. The subclavian was an ideal vessel to use, as it was a systemic artery, lay near the lung anatomically, and could be divided and mobilized to allow its position to be changed. They developed techniques of both end-to-side and end-to-end anastomosis by joining the subclavian to the pulmonary artery in dogs. So it was Blalock's effort to produce pulmonary hypertension that set up the technique of the shunt for the blue baby, and it began to be called the Blalock operation.

Dale: Dr. Blalock always seemed to me a particularly gentle man. If, as you said, it was Prussian in Boston, how was it in Baltimore?

Scott: Dr. Blalock was a very kind individual and a most charming person outside the operating room. In the operating room, he was quite different from Bob Gross, for instance. When I was assisting Bob, on, say, a ductus or a coarctation at Boston Children's, he chiefly wanted me to hold things out of his way so he could do the job. He didn't want a lot of operative help from his first assistant. That caused me some trouble when I started to work with Dr. Blalock. I was used to staying out of the surgeon's way, and Dr. Blalock would get furious if you didn't help him do every part of the operative procedure. During the subclavian-pulmonary anastomosis, he wanted to have the two vessels held closely together. When he used his needleholder to suture through the two vessels, he wanted his assistant to catch the needle, pull it through, and then put it back in his needleholder. If you didn't do every bit of this, he would become unhappy. He had an agonized, paranoid way of saying, "Will somebody help me?"

Dale: What else happened?

Scott: One day in mid-February 1946, when I had just started with Dr. Blalock as a senior assistant resident, Bill Gross, my predecessor as chief surgical resident at Hopkins, and I were helping Blalock on a blue baby procedure. There was also a new intern. It was our first time, and Dr. Blalock took a look at us. Then he looked at the audience standing there observing—an audience including surgeons of great experience like Owen Wangensteen; there was a galaxy of talent there in the audience—and I thought he was going to cry, the way his voice sounded. He said, "I've got a completely green team." And so he had. We felt a little bit discomfited, to say the least.

Eventually Bill Gross got very busy on the general surgical service, and I became the one that helped Dr. Blalock with the cardiac cases. I kept that up through the rest of my assistant residency until I became chief resident.

Dale: After you finished your formal training, did you stay at Hopkins?

Scott: Yes, first I was an instructor in surgery and then I was promoted to assistant professor after about a year. For five years on the faculty, I worked under Dr. Blalock, and it was a most fruitful period. We were busy in the laboratory with a whole variety of things. It was a delightful form of schizophrenia—I would get busy working in the lab and then become concerned about the fact that I wasn't doing enough clinical work. Then I'd get going with clinical work and I'd be worried that I was letting the laboratory work go to pot. It was always one or the other.

Dale: How did you happen to change to Vanderbilt University as chairman of the Department of Surgery?

Scott: The first time I visited Vanderbilt in 1951, I was smuggled around by the dean, John Youmans; apparently he didn't want anybody on the faculty to know that I had been invited to come down and be interviewed. He kept me under wraps from one office to another. I remember meeting Dr. Hugh Morgan, who was chief of medicine, and two or three other members of the faculty, but I didn't meet any surgeons. Dr. Youmans in particular did not want any surgeons to know that any outsider was being considered as a candidate.

Dale: Dr. Barney Brooks was still alive and chief?

Scott: Yes, but he was in bad health. He had retired at the end of June 1951 and my visit was in September of that year. The service was being temporarily run by Dr. Ralph Larsen. So the dean sneaked me around, wouldn't take me to his home, and told me the reason for that was that his wife and Alfred Blalock were enemies, so that she would be very unenthusiastic about me because I was one of Blalock's residents.

Dale: What was the story there?

Scott: I have no idea, but it apparently went back a long way. She and Alfred Blalock were strong, strong enemies.

Dale: Who else was being considered?

Scott: The chief contender was Rollin Daniel. I think they had talked to Bill Longmire about the job, but Bill had already accepted the chair at UCLA.

Dale: Did you know Rollin Daniel?

Scott: Yes, I knew Rollin from the Society of University Surgeons.

I thought highly of Rollin, and I thought he would be a superb person to follow Dr. Brooks.

Dale: How old were you then?

Scott: I was thirty-five.

Dale: Do you think your youth counted against you at all?

Scott: I thought it would count against me. Also, I didn't feel that I was ready to head a department of surgery. I came for the ride and to see Vanderbilt more than anything else. I was flattered to be asked to come for a visit, but it didn't occur to me for the world that anyone would want me to take the job. I came for a free trip to get to see Vanderbilt.

Dale: Is there anything to the story I heard that you might go back to the University of North Carolina at that time?

Scott: They were talking to me about that. I had paid a visit or so to Chapel Hill and was very much interested. The problem at Chapel Hill, though, was that they were starting a new school, whereas Vanderbilt was an established institution with a fine legacy of surgical history.

Dale: How long did the negotiations go on?

Scott: I accepted the chair in November 1951. I came down for several visits. They began talking to Dr. Blalock and asking me to think about this job seriously.

Frankly, I had the feeling that I was not qualified. I definitely wanted to stay at Hopkins with Dr. Blalock and really did not want to leave. I had visited a few other schools, such as Oregon and Ohio State, but I really had no enthusiasm for leaving Dr. Blalock and Hopkins.

Finally, they became quite serious and wanted to make a formal offer; it was done essentially through Dr. Blalock. He put it to me that I had a rich opportunity and that there would be much challenge. He didn't say so, but by implication he made it rather clear that any young squirt who gets a chance at a major chair had better snap it up if he has any sense at all. That certainly came through in his discussion.

Dale: What sort of relationship did you have with Barney Brooks, who was still alive?

Scott: It wasn't until January 1952 that we were able to wind up things at Hopkins and move to Nashville. I had called on Dr. Brooks a couple of times the preceding fall during visits to Vanderbilt. He had recovered from a couple of small strokes but was clearly not a well man. However, he was alert. Just before the Southern Surgical meeting, he noted that somebody had a paper on the program describing his experiences with Henry's operation for inguinal hernia. Dr. Brooks asked me, "What on earth is 'Henry's operation'"? I still don't know what Henry's operation is.

Dale: Was he supportive of you?

Scott: Well, he naturally was disappointed Rollin was not given the appointment, because he wanted one of his own trainees to have it, which is absolutely understandable. I felt a little bit like an interloper, but he was kind to me in that light and wanted to know about Dr. Blalock and what he was doing and how the cardiac program was going.

Dale: How long did Dr. Brooks live?

Scott: Until March. We called on Dr. and Mrs. Brooks in January after we got here, and they were very, very nice to us. When Dr. Brooks came into the hospital, I got to know Mrs. Brooks quite well during his terminal illness. She was there all the time, sitting with him.

Dale: Were there any problems that you inherited with the house staff?

Scott: Yes. We started with a rather small number of members of the house staff and picked up a little bit during the course of the year, so that by July 1 we were doing a lot better. During the first few years, there were problems with the recruitment of house staff which, at times, were serious.

Dale: Well, over the years, you've had thousands of excellent young people apply for jobs as residents, increasingly so as time went on. What is it that you are looking for in a young man or woman to come on the service? All of them have good records.

Scott: I think we all want to see someone who has a good mind, that is, an inquiring mind—someone who wants to know why and how things work, who has an interest in learning the facts about medical problems and delving into the causes of the various and sundry illnesses that we deal with. Also, I look for an individual who has the hallmarks of scholarship—someone who acts as if he or she wants to do something over and above just going through the residency program. We've always asked applicants if they had any interest in research. And those who are well briefed usually reply, "Yes, indeed!" But recently there have been quite a number who've said, "No, I have no interest in research whatsoever—I just want to get my training so that I can become the best surgeon in my town." That kind of individual has never had much appeal for us in academic surgery.

Dale: What about the young person who strongly wishes to be a surgeon but who is technically clumsy? Do you think you can train such a person, or does he or she have to possess manual dexterity from the start?

Scott: You can train people to do the mechanical maneuvers of technical surgery as long as they are not too clumsy. Most people can learn by repetition to do things pretty well. But the person who is naturally dexterous is always going to do it better. I remember more than one person who had trouble with his first circumcision or inguinal hernia but who later became competent surgeons.

Dale: Perhaps you are saying that you can at least teach them to be safe surgeons and to work within their own capabilities?

Scott: One of the aims of surgical residency programs is to train safe surgeons.

Dale: What is the outlook for the young person going into medicine today? Is there still the challenge that was there when you came along?

Scott: No, there is no longer the opportunity that you and I had. The wealth of clinical material in an outpatient department hammering at the door to come in is a thing of the past. The roadblocks that limit time in the hospital for evaluation and study are cutting away many educational advantages that we had. The whole business of same-day surgery, for instance, is an example of it. The surgical trainee now has nothing to do with the initial decision making for such a patient or his evaluation. Even though patients can be handled alright, it's not the best way to teach young surgeons.

Dale: Of the roughly 350 papers that you have published, which one is the best in your mind?

Scott: Every time I have done a paper, I have been most proud of it. I've never tried to make any kind of single selection.

Dale: You've been president of most of all of the important surgical associations and societies. Which of those do you consider the highest honor?

Scott: It would be between the American Surgical Association and the American College of Surgeons. The road to each is different in that I worked as a fellow for quite a number of years before I became president of the College of Surgeons. The American Surgical honor comes from your peers without any knowledge on your part—it comes out of the blue, and your work in the American Surgical itself probably does not contribute much in that direction.

Dale: Which of your overseas trips have been particularly enjoyable?

Scott: Mary and I loved Great Britain and Scandinavia more than almost anything else. We have enjoyed traveling everywhere we went in Europe, except for Communist Russia. We did not enjoy our two trips there.

Dale: Who were your particular friends in Scandinavia?

Scott: Well, to start with, Dr. Philip Sandblom. He was the head of the Department of Surgery at the University of Lund. I first knew him when he visited Hopkins back in 1946. He then became quite a frequent visitor to the States; and later in 1950 I had an opportunity to visit him in Lund. He had a tremendous collection of magnificent art in his home—just every space on the wall was covered with paintings, many by old masters. It was said to be the best art collection in Northern Europe.

Dale: What happened to them when he went to Switzerland?

Scott: He gave the bulk of his collection as the Sandblom Collection in the Stockholm Museum.

Dale: Who else did you know in Scandinavia?

Scott: Carl-Axel Ekman, who had been at Lund, moved to the town of Boras, near Goteborg. He was with us at Vanderbilt for a year's fellowship. He then became associate professor of surgery at Lund and then he moved to the county system; he is surgeon-in-chief of a 1,400-bed county hospital in Boras. He's been doing portacaval shunts there for many, many years now and is an expert in that field especially.

Dale: Who were your particular friends in Britain?

Scott: I'm a member of the International Surgical Group, which includes Sir Geoffrey Slaney, who currently is the president of the Royal College of Surgeons. John Goligher of Leeds has been a long-time friend. Before that, Philip Allison of Leeds was a great friend of Dr. Blalock, and he was an old friend of mine and of Dave Sabiston, who spent a year with Allison.

Dale: How did you become friendly with Maurice Mercadier of Paris?

Scott: That began during his visits to the American College of Surgeons, where I first met him. Later we made him an honorary fellow of the College. He is predominantly a gastrointestinal surgeon, but he is very much at his best with the biliary tract and the pancreas. He does a tremendous amount of work in that area. He is a thoroughly delightful individual. He gave the Barney Brooks lecture at Vanderbilt one year. Recently he was the president of the International Society of Surgery. We had the privilege of being with him at their meeting in Paris last September.

Dale: Your residents always respected and, yes, loved you. Did they ever joke with you about experiences on your rigorous service?

Scott: One of the things my residents did in the way of a wonderful joke on me was to show a movie that I had made on pheochromocytoma. It was made during the days when we thought the sun should not be allowed to set on a pheochromocytoma because some catastrophic thing might happen to the patient—somebody would give him a big dose of histamine and destroy him, or some other disaster would occur—so that we thought we ought to get the tumor out at once. That patient seemed to have a pheo clinically, and the medical people were so persuaded. We thought the patient had it, so we went ahead and operated upon him at night. On the right side we thought we had the tumor—the movie camera was moving along nicely—but it was normal. We looked down into the lower abdomen, but there was nothing. I felt the region of the left adrenal and thought there was a big pheo. In the movie my finger pointed to the left—that's where the tumor was going to be. So we mobilized the spleen and the splenic flex of the colon and reflected them to expose the adrenal gland. But what I had felt was simply the normal kidney and not a tumor. And on the tenth anniversary of my tenure as professor of surgery at Vanderbilt, that movie was shown to the group by John Foster, using the title "Pheochromocytoma, Oh Where Art Thou?"

Dale: Dr. Alfred Blalock was Dr. Barney Brooks's first chief resident at Vanderbilt. He went on to head the surgical department at Johns Hopkins, where you trained. What can you say about him before we end our interview?

Scott: Well, I do recall one funny anecdote about Dr. Blalock. He would become intensely involved in every operation, becoming much accustomed to the team. He knew everybody's name. During one period he had an intern, Glenn Morrow, who later became chief of the cardiac service at the National Institutes of Health. One day he couldn't get the exposure that he wanted—he couldn't see very well, and the light wouldn't work—he was having a hell of a time. In the meantime, Glenn had gone off the service and an old boy named Joe Cox had come on. Blalock didn't notice the change and kept saying, "Come on, Glenn, help me." Joe had about three retractors in his hand, was doing the best he could, and I was retracting everything I could to try to show him what he needed to see. He kept saying, "Come on, boys, help me. Come on. Glenn, you're not helping me, damn it." He finally turned around and looked at Joe, and in the most accusing voice I've ever heard, he said, "No wonder. You're not Glenn!" And Joe said, "I'm sorry, sir. I'm Joe." We all had a big laugh over that.

Harris Shumacker

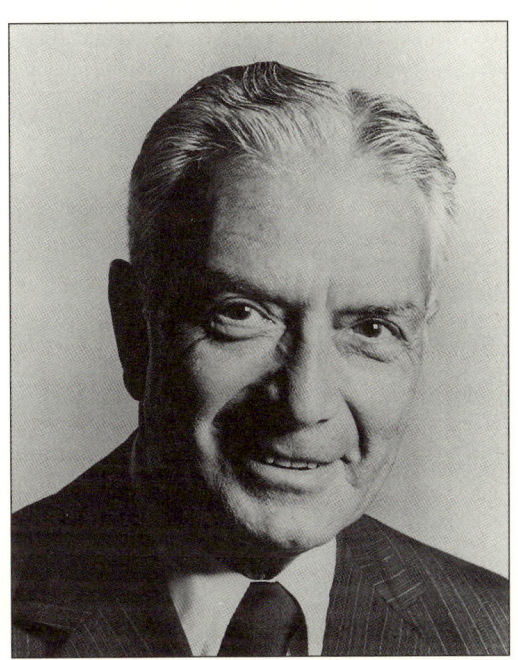

H ARRY SHUMACKER has probably brought more programs
to excellence than anyone else: the South Pacific, Mayo
General Hospital, Yale, Indiana, St. Vincent's, and now the
Uniformed Services University of the Health Sciences. He is a great
historian and a friend to all, as well as being a major contributor to
vascular surgery. He was interviewed April 11, 1987.

Dale: Tell me something about your early life.

Shumacker: Most of my ancestors came from Germany. My paternal grandfather told me that his family came to what was then East Prussia from Sweden after the Swedish invasion long ago. They were in East Prussia a long time, but eventually wound up in Mississippi. My mother's people were from Vicksburg. I was not born where I was supposed to be born, which was in Holly Springs, a small town in north Mississippi. Instead, I was born on May 20, 1908, in Laurel, because my mother happened to be there at the time. Laurel is in Jones County, which is unique because it tried to secede from the state of Mississippi upon the outset of the Civil War.

Holly Springs is the old home of the Shumackers. My grandfather's home is still there. Fortunately, well-to-do people acquired it and restored it and the garden to its beauty as a Georgian antebellum home. When I was about seven we moved to Arkansas, to a little town called Marianna.

Dale: Did you do well in school there?

Shumacker: I went along pretty rapidly, and I was accepted at Harvard College. The high school I went to was good enough and I was a good enough student that Harvard didn't require me to take college boards or anything.

Dale: What did you do in high school, besides study?

Shumacker: I did the usual things: chased girls, dug caves in the hillside, and played on the football team. I was so small that I was really battered in every game. One time, on a rainy day, I was backing the line and it seemed that every pass thrown somehow ended in my hands. On weekends, the *Memphis Commercial Appeal* printed news of all these games. The write-up of this particular game praised a player by the name of Harry Shumacker. I had an uncle who was both a good student and quite an athlete at the University of Mississippi—he was captain of the tennis team and was also on the All-Southern football team. Some of the Ole Miss alumni read the article and because of the peculiar way in which our name is spelled, thought I must be his relative. They wrote that they would appreciate my visiting Oxford and considering it as a school, and that if I had any financial difficulty they could help me. Well, I told them they had made a big mistake, that I'd never make a football player.

Dale: What college did you attend?

Shumacker: There was another relative whose parents were having financial trouble, so that he couldn't go away to college. He went to school where he lived, Chattanooga, where there was a small Methodist college, the University of Chattanooga. Most people feel that I was very foolish, for I gave up my chance to go to Harvard and went to Chattanooga instead.

My high school superintendent said, "Harry, you learn fast and if you don't watch out, you're gonna get in a hell of a lot of trouble in college, so you tell the dean to let you take as many courses as you can and just keep busy." So I told the dean at Chattanooga just that. He allowed me to take more than the usual number of courses. Each quarter when I came in with "A" grades, I would say that it wasn't very hard, so how about my taking some more hours of work. The upshot was that I finished college in two years instead of four.

Dale: So you started early in medical school?

Shumacker: I graduated in 1927 and had been accepted at the Johns Hopkins Medical School. My professor of biology had been urging me to become a biological scientist. In fact, he had obtained a teaching fellowship for me in that field.

This was at a time when chemistry was changing from cookbook chemistry to a real laboratory science. I asked the Hopkins people if I could spend an extra year studying chemistry. They allowed me to do that, so I delayed medical school for a year while I obtained a master's degree at Vanderbilt.

I don't know whether that was a mistake or not. I didn't accomplish what I had set out to do on a research project, but I learned to like research and I learned how to work at it. When I entered the medical school at Hopkins, I began to do some investigative work, even as a first-year student. I didn't find it a great handicap that I hadn't gone to Harvard, but looking back on it, I guess it was something no one else would have thought of doing.

At Hopkins I had a good time, studied hard, and played hard on weekends. It was a wonderful opportunity, because we had half of our time free; we could do what we wanted, and we didn't waste that free time. There were only seventy-five students. I enjoyed every bit of it. Student life was good.

Dale: Was William S. Halsted still the chief there?

Shumacker: He had died in 1922, I began in 1928. Dean Lewis was the professor of surgery. Coming from Chicago, he was different from any other person on the surgical faculty. He added a different touch to teaching. I don't say it was better or worse; it was different. Monty Firor was the one who influenced me most.

Two other men tried to divert me from surgery. Dr. Crowe was the professor of otolaryngology, and he wanted to make me an oto-laryngologist. I substituted on that service a little while, but I didn't want to go into that specialty. Dr. Williams wanted me to become an obstetrician, as he was. He was so impressive, walking down the middle of Broadway every morning after having been driven to the beginning of the street by his chauffeur. He always was beautifully dressed, a big, tall man with a walrus mustache. But I was diverted from that by an opportunity the summer after my third year by going to the Massachusetts General as a substitute intern, or what they call in Boston a "striker."

Dale: How did you obtain the job in Boston?

Shumacker: At that time the Massachusetts General, for some reason, was not taking Harvard students as substitutes. Somebody had suggested me. That experience in Boston opened my eyes, because at Hopkins we were led to believe that there wasn't any good surgery done anywhere except around Broadway and Monu-ment Street. So I learned that this wasn't the case.

Arthur Allen and Leland McKittrick were temporarily running the surgical service. Arthur was happy to have a Hopkins man there, because there had been none since he himself came. I substituted for a man who was ill. I stayed six months. That went over into the school year, so I wrote a letter to the dean and said, "If I don't hear to the contrary, I will assume it is alright for me to be here." I stayed on at Mass General until Christmas. By then Dr. Williams had died, and my interest in obstetrics was gone. One of the surgical house officers told me, although he was not supposed to, that the staff had indicated that I could have a internship at the MGH if I wanted, and that they didn't care what kind of an examination I took. Finally, however, Dean Lewis and I got together and he said, "Stay where you are." I remained at Hopkins for three more years. The last year and a half I was working in the Hunterian Laboratory. While I was in Baltimore as an intern, before I went into the laboratory, I had a week's holiday. It was a big deal at Hopkins, because when we were appointed, the appointments were for a year with no time off. You had a year's appointment at a time. Monty Firor suggested that during that week I stop by Nashville and meet Dr. Alfred Blalock and Dr. Barney Brooks.

Dale: Did you see them?

Shumacker: I vividly remember my conversations with both of them. Dr. Blalock asked me what I was going to do during the next year. I told him I was going into the Hunterian Laboratory. He said, "You are so fortunate. I wanted to do that ever so badly, but Dr. Halsted wouldn't let me."

Dale: What was the next step?

Shumacker: I knew I wasn't going to be kept on indefinitely at Hopkins. Monty Firor wouldn't let me take a job that he didn't think was first-rate. That only included institutions where the professor was either from Hopkins or trained by somebody from Hopkins. I was lucky and obtained a position at the Neurological Institute in Montreal with Wilder Penfield, and at Yale at the same time. Yale was great in Monty's opinion because Dr. Sam Harvey had been trained by Harvey Cushing, and he was more Halstedian than Halsted himself. I went to Montreal for a while. Dr. Penfield said I could come back if I wanted, but I went on to Yale and stayed in general surgery. When I finished at Yale, Dr. Harvey called me to his office and said he would like to keep me there. I asked, "What will I do?" and he said, "I would like to see what you could do with the cardiovascular service."

Dale: What year was that?

Shumacker: That was in 1938. I asked him, "May I think about it a while?" At the time, my wife and I didn't know whether we wanted to go back down south or not. I was thinking of going to New Orleans and had visited the professors at LSU and Tulane and arranged to have a part-time position, thinking of opening an office and entering practice in New Orleans. When I returned to New Haven, there was a letter asking me to come down to Charlottesville, Virginia, to look over a job at the university. Dr. Lehman was the chairman. After my visit with him, I stopped in Baltimore on the way back, where I learned that Dr. Lewis wanted me to return to Hopkins. Now, Dr. Lehman had offered me a position as an assistant professor at $3,800 a year. Dr. Lewis's offer was an instructorship at $1,800 a year. Of course, any surgical fees did not stay with me but went to the Department of Surgery. I had thought I didn't want to return to Baltimore, but I said right away, "Okay, I'll take it," and so I went back there.

Dale: How did you become interested in vascular surgery?

Shumacker: I had hardly arrived before the person who had been in charge of what there was of vascular surgery departed on leave of absence. Actually, he hadn't done much with it. Of course, I really didn't have any particular background in vascular work; who did, in those days? But everyone was helpful. Dr. Walter Dandy, who had many loyal friends and quite a few enemies, was always nice to me. His neurosurgical service was doing all the sympathectomies. I went to see him, saying, "Dr. Dandy, I am in a dilemma. I've been asked to run the vascular service. Most of the peripheral vascular problems are such that there is no other treatment to offer except sympathectomy, which is your business." He put his arm around me and said, "Harry, you can have the whole works—the private patients, everything." He was an extraordinary man. There were others, such as Curt Richter, who was very much interested in cutaneous resistance. We were able to come up with a few new observations.

Dale: When did Alfred Blalock become the chief?

Shumacker: In 1941, after a hiatus during which Monty Firor ran the service, Al Blalock arrived as professor. As was customary at that time, we had all put letters of resignation on his desk. He accepted most of them, but he asked me to stay on. I was delighted and he and I became very good friends. I was really sort of a child on the faculty, but he wasn't much more than a child either. I think he was only about forty, and I was his senior full-time associate. We got along just fine.

He did me a great favor. He called me to his office and said,

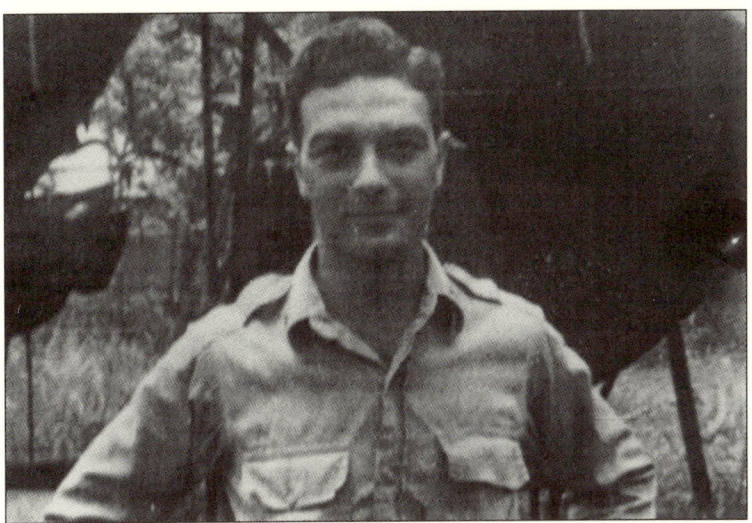
Harry in the South Pacific in 1943.

"Harry, you are so interested in trying to find a solution to problems you meet that you are doing investigative work first in this area and then in another one. I think you would be smart to concentrate in the field of cardiovascular surgery. If you have an idea outside that field which you think is really good, give it away, give it to somebody else." That was one of the best pieces of advice I ever had. Although I didn't stick to it rigidly because of the obligations of running a department and training young people, I stuck to it fairly well after that.

Dale: How long were you at Hopkins before World War II started?

Shumacker: I came back in 1938, by which time the war was already underway in Europe. Before we got into it in 1941, the university units began to be formed. Both Yale and Hopkins offered me a place—as a major in the Yale unit and as a captain at Hopkins. It was a hard decision, but I accepted a captaincy in the Hopkins unit. Then Dr. Blalock called me to his office and said, "Harry, I am allowed to keep one man who is not going to go into the service at all, and I want that person to be you." I asked him what he would do with my commission and he said, "It is on General Rankins's desk, but it will be in shreds in the waste basket if you accept my proposition." Well, it was the best university career development offer any-body ever had. At the same time, I had a rather queer feeling about it, so I said, "Dr. Blalock, I can't tell you how much I appreciate this, but would you mind if I think about it for a little while? I would like to talk it over with my wife." He said, "Of course." So I went home and my wife hugged me and said, "This is marvelous. You're not going to get killed and you can just stay home with our son and me." The next day when I came home she exclaimed, "What's wrong?" and I said, "Nothing." She said, "Don't tell me, I can see it in your face. You don't want to stay. You want to get into a uniform," and I said, "Well, I guess you're right." She said, "Go to Dr. Blalock and tell him." That was the first time he ever said, "Harry, you are a damn fool, but if you must, you must, so I accept your decision." He told me I was a damn fool a couple of times later.

Dale: Where did the Hopkins unit serve?

Shumacker: The Hopkins unit split into two parts. I was with the 118th General. After we had been activated for fifteen days, we went to the Pacific theater. It was a good assignment; we were busy and stationed in a wonderful city, Sydney, Australia.

After about a year and a half, we received our first surgical consul-tant. He was a wonderful fellow, Barkley Parsons, who was on the clinical faculty at Columbia. He told us, "Some of you people have to volunteer to leave. There aren't enough patients to go around." So two of us volunteered, and I was one of those two. Once again I wondered whether I was, as Blalock said, a "damn fool." The next day I received orders to become chief surgeon at a station hospital in Sydney, where I was happy and busy. A few months later, much to my surprise, we were ordered out of Sydney because many of our personnel were not on full duty but limited duty because of wounds or illness. Of course, we didn't know where we were going. The com-manding officer pulled a fast one on me. He appointed me "move-ment officer" and told me that he himself would have nothing fur-ther to do with the move of our five-hundred-bed station hospital and an auxiliary five-hundred-bed tent hospital. I didn't like it, but what could I do? I couldn't follow the orders strictly, because it was impossible. The orders simply said that we were to go via something with a code number to a place somewhere with a code number. I found that it was a ship, but didn't learn where it was going. It was a hospital ship and couldn't take the whole outfit, by any means. So I had to disobey orders. I just went from one freighter to another and asked the captains whether they could take anything for me. I got that hospital up to New Guinea on eleven ships instead of one. I couldn't have gotten those orders changed; the war would have been over before anybody in General MacArthur's headquarters had time to look at them, much less change them.

Dale: What type of surgery were you personally doing?

Shumacker: All kinds. We had a big hospital. The first year we shared the Royal Prince Albert Hospital with the university staff, but later we were out in a 5,000-bed hospital center.

Let me tell you a funny story. The military didn't know just what the demand would be for services in general hospitals. We had only one otolaryngologist in the 118th General, John Bordley, who subsequently became chairman at Hopkins. He asked me to start my operative work early in the morning and help him in the afternoon. I wasn't very keen about it, but I did it, every afternoon. One day he said, "Harry, will you teach me how to straighten noses? I don't know how." I looked around the various wards until I found a big fellow with a flattened nose: "Soldier, how did you get that?" He said, "A friend hit me a long time ago." I said, "Would you like to get it fixed? What are you in here for?" He replied, "I have hookworms, malaria, amoebiasis, and some dermatitis and a few other medical diseases. My wounds have healed and they tell me that I am going to be here for a long time." I repeated, "Would you like to get your nose fixed?" He said yes. I did show John how to fix his nose, and I gave him the most beautiful nose you ever saw. He used to admire it. After the medical people were finished with him, he said, "Sir, could you get me changed back to full duty? I want to fight some more." I said, "Well, what section do you want to go in?" He said, "I want to go back to the small ships section." That was the most dangerous organization in the service, because they were carrying ammunition up to the islands in little launches borrowed from the Australians. The Japs controlled the sea and the air, so it was dangerous.

By and by, up in New Guinea, I got a paralysis of my right leg, probably a viral thing. They sent me down to my old hospital in

Sydney and a medical board ordered me back to the States because it took a long time for recovery to take place. We were sent by hospital train to Brisbane, spent the night in the hospital there, and then we came home by ship. As we were entering the hospital in Brisbane, they brought in a bunch of wounded from the small ships section. They had just been shot to pieces by the Japanese air force, and one of them was my patient with that beautiful nose. He recognized me and said, "Sir, I wish you had left that damn nose of mine flat. I would be home with my wife and kids now. Take a look at me." He was literally peppered with wounds from top to bottom.

Dale: What happened next?

Shumacker: I don't know how Dr. Blalock found out everything almost before it even happened. I couldn't even tell my wife that I was being sent home, but he knew I was coming home and so asked General Rankin whether he couldn't have me back: "I understand the poor fellow is in a cast." I was in a cast because we didn't have any braces in the Pacific. I didn't need a cast, but I did need a brace. General Rankin said, "No, if he is any good to you he is better for us, but I will get him a good job." And so he gave me direction of one of the three vascular centers. The whole war turned out to be a good experience for me. I was never sorry about it and it was one time when I don't think I was a "damn fool."

Dale: Which hospital was it?

Shumacker: First it was the Percy Jones in Battle Creek, Michigan, but we didn't have room enough there, so we moved to the Mayo General Hospital in Galesburg, Illinois. I remained in service for about a year after the war was over, because I couldn't desert those poor soldiers. Mike DeBakey was in the Surgeon General's office and he asked some of us to stay longer, so I did.

Dale: What was your final rank?

Shumacker: I was just a lieutenant colonel. The hospitals all had a fixed table of organization, and the only way you got promoted would be for somebody to die or leave. Jack Gibbon was chief of the surgical service, and when he left at the end of 1945 I became chief of the surgical service as well as head of the vascular center.

Dale: Where did you go after your discharge?

Shumacker: To Hopkins. By that time it was practically blue with blue babies. We were having a great time operating on congenital hearts. A few days after I returned, I had a message from Yale asking me to come up there and start up a surgical cardiac unit. I thought I would like to do something on my own, so I told Dr. Blalock that I was going to Yale. Once more he said, "Harry, you're still a fool and I don't understand it, but if you want to do it, do it."

Dale: What year was that?

Shumacker: That was in the fall of 1946. I had only been back at Hopkins for a short while, maybe two or three months before I went to New Haven. I stayed there a couple of years. Things were going along just fine with a busy surgical cardiac service. A Hopkins pediatrician, Ruth Whittemore, was there as an important helper. We got along splendidly. I was considered for a few chairs, and then was offered the one at Indiana.

Dr. Harvey was retiring at Yale, and Gus Lindskog had been appointed chairman. Dr. Winternitz, who had built Yale into a great medical school, called me to his office and said that he had talked things over with everybody and that they didn't want to lose me and would I stay on and share the chairmanship with Gus. I told Dr. Winternitz, "You know that won't work. You can't share a position like that." Furthermore, I was impressed with the president of Indiana University, Herman Wells. He is still living, and still has a keen mind. He was, and is, a great man. He appointed me, and I was never sorry that I went there; I was never interested in any other position. I suppose one would say I had moderate success. I gave up the chairmanship a couple of years before I had to do it.

Dale: Why did you step down?

Shumacker: I have often asked myself whether I was a "damn fool" to do it. The reason was that the dean came to me and said, "We have quite a bit of money that we can let your department have. You can fill some new positions with young people." I went home and told my wife, "I don't like the idea of bringing young people with their wives and children here with only a few years left to run the department. My successor might not want those people, and then I would have moved them and they would be left in a bad position. I just don't think it is morally right."

Dale: What year was that?

Shumacker: I went there in 1948, so this took place in 1968. I had a few more years to go. Anyway, the dean didn't like it but he understood. He promised me that he would fill my position within six months, but it took longer than that.

Dale: When did you begin your work at St. Vincent Hospital?

Shumacker: At one of our cardiothoracic meetings, a man who seemed to find out all kinds of secrets said, "They're going to establish a heart service at St. Vincent Hospital." They ran the best private hospital in town. I had used it for student teaching and I sent my residents there. I talked it over with the dean and, although he didn't want me to leave the university, he saw no reason why I shouldn't make the change. So I established a heart service there. It is one of the largest medical and surgical cardiac outfits in the country now.

Dale: How long did you stay there?

Shumacker: I did the first heart operation there in 1973, and I have been in Washington since 1981, so I was there for quite a while. I began with one young surgical associate; later we increased to seven. Today they have eleven. Again, I don't know whether I was a "damn fool" for leaving St. Vincent or not, but I did stick with my belief that one should not stand in the way of young people, and they really didn't need me.

Dale: It is unusual for a man to retire to a new position which requires a long commute by air each week between Indianapolis and Washington. How did that happen?

Shumacker: Norman Rich had discussed with me whether he should accept the chair of surgery at Bethesda in the new Uniformed Services University of the Health Sciences. He had often said, "Why don't you quit what you're doing and give me a hand? I am desperately in need of help." After I made the decision to leave my practice group at St. Vincent, he repeated the same thing. I said, "Are you serious?" and he said, "Yes." Much to my surprise, my wife was delighted, because she had a dreadful fear that I would just quit and die. So I came to Bethesda as visiting professor for some months, met the people, and decided I would like to take it on. That is what I am still doing.

Dale: Are you still commuting?

Shumacker: I don't really commute. We have an apartment here.

We also keep our home in Indianapolis—that is where my family is, that is where my friends of nearly forty years are. I am here through the week, full time.

Dale: So you don't go back and forth every week?

Shumacker: My wife is in Indianapolis more than she is here, because she has obligations, friends, and family. Sometimes I go back to Indianapolis on Friday afternoon and return to Bethesda Sunday night or Monday morning. Sometimes she comes to Bethesda instead. So, in a sense, it is a commuting job. But I have loved it because I have been interested in the military since I was a child. I joined the National Guard when I was far too young and had to go to the regimental commander, who was a friend, and ask him whether he would overlook my birth date because I was going to falsify it. He said he would and so I had several years of service in the National Guard. I was in service during World War II for a fairly long time, more than four years. Later, I became a consultant to the Surgeon General, served on all kinds of military committees, and went to Korea for a while.

Dale: Harry, you belong to everything, all the prestigious organizations, and have served as president of most.

Shumacker: Becoming president of a lot of groups is another reflection of the fact that I really had good luck and good friends. I didn't deserve all the nice things that happened to me.

Dale: What was your philosophy of teaching students and residents? Your outstanding reputation is clearly deserved.

Shumacker: I suppose my philosophy of teaching was influenced by what occurred at Hopkins when I went there as a student, and by Yale. I believed in small-group teaching. I tried to interest students in thinking for themselves and in trying to make the most of themselves. I tried to give them confidence that they had greater potential then they realized. Everyone in the medical field should attempt to make himself or herself the very best possible doctor. There has developed a decided change in teaching, away from the bedside, to conferences in a nook without a patient being present. I think we have made a mistake in ending the weekly surgical clinic whereby all the students come to know the professor well. Every week he appeared before the students; patients were presented to him; he discussed them with the students. I think that the teaching session should have been continued.

As long as I was chairman, despite the fact that we were a large institution, it was mandatory that one-fourth of the students take vacations in a given season. With that maneuver, and by using a number of institutions, including the university hospitals, the VA Hospital, the City-County Hospital, and St. Vincent Hospital, we could divide the students so that we always had small groups. Our teaching was almost exclusively at the bedside.

That form of bedside discussion is not always possible here at this university. Our students are scattered, primarily at Walter Reed Naval Hospital in Bethesda, a few are over at Andrews, a few are at the Naval Hospital in Portsmouth, and a few are at Brook in San Antonio. Our teaching often has to be seminar sessions without patients present.

Dale: What is your concept of research during surgical residency? Does this slow the young surgeon? Should everybody do it, or just a few? You did it and I did it, but is it in order today?

Shumacker: At the beginning, I told you that Al Blalock said one of his greatest disappointments was that he had not had a year as a fellow in the surgical Hunterian Laboratory. It was certainly one of the best experiences that I ever had. I believe that research experience is not only good for the person, to find out whether he likes it and whether he has any ability in it, but also because it provides the proper atmosphere in which young men and women should be brought up in medicine. It makes them think, it teaches them that problems do exist, and that if they have an idea and try to test the idea appropriately and draw valid conclusions, they can produce new knowledge. I always had most of my residents spend a year in the laboratory.

Dale: What about today's world? Has science passed beyond the young surgeon's ability to study, and does it now require more of a basic science approach?

Shumacker: I am concerned about it. But much to my bewilderment, wonder, and admiration, some surgeons seem to be able to master cellular biology, for example. I don't like the idea that surgeons should be supplanted by basic scientists in their research laboratories. I do think that our research activities should be directed toward problems which have some potential clinical orientation. During my time, I was very lucky: You didn't have to be very good to conceive a decent research project and work it out. Compared with the complex ones of today, they were simple, so we could be productive without being clever in the basic sciences.

Dale: Let me ask a question in regard to cancer. Have we made any real progress against cancer in the last twenty-five or thirty years, or is it all media talk and improvement in small details?

Shumacker: We have definitely made some progress. For example, when I was a youngster, everyone with Hodgkin's disease died, whereas now the prognosis in the early stages is so good that many people feel that properly treated individuals may be cured. I personally don't ever use the word "cure" with regard to cancer, and the reason I don't is that I have had the experience of having to reoperate on many patients years after they thought they were cured.

Dale: Let me pose another question. Perhaps surgical procedures have now been standardized to the point at which there is little room for improvement, so that all we are doing is teaching standard techniques. Is that correct?

Shumacker: You are absolutely right in stating that we have learned good ways of doing most operations, although as I wander around the world and watch people operate I find that there are still wide variations in the way operations are done. The end result is essentially the same. That is, the technique of getting the procedure accomplished may differ a bit, but the objective and result are the same.

Dale: Would it be worthwhile if a surgeon's results were published and if the consumer knew the percentage of infections, the good and bad results that individual surgeons have? Do you believe, as I do, that some surgeons are better than others?

Shumacker: I personally think that the patient deserves the right to choose the surgeon that he or she wishes. I hope that patients do seek advice and get the best possible surgical care, because there is no doubt that some surgeons are more competent than others. I am concerned about new social and economic ideas of the collective care of patients from the standpoint that we may be seeking arrangements with surgeons on the basis of the least cost rather than the best results.

Dale: Let us close with a few words about Dr. Alfred Blalock. What sort of man is he personally?

Shumacker: He was just the greatest fellow—he was fun, he always had a smile on his face, and he really cared about the men who were associated with him and the men he trained. He followed them all of their lives with great interest and affection.

Frank Spencer

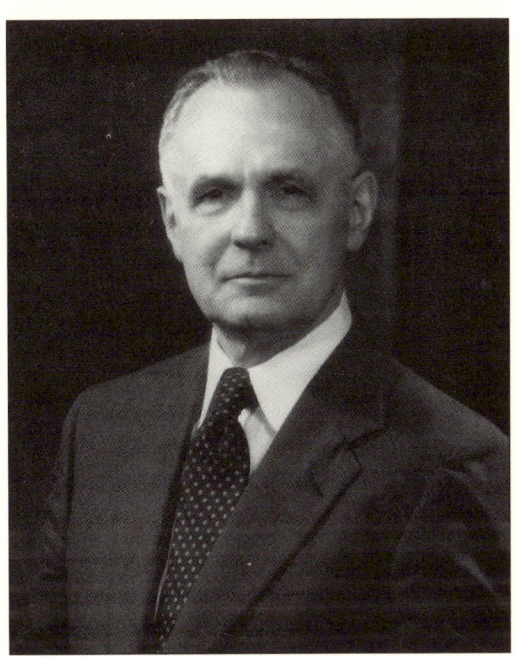

F RANK SPENCER, like many of the great surgeons of his era, was a rural, intelligent southerner who, with a little luck and a lot of support, made it to the big city. He took advantage of every opportunity afforded him and became one of the giants of surgery. Elected to numerous offices, he has achieved international fame as a surgeon. He was interviewed on October 14, 1987.

Dale: Frank, let's start with your early days.

Spencer: I was born on December 21, 1925, in a farmhouse between Haskell and Weinert, Texas, about 150 miles west of Fort Worth at the base of the Texas panhandle. The nearest house was a half-mile away, so I learned early that if a problem occurred there was no one but oneself to fix it.

I also learned the value of public education. The roads were impassable in winter, but no one had to walk more than three miles because the country schoolhouses were six miles apart. I received my elementary school education in a country schoolhouse in the Gilliam community, where a teacher in one room taught the first four grades and another teacher had the fifth, sixth, and seventh grades. The dedication of these teachers was remarkable. I have never been aware of getting anything but an excellent foundation in mathematics and English as well as the basic sciences.

Dale: Did you always walk?

Spencer: My father thought that walking might be a little far, so he provided me with a pony. He knew that one hazard of a small child riding a pony with a saddle was that if he fell from the saddle and his foot hung in the stirrup, it was usually fatal. The solution was to have no saddle, so I rode bareback with a blanket six miles a day, rain or shine, tying the pony to a mesquite bush at school. After gravel roads, which were passable in the winter, were laid, all of those schools were consolidated into a central high school in Haskell, Texas, about seven miles away. I had my high school education there, in a class of about forty students.

Dale: Did you do well academically?

Spencer: Yes. I was the valedictorian.

Dale: What else did you do in high school?

Spencer: In high school it was mostly track. My father vetoed football as too violent, but basketball and track were okay. I took a course in typing in high school and developed skills as a speed typist, and I competed in the regional typing championships. Incidentally, I have never encountered anyone who could learn to use a typewriter with a speed-touch system without taking a formal course.

Dale: I tried it without a teacher and didn't succeed. So you have to have a teacher?

Spencer: Yes, you must have a teacher. It is an interesting model of dexterity training, because at an early age it sets a permanent pattern in your brain.

Dale: Do you still "know the board?"

Spencer: Yes, I still know it, but I don't type now. The other aspect of that rural background was that all farm children worked. The work ethic was a badge of honor. No one would have dreamed of not working, any more than he would have been caught not wearing clothes. From the age of eight or nine the mark of masculinity was to be able to work a full day on the farm with the adults. The work ethic was imprinted quite early on me. It was valuable basic training for a surgeon.

Dale: Where did you go to college?

Spencer: North Texas State University in Denton, Texas. It was a school primarily for training teachers, with a student body of about fifteen hundred, and a marvelous faculty who related closely to the students.

Dale: When did you decide to go to medical school?

Spencer: My grandfather, Frank Sutton Spencer, was largely responsible, although he was gone before I knew him. He was a horse-and-buggy general practitioner near Sherman, Texas. His death was sad but interesting. At that time, the use of chloroform as a sedative was popular. After a fatiguing day with a lot of responsibility, he would wet a handkerchief with chloroform, put it over his nose, and lie down to sleep. Liver toxicity led to his premature death, and my father couldn't complete college because of the family's finances. He became a frustrated farmer with a long-term goal that I would go into medicine. He had the wisdom, however, to say that I didn't have to, but must make my own decision, but that he would be most pleased if I did. In college I majored in mathematics and physics with an uncertainty of which to pursue. By the time the decision was finally made, there was World War II.

Dale: What year did you graduate?

Spencer: I only attended college for a total of about twenty-eight months, ending in 1943. The government then decided that if one were accepted to medical school and applied for a commission in the army or the navy he would be assigned to the school at which he was accepted and given a commission. His tuition would be paid and he would receive a salary. The financial support was important for someone like me with limited finances.

Dale: In which service were you?

Spencer: I joined the navy V-12 program. They commissioned me in Dallas, waiving the age requirement because I was only seventeen. I had no intention of going to school anywhere except in Texas. However, I was rejected by both medical schools in Texas as too young at seventeen, but they said they would accept me for the following year.

Dale: How did you become accepted?

Spencer: Unless I went to medical school by age eighteen, I would be drafted into the army or the navy, so admission to medical school became an urgent priority. Someone in my class had been accepted at Vanderbilt University in Nashville, Tennessee. I inquired briefly about its background and was told it had adequate credentials, so with the naiveté of a seventeen year old boy from the farm I wrote for an application. To my amazement, without interview or further comments about my age, I received a note that I had been accepted! Those events are astonishing in retrospect, because there were only two students from the state of Texas who were accepted in a class of forty-five from one thousand applicants. It was probably because I had all A's in college.

Dale: When did you start at Vanderbilt?

Spencer: December 1943. I saw you then on a tennis court.

Dale: Yes, I remember; I was starting my fourth year. Did you like it at once?

Spencer: Medical school was a delightful time, with a warm congenial arrangement between a small class and the faculty. Undoubtedly the close relationships between the faculty and the students molded my career.

Dale: Who was your best teacher? Maybe there were two or three.

Spencer: There were several. Sam Clark was not an articulate teacher, but he had a manner about him that made anatomy an exciting adventure. I had never seen anything like a cadaver before in my life and do recall a wave of nausea when I first saw a student with a sandwich and a glass of milk sitting adjacent to his half-dissected cadaver. That disappeared within a few weeks.

Billy Orr was a neurologist who at first could not get a regular faculty appointment. Ultimately, he became head of the psychiatry department. Many of the surgical faculty were away in World War II.

Dr. Barney Brooks was the chief of surgery. He had an aloof personality unlike any that I have seen before or since, but his lectures were vivid. Maybe it was from clarity, or from sheer terror, that forty years later I can remember some of the contents of his lectures. By one method or the other, he was a good teacher. There was certainly nothing of the modern in him.

Dale: Did you have any particular relationship with him?

Spencer: I don't recall any personal conversations. Some people later said that they had never seen a student who had the courage to ask Dr. Brooks a question.

Rollin Daniel was a junior person but a warm figure with the students, as was Barton McSwain. I wrote my first medical paper with Barton McSwain, as he gave me a case of literature research to do about carotid body tumors.

During my first two years in medical school I was certain that I wanted to be a psychiatrist. In retrospect, it was because I had a charismatic teacher of abnormal psychology in college who convinced me that psychiatry was absolutely *the* field. I had purchased a half-dozen textbooks and in my mind the decision was settled. When I was a third-year student, I saw my first psychiatry patient without any medication. My interest disappeared quickly.

Dale: Who was your faculty advisor?

Spencer: My advisor was Dr. Cobb Pilcher. By good luck rather than sound planning, my first meeting with him was a significant episode. He sent me a note to appear in his office the following Thursday at 4:15. When I appeared, he said, "Come in, you must be Spencer." That was the extent of our introduction; the conversation lasted less than fifteen minutes. He asked me what I wanted to do and I said I wanted to train in surgery and that I had heard that there were some good places in the East. He asked, "Why not stay at Vanderbilt?" I said that I enjoyed Vanderbilt very much but I knew there were some good institutions in the East and I thought it would be worthwhile to train there. He admitted that there were and asked me what I had in mind. I told him that I had no idea because I had never been east of Nashville and that I thought he was better qualified to advise me than I was. It was a presumptive statement for me at age nineteen but was quite correct and showed my confidence in his advice. He smiled and said that I was probably correct.

He advised me to apply to Hopkins, Yale, and Rochester, and said they probably would have a position at Hopkins. Dr. Blalock was his personal friend, so he told me not to accept without talking to him first. I wrote all three places, obtained applications, and returned them by mail. It was an efficient way to obtain an internship because there was no correspondence, no visits, no nothing. I was accepted at Hopkins, along with the other institutions, and I went there. It all stemmed from that one short interview with Dr. Pilcher.

Dale: You graduated then in 1947 and went on to Hopkins?

Spencer: I was Founder's Medalist of the class. When I arrived at Hopkins in 1947, the program had a fierce competitive system. There were ten or twelve interns, two of whom they kept for further training. My group reflected both the competition and the attraction of Hopkins because it included Dave Sabiston, later chairman of the Department of Surgery at Duke, and Jim Maloney, later chairman of the Department of Surgery at UCLA. Henry Bahnson, later chairman of surgery at the University of Pittsburgh, was in the assistant resident group ahead of me, along with Glenn Morrow. The junior faculty included Mark Ravitch, later chairman of the Department of Surgery at Pittsburgh, and Bill Longmire, later chairman of the Department of Surgery at UCLA, and a young man back from the navy called Rollins Hanlon, later chairman of surgery at St. Louis University. So it was an outstanding place with a lot of good people. But just after World War II there were many uncertainties. I was not offered a continuing position but was not told to leave; it was somewhat vague.

Dale: What did you do?

Spencer: At the end of a year I went into the catheterization laboratory for a year of research with Richard Bing. Jim Maloney went for a two-year training program in public health. We were both in limbo, neither hired nor fired. The uncertainty remained, since there were more people coming back from the war than there were positions available; Denton Cooley and Harry Muller returned from military service a short time later to resume their positions on the house staff. Bill Longmire accepted a position at UCLA and asked me to go with him. Harry Muller was also going with him. The attraction of California and the uncertainty at Hopkins led me west. So Connie (my wife, from Manchester, Tennessee) and I went on to California in 1949.

UCLA at that time was a collection of frame huts and blueprints, but they had a marvelous facility at the Wadsworth Veteran's Hospital, with over a thousand beds and an outstanding faculty. After a year and a half Bill Longmire obtained a grant to start a cardiac research lab. He asked me to drop out of the training program to help start this new venture, where Harry Muller and I worked closely for about six months to the spring of 1951. Then the Korean war started and, as I had not previously served, I was quite eligible for military service and was promptly drafted into the navy.

Dale: What year was that?

Spencer: It was June 1951. I was assigned for the first year to the U.S. Naval Hospital at Oakland, California.

I've often thought that the opinions that other people have of your potential often influence your career more than what you do yourself. John Beal wrote ahead about me. He had been my immediate chief at the Wadsworth Hospital during my clinical training there, and I had worked with him doing research on hyperalimentation with 25 percent glucose—which produced elegant venous thrombosis in the arm vein but nothing further, but did eventuate in a publication. Unbeknownst to me, he wrote the chief of surgery at the Naval Hospital that Lt.(jg) Spencer was reporting for duty and he thought I had adequate training and potential. I never saw Dr. Beal's letter, and didn't know that he had written it, but because of it, I received a good assignment.

The chief of surgery, Captain Everett Dickinson, was a marvelous man trained in neurosurgery. He proved to be a volatile, enthusiastic person. He assigned me to a ward for vascular surgery. We were on the evacuation chain from Korea. There were many injuries, traumatic aneurysms and the like. At first I didn't realize the uniqueness of this assignment, until later I found that most jg's were assigned to the dispensary or the outpatient areas. There were senior officers (often of the commander or three-stripe rank) about, and, oddly enough, I was supervising them, rather than vice versa. It was somewhat delicate, but we were harmonious.

I had a delightful year there with Captain Dickinson and a very supportive faculty that was enlarging the research activities. Someone named Jack Wylie was performing aortograms over at the University Hospital at Cal, so we obtained some needles and proceeded to do aortograms. After the first injection I couldn't see anything, so I put in two needles to get a picture.

Frank Gerbode was a consultant, and we formed a warm, lifelong friendship. He was thoughtful about young surgeons and invited us to the medical school at Stanford to grand rounds, made us special members of the Laennec Society in San Francisco, and made us at home in the academic community around Stanford. That thoughtfulness was typical of him. The year at Oak Knoll constantly gave me new things to do.

They wanted to start a catheterization laboratory and said, "Spare no expense; order the best." I asked who was going to run it, and they said, "You will be in charge." We ordered about $250,000 worth of equipment. I was puzzled by all of this, because the standard two-year tour of duty in the navy was one year in the hospital and then one year afloat in the fleet, usually aboard a small ship, or assignment to the Marine Corps. The Marine Corps was the least desirable because, regardless of background, one went to an aid station for four to six months. Even though surgeons were sent, they went to an aid station for six months. In the midst of ordering all of the equipment, I was repeatedly assured that arrangements had been made that I would remain at Oak Knoll for my full two years tour of duty.

Dale: Where was Oak Knoll?

Spencer: Oak Knoll was in Oakland, California. The hospital was rapidly expanding. Of course, nothing could please me more because it was an invaluable experience, with pleasant colleagues along with clinical opportunities and research opportunities. Suddenly, I received an official-looking envelope from Washington with a letter stating that I was detached from this facility within the next thirty days and would report for training to the Marine Corps at Camp Pendleton, California, for basic training to go to Korea!

That is what I had been assured would not happen. I went to see the commanding officer (whom I did not know). He granted me about a thirty-second hearing, saying that it was great to have me and it was a wonderful opportunity for me to see the world: Goodbye and good luck. I was seething with indignation over the prospect of going to an aid station in Korea, not to mention money wasted in purchasing the equipment, with general outrage at being unable to do anything about the circumstances. So I thought I would send a letter to the secretary of the navy. In the military you can always send any official letter that you wish. It goes through your commanding officer and through the district commanding officer and on to Washington and becomes part of your permanent record. Anyone can comment on the letter. I wrote out a four-page letter and put it in the mailbox.

Within twelve hours I had a telephone call from a corpsman who said the admiral wanted to see me immediately. He greeted me on a first name basis, "Come in, Frank, my boy, sit down, have a cigar. There is nothing to worry about, no need to send any letters." (He had it in his hand). "I telephoned Admiral Bach in Honolulu this morning and you will be assigned as chief of surgery in the Easy Medical Company in Korea and can operate all you want to." I told him that of course I would be pleased, and I would have nothing to write about if this happened, so I wouldn't send the letter.

My training in the marines included combat duty as a corpsman and learning how to assault a building, run a machine gun, and crawl through an infiltration course. But I was the first surgeon in two years who was assigned directly to a unit in Korea rather than going to an aid station.

Dale: There was not a MASH hospital there?

Spencer: No. Marine hospitals were never designed to be permanent. The marines are a mobile organization whose mission is to assault an island or other area, establish it, and leave it for more permanent troops. Where we were in Korea there was a six-mile circle in which it was agreed there would be no bombing or gunfire as long as the truce continued. The result was a blood bank and an operating room *that* close to enemy lines. In World War II it was eight or nine hours before an injured soldier would come to an operating table. In Korea it could be less than an hour.

Dale: What kind of wounds were there?

Spencer: One of the first patients I saw was a twenty-year-old marine who had suffered a small penetrating injury of the femoral artery. The vessel had been ligated and the leg was gangrenous and was to be amputated the following day. The obvious question was why the artery wasn't repaired instead of tied off. I soon learned that it was contrary to orders: The policy book clearly stated that arterial injuries would be ligated and no attempts at repair would be made. That came from the old study of DeBakey and Simeone in World War II, at which time it was a sound policy because evacuation times were long and there was not expertise for vascular repair. But after two or three years of war in Korea that dictum had not been changed. There were some MASH surgical teams evaluating a change, but the official policy continued to be ligation. I found out that violation of the policy would result in a court-martial.

My basic instinct from student and house officer training was to do what is right for the patient and don't consider your own interest first. Of course, I had not completed my surgical training, but I had acquired ample experience in the animal laboratory and also the preceding year in Oakland, so that I had no uncertainty about what could be achieved. For three or four weeks we tried unsuccessfully to obtain permission to repair arterial injuries. Finally Roland Grant, who was an advisor with no authority, suggested we go ahead and do it anyhow. He said he didn't have the authority to approve it, but he thought that although we would never get the approval no one would be upset by an effort. So the vascular repair program in Korea was begun, in direct contradiction to orders. I said at the time, if it succeeds we will get a decoration, if it fails we will be court-martialed. So we began to remove femoral arteries from dead soldiers to stock an artery bank.

Dale: How did you preserve them?

Spencer: We removed them with aseptic precautions, placed them in blood plasma, and cooled them in the blood bank refrigerator.

That launched the vascular repair program. It was an instant success for the simplest of all vascular trauma.

During the next months we operated on about one hundred people with a success rate approaching 90 percent. There was only one loss from an inadequate repair. The other failures were gangrenous legs where a last-ditch effort was made to save them. The navy people became supportive, and there were national press releases. I would periodically be called to board a helicopter, carrying my blood vessel bank to repair an artery. One of these was on a hospital ship lying in Inchon Harbor about fifty miles away. With a carbine on one arm and the bottle of blood vessel grafts on the other, I was carried by helicopter to repair the artery and then returned to base. It was an exciting time.

Dale: It must have been a rewarding experience.

Spencer: It was the first time in military history that the repair of vascular injuries had been firmly launched. Like the advent of penicillin for infection and streptomycin for tuberculosis, our work was adopted overnight and became a standard policy at once. Ten months later I received the Legion of Merit. When I see that award hanging in my office I always imagine the court-martial that would have occurred if the program had not succeeded.

We found that if an injured man arrived alive with a pulse, was breathing, and did not have a neurological injury, we could resuscitate between 90 percent and 95 percent. Some of these patients would have fifteen or twenty wounds, mostly of the extremities, from mortar and shrapnel. We seldom saw a patient alive with a chest injury because armored vests would stop anything short of fifty caliber, but that would destroy anything.

The bulk of our work was in extremities, with a moderate number of abdominal injuries. All wounds were debrided, packed open, and sutured about three days later. The infection rate was low, probably about 5 percent. The key concerns with vascular surgery were two: getting them early enough and preventing infection. The wounds were terribly contaminated with organisms and impregnated with exploding grenade particles. We would do a radical debridement to clean it, and then an arterial repair with a vascular graft. These were successful in about nineteen in twenty if you could obtain soft tissue coverage of the graft. The failures were primarily around the knee joints, which, with the loss of soft tissue, you could not cover. Free graft of fascia lata would slough. If you covered it and didn't debride, it became infected. If you covered it with a foreign substance, that would separate. If you left it open, the graft would soon disrupt. The one area where we did not make progress was with a popliteal injury.

There were some remarkable human interest stories. A Korean marine who could not speak English arrived one night. He was a wrestler with enormous strength, and he was shouting and talking incoherently; he had two small mortar wounds over his left chest about the eighth interspace. We couldn't examine someone who was shouting and pulling about; we couldn't take his blood pressure, or feel his pulse. Our reaction was that if he was well enough to shout, he couldn't be very sick. We restrained him on a cot, and held an oxygen mask to his face.

About fifteen minutes later he became much too quiet, obviously near death, as he dropped into a coma. I thought he must have an injured spleen. We rushed him to the operating table and splashed some antiseptic on the wound. A long abdominal incision was made. There was nothing wrong inside the abdomen. The anesthesiologist said he could no longer feel a pulse. I thought that if he was dying and was not injured within the abdomen, it must be in the chest. I pushed up the drapes and hurriedly made a left lateral incision in his chest. His heart had arrested. With manual massage, the heart at once recovered and began to spurt blood all over the theater from a hole in the left ventricle. We secured that with sutures but could find only one hole. There was not an exit wound. The following day an x-ray showed that the missile had embolized the subclavian artery. We removed that and subsequently reported him in a surgical journal.

It was explained to this Korean that his heart had stopped but that we were fortunate in restarting it. In their religion, if the heart is stopped, you're dead. If you've been brought back to life, you have been resurrected, and hence you belong as a slave to the man who saved you. This patient came to me and said, I'm now yours, master, what will you have me do? To get rid of him graciously, without being harsh or brutal, became an embarrassment. It was sort of humorous, as I wanted to treat him with dignity and not embarrass him for his gratitude and yet not be ridiculous about it for being more fortunate than skillful. He was reported widely in the U.S. newspapers, with photographs and the like.

I received a letter from him in English about a year or two later. He had gone to a Catholic mission school and learned English so he could write and thank me. It is one of those little things that you remember with a rosy glow.

That was my first contact with the press. One night a reporter came by to visit us on what we thought was a social basis. We chatted and had him to dinner and some drinks afterward. Naturally, we talked about arterial repairs. To my embarrassment and consternation, what we told him went out to all three wire services as something like "Boy Hero Saves Marines' Legs," with photographs and the like which he had obtained from somewhere. I apologized to my colleagues because of the circumstances. If you're talking with a newspaper reporter, say nothing that you wouldn't want on television.

Dale: How long did you stay in the marines?

Spencer: My tour was for two years. I was then assigned for my last six weeks to the Naval Research Institute at Bethesda. UCLA's buildings were still not constructed. There was a vacancy at Hopkins, where I returned to finish my residency, about a year and a half.

Dale: What about California?

Spencer: I was very fond of California and had no intention of doing anything except returning to UCLA, and I would have if they had had a hospital, but the hospital buildings didn't actually open until 1955. So I accepted the Hopkins offer and resigned from UCLA. In 1955 I finished as chief resident in Baltimore and joined the faculty there.

Dale: Frank, how long did you stay in Baltimore?

Spencer: For six years. I started with Henry Bahnson in the open heart work. The surgery on thoracic aneurysms had evolved during my years away and Bahnson was a pioneer. We were very close and became lifelong colleagues and friends working with peripheral vascular surgery and cardiac surgery.

Dr. Alfred Blalock was a remarkable chief at Hopkins in that he was an aloof aristocrat who gave orders but didn't communicate much. We never had a departmental meeting. His pride was in training young men to step into the forefront of American surgery. He thought that if you were not up at the front you were not working hard enough.

At the outset of the open-heart surgery program in 1955, he asked Henry Bahnson and me to launch it clinically at Hopkins. Although he was chief and only fifty-five years of age, he said that it was for younger people: "I will watch." Cardiac and vascular were still close together, so he made Henry Bahnson the senior for the cardiac cases and me the senior for peripheral vascular. We worked together. If one of us couldn't do the operation the other one would.

At the meeting of the American Surgical Association in 1957, I heard Champ Lyons's paper on four cases of carotid artery surgery. Returning home, I told our chief resident, Rainey Williams, later chairman of surgery at the University of Oklahoma, about it. We told him to find a patient. One night a few months later he called to say there was a man in the emergency room who had lost control of his right hand while playing cards. That was the first carotid endarterectomy at Hopkins.

Dale: Did he immediately regain use of his hand?

Spencer: He immediately regained control. It was a tough case to start with. At the time there was bitter resistance to angiography by the neurologists. The wanted to send the patient for operation after ophthalmodynamometry and clinical evaluation, but without an arteriogram. To get started I agreed. I well remember that I reported the first ten cases to the monthly meeting of the Johns Hopkins Medical and Surgical Society; Earl Walker, the distinguished professor of neurosurgery, was quite complimentary. He said it was a remarkable development, because two years before he had done a worldwide survey of carotid surgery and found only a few successful cases, but he said he could not believe it wouldn't be better to have an angiogram beforehand.

We also launched the bypass grafts for renal artery surgery at Hopkins. The first patient presented with a blood urea nitrogen of 90. One kidney was missing from a previous nephrectomy. There was a high-grade stenosis in the remaining renal artery. My first renal revascularization was a splenorenal anastomosis via a left thoracoabdominal incision. There was at once remarkable improvement with a massive diuresis and a fall in the BUN to 40. So it was a busy and productive six years in cardiac and vascular work.

Dale: And then you moved to Lexington, Kentucky?

Spencer: In 1961 Ben Eiseman became chief of surgery at the new medical school in Lexington. He was a graduate of Yale and had trained at Barnes in St. Louis with Dr. Evarts Graham. Ben and I knew each other slightly but not well. But Ben is a very persuasive and insistent man and kept calling me to come see him. I was busy, but I wanted to be polite. He wanted me for three days and I said that was impossible, so we finally agreed on a single day. I asked him, by the way, where is Lexington? I knew it was in Kentucky someplace, but I didn't have a map at hand, which reflects my ignorance.

I spent twenty-four hours looking at one of the best-designed medical school plants in the United States. It was a marvelous combination of a university hospital, medical school, and dental school, with a nursing school on the same campus. It was functional. I returned and told my chief, Dr. Blalock, about it, and he said that it sounded so interesting that I should look into it closely and get several people's opinions about it. After about two weeks, on the basis of that one visit, I accepted the position, which led to my transfer to Kentucky in the summer of 1961.

Dale: What was your position there?

Spencer: Dr. Blalock had always cautioned against sub-specialization too early. He thought that big ideas derive from a broad background of experience. He personally continued doing some abdominal surgery throughout his life. I became vice chairman and professor of surgery, with the goal of developing the cardiac and vascular programs. Ben and I were alone at first, and then Rene Menguy joined the staff. We worked in the laboratory and opened the hospital about nine months later.

Dale: Did you have a fast start?

Spencer: It was a challenge. While the facilities and the plant were magnificent, Lexington as a community of 70,000 already had superb physicians and surgeons. There were three first-class hospitals within a mile of the university hospital. At the Lexington Clinic, the senior figure was Dr. Francis Massey, who became a strong supporter of our school as well as a close friend. Lexington actually didn't need additional medical facilities. Where would the patients come from? You have to have patients to run a medical school and you also have to take care of them yourself until you recruit a house staff, and you can't recruit a house staff without patients. So finding patients was the primary consideration. Appalachia was the only likely source, so we quickly became circuit riders over the hills of Kentucky. If there were four doctors together we'd take slides and go talk to them about Lexington. It got the university hospital off to a rapid start, because of the many indigent people, particularly in eastern Kentucky. That missionary effort led to the rapid growth of the hospital. The new hospital opened with something like seventy-five beds, so you wouldn't think that doing open-heart surgery would be the first priority.

Dale: But you started the cardiac work immediately?

Spencer: Ben Eiseman was enthusiastic. He thought that if we didn't start at once, there would always be a reason to put it off, so we began doing open-heart surgery within the first few months. The first patient was an interesting adventure for us. In 1962 the bulk of cardiac surgery had been done on congenital lesions. In Kentucky we could not get state approval and money for this until we had been working for a while. The state wasn't interested in how you started. You had to demonstrate your ability before they would send their patients to you.

The chief of medicine had a patient with cardiac failure from aortic insufficiency and some mitral insufficiency. This was not what we wanted for a start because aortic valve replacement was in its infancy. The prosthetic aortic valve had not been invented. Henry Bahnson and I had developed some Teflon valve cusps, which we had used a bit at Hopkins. They worked well initially, but later became stiffened too much. Operative mortality for aortic valves was prohibitive.

At the time I left Hopkins in 1961 we had no patients who had survived total replacement of the aortic valve. After postponing this

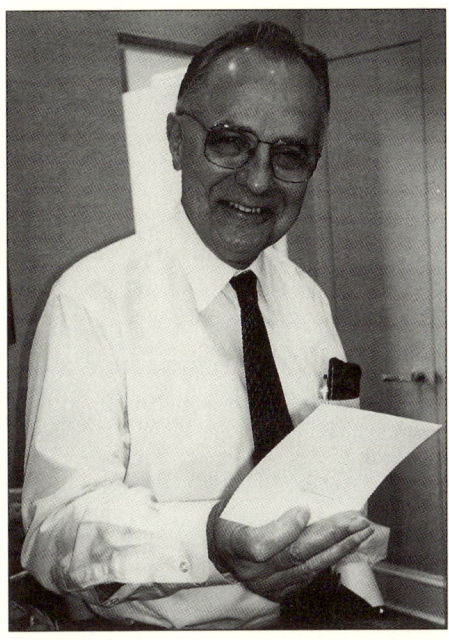

bad risk for a week, the chief of medicine threw down the gauntlet and said, "He's very sick. If you're not going to do it, I will send him elsewhere." The patient had a lot of courage. I replaced all three aortic valve cusps with Teflon valve cusps and plicated his mitral valve, and he had an uneventful recovery. So we launched upon cardiac surgery. It was an exciting three or four years there.

Dale: How did you decide to move to New York?

Spencer: New York was similar to many of my experiences looking for opportunities. Kentucky was most enjoyable to me, but there was the usual stress, which bothered others somewhat more than me, that all of the school was at the mercy of the state politicians. They changed legislatures every two years, so the budget was never a certainty but depended upon who was elected.

If someone honors you by offering you a significant position, you should have the good manners to go look at it and at least pay a personal visit to say thank you. You can do this in less than twenty-four hours, so you don't consume a lot of their or your time. In 1965, for some reason, my credit rating was unusually good as a candidate for a chairmanship because I looked at something like six offers with three serious invitations, including one from Yale, one from Cornell, and one from NYU.

NYU had been in the process of rejuvenation for the previous ten years and had built a new university hospital for the first time in history. Bellevue was the oldest hospital in the United States, originally started as a very small building in 1736, but it had never had a facility for private patients. The faculty would come and see patients in Bellevue and then would go back to their institutions, so the place was like a bus station as people came and went. As it aged, each crisis would trigger some rejuvenation. In the 1880s Bellevue was in the forefront of American medicine, but it declined after that.

Had I listed fifty cities for my preference for living, I don't think New York would have been on the list, because as a southerner with a rural background I had been to New York once in the 1940s, didn't like it, and decided I would never go back. I went to New York to be polite, to visit NYU, and I asked them where Bellevue was. I was intrigued with that old ruin. The new hospital had been started.

I liked the new Bellevue, with its attractive group of faculty, all strangers to me, and a bright student body. There were twenty million people within one hundred miles, in contrast to Kentucky, where less than three million people were scattered over the entire state. So the opportunity was there. Building it was a job, because they had less money than they did at Kentucky.

Dale: Let me ask you one more question before we close. Who was chief of surgery when you came?

Spencer: It was John Mulholland, who was retiring. Within a year we had more patients than we could handle. The only thing that limited us was how many cardiac operations we would do. It became so popular that I put a limit on it. It would have flooded the hospital, so we restricted the number.

Emerick Szilagyi

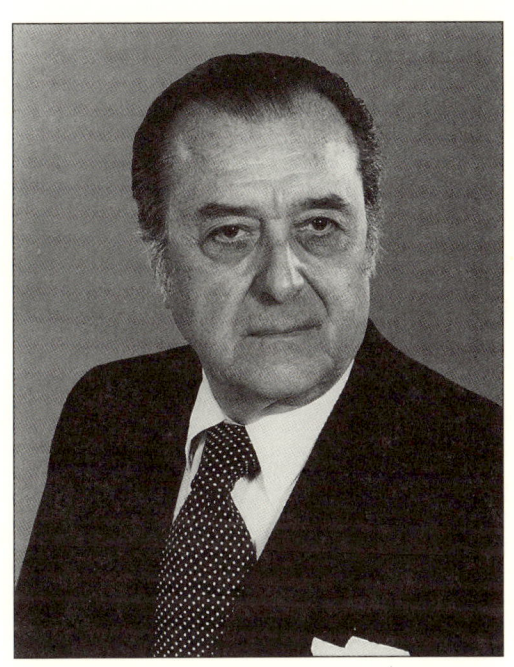

E MERICK SZILAGYI is one of the grand old men of vascular
surgery, firm in his convictions of right and wrong. His contributions to excellence in vascular operation, training of vascular surgeons, and the ethics in reporting data will long be remembered. He established the *Journal of Vascular Surgery* as a journal
that stood strong among its peers. Szilagyi has retired from practice,
but his contributions will continue to influence vascular surgery. He
was interviewed December 3, 1986.

Dale: Where was your original home?

Szilagyi: I was born on June 20, 1910, in a town in Hungary that was annexed to Romania after the First World War. Actually, Hungary was severely partitioned after the war because of its role as an ally of the Germans, and lost about half of its population and two-thirds of its territory. Fate dislocated my family into a very hostile environment politically. The Hungarians who had ruled Eastern Hungary, or Transylvania, the land where I was born, became a ruthlessly suppressed minority. My father planned to take his family to the United States, more or less as political refugees, but he died before he could make the change. It was an unexpected turn of fortune that my mother met a Hungarian/American businessman on vacation in the Old Country and eventually married him. My mother moved to the United States with her husband but left my brother and me in Europe to finish our secondary education. So my early education to the level of gymnasium and the premedical studies were obtained in Europe. The European system of education was extremely discipline-oriented, but broad and very well taught. After completion of the gymnasium, I took premedical courses at a provincial university in Hungary and at the Sorbonne in Paris. Eventually I joined my parents in the United States and entered the University of Michigan Medical School in the fall of 1931. After graduation in 1935 I spent four years as a surgical house officer at the University of Michigan Hospital and in 1942 finished my residency training at the Henry Ford Hospital in Detroit.

Dale: I believe your wife was a native of Franklin, Tennessee, which is only eighteen miles from my home in Nashville.

Szilagyi: Yes. Her name was Martha Evelyn Fowlkes, but since her mother had remarried she assumed her stepfather's name, and I knew her as Eve Harper. She came to visit her brother, who was a neurosurgical resident in our hospital, and I met her at a party. It was a long courtship, and by the time I married I was thirty-five. I was brought up in the old school of belief that a man does not marry until he can support his wife.

Before my marriage, however, the Second World War intervened, and after I finished my residency in 1942 I was assigned to a para-military post in Brazil as medical director of the rubber plantations owned by Henry Ford. I ran the medical establishment for about two thousand employees from 1942 to 1945.

Dale: What did you do? Were you deferred from military service?

Szilagyi: I was the administrative head of the two hospitals on the plantations and head of the medical staff, which consisted of four Brazilian doctors and a dentist. I was assigned this post after the army released me for a duty that was considered to be essential for the war effort. As you may recall, the United States lost access to the rubber plantations in the East Indies and rubber became a vital war material. I should mention that from the point of view of my professional growth, the two and a half years spent in the jungle were invaluable. I was called on to perform operations on every part of the body except the heart and the brain. I even performed cataract extractions. In addition to my professional duties, I had a somewhat minor role in some undercover activity for the U.S. government.

Dale: How did you become interested in vascular surgery?

Szilagyi: My interest was aroused when I was an intern at the University of Michigan in Ann Arbor. Doctor Walter Maddock had a special unit in the old University Hospital, which is now torn down, for people with peripheral vascular disease. There was not very much that we could do for them.

At that time we thought that the most effective treatment was the Pavaex boot, an apparatus that applied alternating suction and pressure on the leg and foot. The boot had been invented by Louis Hermann of Cincinnati, a pioneer in vascular surgery before the era of reconstructive procedures. Some time later when I had become a staff man at the Henry Ford Hospital in Detroit, every time I had a case of peripheral vascular disease I remembered that large ward and the frustrating inability to help the patients beyond amputations.

In 1947 I happened on a French paper that described a new method of approach to arterial disease. The author was João Cid dos Santos of Lisbon, Portugal. As is well known by now, he successfully performed the first superficial femoral endarterectomy. After my first femoral endarterectomy in 1951, I became more and more involved with aortic occlusive disease. The early results of femoral endarterectomy were encouraging, but after two or three years recurrences became common. The next step was to dissect free the diseased arterial segment and replace it with what we thought to be a normal human artery; that is, an allograft obtained from a cadaver.

At first we obtained the grafts through extremely cumbersome aseptic autopsy, but eventually a sterilization method was worked out and the grafts were stored in a freeze-dried condition. After about two years of observation, I reported that allografts were not suitable for arterial substitution. Fortunately, in 1952 Voorhees reported the feasibility of the use of a porous textile material as an arterial substitute for replacement of the canine aorta.

We began to search for appropriate arterial substitutes made of various synthetic materials. We began with Teflon, but it was difficult to fabricate and had undesirable physical properties as a textile tube. Eventually it became generally accepted that Dacron was a suitable synthetic material for textile conduits. We evolved a special Dacron yarn which was elasticized. The individual fibers of this fabric were processed in such a way that they became wavy and obtained the capability of stretching and recoiling. I used this so-called Helanca Dacron prosthesis from 1956 to the very recent past. After 1957 its use was limited to aortoiliac reconstruction.

Dale: Who makes the prosthesis?

Szilagyi: The original fabricator, Mr. Sidebotham, reached an advanced age and gave up his business a few years ago, and the manufacturing process was transferred to the Meadox Medical Company, which manufactures it as of the time of this interview.

Dale: What do you now use for femoropopliteal grafts?

Szilagyi: At the present we are using the PTFE (polytetrafluoroethylene, or expanded Teflon) prosthesis made by Gore-Tex. But we try to avoid using any kind of synthetic prosthesis if the distal anastomosis has to be placed below the knee.

Dale: When did you do your first repair of an aortic aneurysm?

Szilagyi: The date stands out clearly in my memory. It was the day before Christmas in 1952. Ormand Julian in Chicago had performed an aortic aneurysmectomy about a month earlier. It is, of course, well known that the first aneurysmectomy had been carried out by Charles Dubost approximately a year earlier in France.

Dale: Did you know Charles Dubost personally?

Szilagyi: I met him early in my career. In 1964 the French Surgical Society had invited me to lecture on peripheral vascular disease. They had a reception at which I met Dubost. After the first aneurysm operation that he reported, he did not do another for several months. He attended a meeting in our hospital in Detroit in 1964 and was asked to discuss aneurysmectomy. He stepped onto the platform and said, "Gentlemen, I do not know how much I can tell you on this subject, because I am followed by Dr. DeBakey, who has done 160 of these operations, and I have only done 6 since I did the first one." He went on to say that his small experience was due to the fact that the French people do not drink milk. They drink wine, he said, and therefore, they do not develop aneurysms. Obviously, this was meant as a joke, because aneurysms are as common in France as anywhere else. It so happens that Dubost's interest in the meantime had turned to cardiac problems.

Dale: Whom else did you meet in France?

Szilagyi: Jean Kunlin was there. He had reported the first femoropopliteal bypass vein graft in 1949. Kunlin was a rather unimpressive fellow with very few words. Apparently the only important thing he did in his life was the great achievement of using a saphenous vein as a long bypass.

Dale: Was he a vascular surgeon after that, or was he a general surgeon who happened to do it?

Szilagyi: He limited himself to some degree to vascular operations. He was a provincial surgeon in Lyon, which is out of the mainstream. During the German occupation he was thought to have cooperated with the Nazis, although this may have been a baseless rumor; I obviously never asked him. He apparently was investigated and was largely cleared, but that this blemish on his past prevented his promotion beyond the provincial position he held.

Another interesting personality was René Fontaine. He was a true pioneer, a direct descendant of the Leriche school of vascular surgery in Strasbourg and a great admirer of his teacher. He visited our country quite often and spoke English well. He actually was not deeply involved in reconstructive arterial surgery and belonged to the group of early vascular surgeons who were mainly preoccupied with venous disease and sympathectomy.

Dale: What about Louis Hermann? Did you know him?

Szilagyi: He and one of my chiefs, Laurence Fallis, were good friends. I visited Louis Hermann several times in Cincinnati. He spent a good deal of time in France and spoke French fluently.

Dale: Do you have any comment on my observation that the French surgeons made great clinical advances that were not based on experimental laboratory work, whereas in our country most things have been based on experiments in the animal laboratory?

Szilagyi: I think that is correct in a general way. The French are extremely inventive, but often do not follow through and often lose their initial inspiration. They do not seem constitutionally to be suited for dreary laboratory routines. The meticulous laboratory background as an underpinning structure for clinical experience was a German tradition that our grandfathers avidly adopted but that the French do not seem to like. It is strange that most of the great innovations in vascular surgery that started in France were later fully developed in this country rather than in their place of origin.

Dale: What about your own personal experience? Did you operate extensively in the laboratory, or were the experiments you reported performed by residents or technicians?

Szilagyi: My approach to laboratory experience was that I would go to the laboratory with the research resident, propose or accept a research problem, discuss its details, and perhaps perform the first experiments. Then I would leave the resident to his own resources to carry on. He could consult me anytime he wished. I would periodically visit him.

In actuality, I never had much time for the laboratory. I was too busy clinically. I grew up in the era when laboratory experimentation for the surgeon was a luxury. Dr. Roy D. McClure, who was my chief in Detroit, used to say, "You can use all the time you want for laboratory work after 6:00 p.m. and during the whole weekend." During the forty-seven years I have spent at the Ford Hospital, I never had any time set aside for laboratory or any kind of research work.

Dale: So your chief discouraged that. He thought that clinical experience was more important.

Szilagyi: He was not antagonistic towards research. Clinical surgeons simply did not at that time believe in research for the sake of research. Experimentation was supposed to be stimulated by clinical experience. If you ran into a puzzling clinical problem for which there was no answer in your or your colleagues' experience or in the literature, you tried to find the solution through clinical or laboratory investigation. If you found the solution, you reported it; if not, you tried something else.

Dale: Last night we were talking a little bit about Al Humphries, your friend who decided to retire at age fifty-seven. Why did he get out so early?

Szilagyi: He had made up his mind to retire at age fifty-six. He actually retired a year later and told me that he simply lost the zest for operating room work. He also very seriously said that he wanted to prolong his life by early retirement, since he was convinced that surgeons who worked beyond fifty or sixty shortened their life expectancy by five years.

Dale: We both disagree with that. Do you think that can be documented?

Szilagyi: No. Work done when you feel up to it has never shortened anybody's life. I suppose if a man who has, for instance, angina, continues to push himself and pops nitroglycerine tablets into his mouth while he is performing an operation is doing the wrong thing. But if you are fit, I do not believe that work shortens your life.

Dale: Do you still like to operate?

Szilagyi: I enjoy operating very much. I do feel fatigue after an operation that lasts more than four or five hours. When we turn over most of our surgical work to the residents to teach them, it does prolong the operation, so I have a little problem with such long procedures.

Dale: Do you find a feeling of stress, as though you have been to the well too many times and wonder why should you go again?

Szilagyi: There is undoubtedly a change in one's approach to the routine type of surgical procedure; when you have done something so many times it becomes sort of rote without much interest. When I get involved with a complicated procedure that demands more and takes longer than the others, I feel a whole lot more enthusiastic about doing it.

Dale: When you help the residents, do you stay on the case the whole time or can you take a little rest? Do you drop out here and there, or how do you work it?

Szilagyi: It depends on the procedure and on the stage of training in which the resident finds himself. Let us take, for instance, an average femoropopliteal problem where there is a reasonable outflow below the popliteal artery, so that the graft can be placed between the common femoral artery and the popliteal artery, and the first assistant has at least five to six months of experience with the vascular procedures. We go over the angiograms carefully first of all and make a plan. In the operating room, the resident can expose the vein, obtain it, and process it for transplantation without any help, because it is a routine procedure that he learns very early in his training. It doesn't require a lot of experience. Once this has been done, the popliteal space is explored by the resident to see the condition of the popliteal artery and its branches. At this point I always scrub in because the decision of exactly where to place the distal anastomosis does require experience and judgment and I want to be there when the decision is made. I usually also help the resident make this anastomosis since it is technically rather demanding. The remainder of the operation will be done by the resident, but I will stay close by, scrubbed. In essence, after the early indoctrination of the resident, my role is that of supervision. I perform the operation only when there is some unusual situation or in instances where a patient overtly asks for it. Rarely some people will say, "I want you to do this operation from beginning to end." Obviously, when this happens the surgeon is obligated technically to comply.

Dale: How long does it take you to do a straightforward femoropopliteal graft, skin to skin, with or without a resident?

Szilagyi: If I do it myself, it takes between two and two and a half hours, and with a resident, about another hour will be necessary.

Dale: What about an aortic aneurysm? Let us say that you put a tube graft in; how long would you figure skin to skin for that?

Szilagyi: This is an interesting question, because I have virtually never used the tube graft. It is my conviction that every aneurysm which involves the distal abdominal aorta is associated with a certain amount of iliac disease, and my experience has been that there is always a progression of the iliac illness if left in situ. In the early years of aneurysmectomy, we did limited operations, but we learned that the patient with such procedures would come back in two or three years, if he lived that long, for the correction of the advancement of the atherosclerotic involvement originally left untreated.

Another aspect of the technique I use in aneurysmectomy is that I attempt to remove virtually all the aneurysmal sac, and certainly all the sac that is not involved in adhesions with vascular structures or the duodenum. I have two reasons for this: I am anxious to make the upper anastomosis under direct vision between the end of the bisected aorta and the proximal end of the prosthesis and I do not want to leave behind diseased aortic tissue that will hamper or prevent the incorporation of the prosthetic implant. Since I have been doing this type of aneurysmectomy for many years, I can carry it out with reasonable expeditiousness, with very little blood loss, and no more postoperative complications than observed by those with more restricted surgical corrections.

To some degree, we are all prisoners of our early experiences. I was led to the relatively radical removal of aneurysmal sacs because in some early experiences the sac left in situ led to complications. Moreover, aneurysms in the early years were brought to the surgeon when they had reached large sizes and it seemed the correct approach to remove as much of the voluminous aneurysmal sac as was technically feasible. At the same time, the size of the aneurysm also required the dissection of the bifurcation. As time has gone on, the size of aneurysms deemed suitable for resection has persistently shrunk, and undoubtedly many of the lesions removed currently, if at all worthy of resection, can be handled with sleeve grafts.

Dale: Emerick, what are your additional goals as editor of the *Journal of Vascular Surgery?*

Szilagyi: In the next few months I shall discontinue my work in the operating room. I am within a year of obligatory retirement from operating practice and the demands of the editorship of the *Journal of Vascular Surgery* have already convinced me that carrying on a busy surgical practice and maintaining the quality of editorial work I believe is necessary for the maintenance of excellence in the *Journal* are not compatible. I shall, however, continue to see patients, referring them to my younger associates when they need surgical treatment. I hope circumstances will allow me to stay with the *Journal* until it is well established as a periodical of high quality.

Dale: Do the young surgeons need an extra or a special year of training in vascular surgery beyond a six-year residency in general surgery?

Szilagyi: This question in difficult to answer in the form in which it is put. In a few surgical centers, a resident may acquire enough experience in instruction and skill in the treatment of surgical diseases of the blood vessels so that in six years he may be equipped to practice vascular surgery in its full extent. I can think of only five or six such centers in the country. It is obvious that this system of training surgeons in vascular surgery is grossly inadequate. Ideally, a year should be added to a five-year training program in general surgery to provide the necessary experience in vascular problems. One could even argue that to acquire full competence in vascular surgery, two years of special training are needed.

Dale: Are the regulations imposed by government and insurance companies changing the quality of surgical care?

Szilagyi: The restrictions imposed on all branches of medical practice from several directions undoubtedly are lowering the quality of care. For a number of reasons, however, many of the regulations that place constraints on the physicians cannot be lifted and the physicians must learn to live with them.

Dale: Are residents overworked to the extent that they may make errors due to fatigue?

Szilagyi: It is difficult for me to answer this question, because when I reported for internship duty in July 1935 at the University of Michigan Hospital, the administrative chief resident outlined my work schedule, saying, "You are on duty twenty-four hours a day and seven days a week for eleven months. You are off duty when you take your vacation, when you are sick, or when you make arrangements for someone else to do your work."

I was twenty-four years old, single, and healthy. The arrangement seemed entirely acceptable. I never felt more alive with a feeling of constant growth than during my internship and residency years.

We now live in a different world. The tasks of the house officer, because of the complexity of the technological changes in patient management, have become far more demanding. And frankly, the old exploitative system was never justified. From what I have observed at the present time, however, the residents are not overworked to the extent that their efficiency could be impaired. If they make errors, it is seldom due to fatigue.

Dale: How do patients find a competent vascular surgeon?

Szilagyi: As one finds a competent lawyer or architect. Ask for the recommendation of someone who understands what proper qualifications are. In the case in question, that would be the internist taking care of the patient, but, unfortunately, this approach occasionally fails.

Dale: Most specialists in peripheral vascular surgery have ceased to perform cardiac surgery. Should the latter stop doing vascular surgery?

Szilagyi: I do not believe that a surgeon, unless he is supernaturally endowed, can practice both cardiac and vascular surgery at an acceptably competent level.

Jesse Thompson

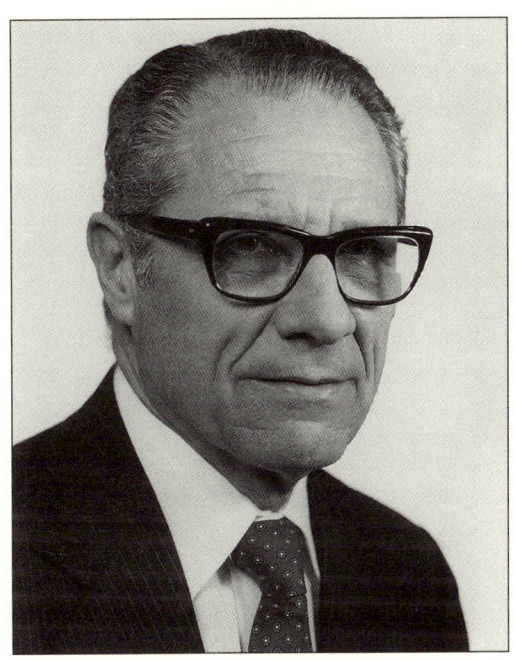

M ADELEINE AND JESSE THOMPSON have done more
to make vascular surgeons a "band of brothers" than
anyone. The road runner of vascular surgery, as Jesse
Thompson's fellows so fondly call him, is a scholar who continues to
search for knowledge about vascular diseases, especially as applied
to the carotid artery. You can always find Jesse on the front row of
vascular meetings, attentively listening to the presenters and absorb-
ing new knowledge. He was interviewed October 17, 1987.

Dale: Let's start out by talking about your hometown, your parents, and maybe elementary school briefly.

Thompson: Well, my parents came from the Deep South. My mother was born in Mississippi and my father was born in Arkansas. I was born April 7, 1919.

Dale: What was your mother's maiden name?

Thompson: Her maiden name was Sara Bolton. After they were married, they moved down to Texas from Arkansas. My father was doing ranching out of Laredo for a while. When the activity down in the lower Rio Grande Valley of Texas came about in the 1920s, we moved from Laredo to San Benito. I was about four years old, so I was brought up in the lower Rio Grande Valley of Texas. I went through school, my entire elementary and secondary high school, in San Benito.

Dale: Did you want to be a doctor when you were in high school?

Thompson: Well, I had two ambitions, either to be a doctor or a lawyer, but as I got out of high school it was clear to me that I was more interested in science than I was in law and history and that sort of business. When I went off to the University of Texas, I decided that I would probably be premed. At the least I was going to take science and see whether premed interested me.

Dale: What else did you do in college besides get ready for medical school?

Thompson: Those were in the days of the Depression and things were pretty tough all over the place, so I worked my way through college.

Dale: What did you do?

Thompson: The first year I was on the NYA (National Youth Administration) and did janitorial work at the student union.

Dale: How much did they pay you—do you remember?

Thompson: I got thirty dollars a month, enough to take care of our room and board at the University of Texas. I got interested in biology and chemistry, and at the end of my first year I got an assistantship in biology. From then on, during my sophomore and junior years, I was an assistant in the biology department all the time. I worked there for the last three years of college. I was interested in athletics, but I really wasn't big enough or good enough to play football. I was also interested in track, so I went out for both track and cross-country for all four years that I was at the University of Texas.

Dale: Were you basically a quarter-miler?

Thompson: I used to run the mile and two mile and cross-country.

Dale: So you were long in distance?

Thompson: Yes, distance.

Dale: I remember a picture of you in a track suit.

Thompson: Actually, I was captain of the cross-country team at the University of Texas. Most of my extracurricular activities had to do with track and cross-country. As a result of that, and my grades, and this other business, I got my Rhodes scholarship at the University of Texas.

Dale: So what year did you graduate at Texas?

Thompson: I finished at Texas in 1939.

Dale: Did you take the Rhodes scholarship then?

Thompson: I was going to take it beginning in September of 1939. I had already been accepted at Galveston, Pennsylvania, and Harvard for medical school. Then when I won the Rhodes scholarship I wrote them all and said I would have to postpone this, and the Harvard people said, Well, we will be glad to take you back after you finish your work at Oxford, and if you take three years over there, why, we will take you in our third year class up here. I was on my way to catch a boat in New York to go to Oxford with my scholarship in premed for physiology when Hitler invaded Poland on September 1, so they canceled my passport while I was en route to New York.

Dale: What did you do, just turn around and go home?

Thompson: No, I went on to Swarthmore, because the American secretary of the Rhodes scholars was in Swarthmore, and everybody just sort of congregated at Swarthmore to see what we were going to do. Well, the first thing I did was to wire the Harvard Medical School. I got another wire back from them that said a "vacancy" had appeared, and I was accepted into the first year class of the Harvard Medical School.

Dale: And that was already in September?

Thompson: This was the first week in September.

Dale: So you went right on?

Thompson: Yes. The other thing that happened at that time, though, was that the American secretary, a man named Frank Aydelotte, a very prominent educator at Swarthmore, also arranged it that if we wanted to go the University of Chicago we could go there on scholarship. It was a four-year scholarship to medical school. He arranged that for several people. I decided to go to Harvard. They gave me a scholarship and I went on up to Boston.

Dale: Who was the chief of surgery in Boston when you were at Harvard?

Thompson: Well, as you know, they don't have a single department chairman, but at Peter Bent Brigham it was Elliott Cutler and at the Massachusetts General Hospital it was Edward D. Churchill. They were still there then because they hadn't gone off to war at that time.

Dale: What sort of relations did you have with them? Did you get to know either one of them?

Thompson: Well, only casually. We didn't get to know them very well because when we started into our clinical years they both went off to war. Francis Moore was the resident at Mass General when I finished medical school, so he was one of the first surgeons with whom I came into contact. But the man that I came into contact with during my internship at Massachusetts General, after finishing Harvard Medical School in the spring of 1943, was Reginald Smithwick. I was assigned to his service; this was the time when splanchnicectomy was just being developed. He and I developed a very close relationship, because I was interested in the sympathectomy. This was something new to me, and a fascinating business. He was working with hypertension; patients were coming in from all over the United States and we were just swamped. I got very interested in it.

Dale: How many cases were you doing weekly or daily with hypertension?

Thompson: At the beginning we were doing about three a day, and then later on, when we moved over across town from Mass General to the Mass Memorial at BU, we were doing six a day, every day, five days a week.

Dale: That was a physically demanding operation, wasn't it?

Thompson: Yes, but it wasn't as hard as aortic surgery.

Dale: How long would you take?

Thompson: About two hours. There was a nice anatomic dissection, so it was really a very fun operation.

Dale: And then what happened to that operation?

Thompson: Well, about that time the various drugs came along— first the low salt diet; then the rice diet to treat hypertension; then the thyazide drugs, the ganglionic blockers, and reserpine. All these developments spelled the demise of doing sympathectomy for hypertension.

Dale: Does it have any place today?

Thompson: I don't think so; it doesn't have any place. The only place I know for a splanchnicectomy at the present time is in treatment of an occasional patient who has pain from pancreatitis and doesn't have a carcinoma and can't be cured for some other reason. You can do a splanchnicectomy to cure his pain. That is about the only place for it that I know of at the present time.

Dale: What sort of a guy was Smithwick personally?

Thompson: Smithwick was really a great man. He was popular with the residents because he was a very quiet sort of man, thoughtful, smart, and an excellent surgical technician. He wasn't very fast, sort of a slow operator, but a beautiful technician and very careful. He insisted on perfection at all times and was a very original thinker. He didn't say much, but he was always thinking. He was the person who actually developed the three-stage treatment of acute diverticulitis of the colon, colostomy and then resection and closure of the colostomy, which revolutionized the treatment of diverticulitis. Then he developed dorsal and lumbar sympathectomy as well as splanchnicectomy. He was always developing new instruments of various sorts to facilitate the performance of these operations. He was the first, after the vagotomy came, to do the combination of the vagotomy plus hemigastrectomy that antedated that of Dr. Edwards of Nashville by a few months. So he had made significant contributions in many areas of general and vascular surgery.

Dale: Did you stay on with him?

Thompson: After I finished my residency at General, I went over to be chief resident with him when he became professor and chairman at BU, and after a year as chief resident I took up my Rhodes scholarship. They opened it up again after the war ended.

Dale: What year was that?

Thompson: I went over in 1950 and spent a year. I got it in 1939, and by the time the war ended I had finished the residency. I went over and took a year doing research at Oxford in 1950.

Dale: Who did you work with?

Thompson: I worked with two guys. One was the chief of the Nuffield Institute for Medical Research, a guy named Geoffrey Dawes, who was a young pharmacologist. Lord Nuffield was the guy who developed Morris Cars and he was a great benefactor of Oxford University, so he set up the Nuffield Institute. The other young fellow I was assigned to work with was John Vane, who was working on his doctorate at that time. We spent a year working together; subsequently, John Vane won the Nobel Prize for his discovery of prostacycline. We had a very nice working relationship. He was one of the brightest guys with whom I have ever been associated. I worked on vascular physiology, gastric blood flow, arteriography of vessels, and peripheral vasospasm problems.

Dale: Were you and Madeleine married then?

Thompson: Yes, we were married—we got married in 1944 and actually had two kids when we went to Oxford; we took the kids along.

Dale: Where was Madeleine from?

Thompson: She was from Pennsylvania but was working at the Massachusetts General Hospital.

Dale: As a nurse?

Thompson: Yes, a nurse in the operating room. That's where we met.

Dale: So you took two children with you, then?

Thompson: Took two children with us, had one over there, and brought three back. Back in the United States I joined Dr. Smithwick full time in the Department of Surgery at Boston University in January 1951 and then moved to Texas in 1954.

Dale: How did you happen to go back to Texas?

Thompson: I had always wanted to go back to Texas. That was my home and I figured that vascular surgery was just getting underway

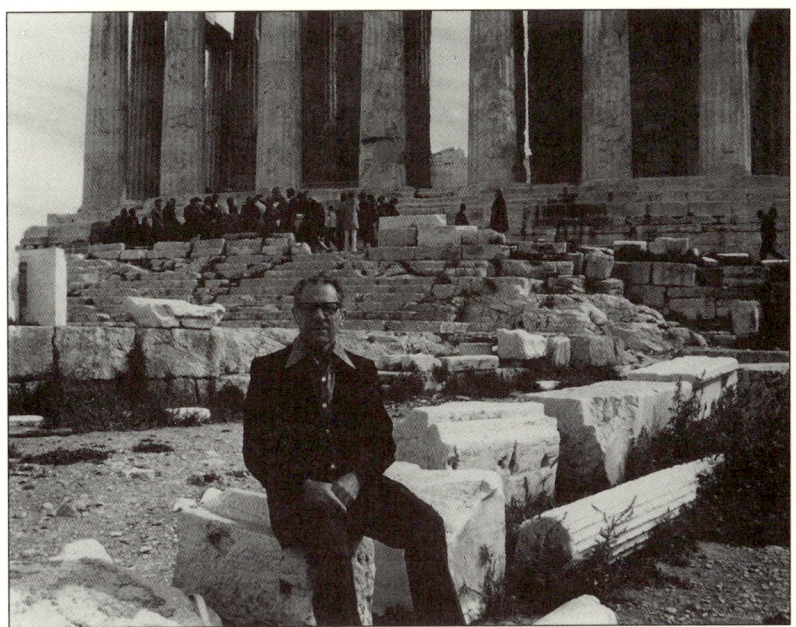

Madeleine and Jesse have traveled all over the world.

at that time. Mike DeBakey had just recently moved to Houston, vessel banks were being established, and I figured there was a lot of opportunity in Texas. That was the main reason I wanted to go back. So we went back and looked over the Houston scene and Mike said, "Well, I think we would be glad to have you come down here to Houston, but Denton Cooley has just started, and I have already promised Stanley Crawford a job, so I don't have any openings at the moment. But if you want to come to Houston and just set up and get going I will support you." I said that was a little bit indefinite, so I looked around at Austin and Dallas and there was a great opportunity in Dallas. There wasn't anything going on there and they offered me a position at the medical school in Dallas. So I got to talking to various people, such as Dale Austin, who was a vascular surgeon there. He was interested in doing vascular reconstruction and setting up an artery bank at Baylor Hospital and wanted a partner. I thought it over and it seemed like a good opportunity, so I joined him and went into private practice and joined the clinical faculty of the medical school. Carl Moyer had just left as chairman and Ben Wilson was the chairman at that time. That is how we got to Dallas. That was in 1954, and I have been there ever since.

Dale: Where did you do your first aneurysm?

Thompson: My first aneurysm was done at Baylor Hospital in 1955.

Dale: What did you replace it with?

Thompson: A homograft. We set up an artery bank at Baylor Hospital. There had been a place during the war where the army got lyophilized blood plasma. We already had the facilities for lyophilization, freezing, and freeze drying; a technician; and the whole bit. It wasn't too hard just to transfer over to procuring arteries and doing lyophilized homografts. That's what we used first.

Dale: When did you start doing vein grafts?

Thompson: I don't remember the exact date, but it was after you were doing them. Bob Linton was doing them while we got interested in it, too. As I recall, we were putting in some nylon grafts after Sterling developed his nylon graft and then his Teflon. It was obvious that those weren't working very well and so we started doing the vein grafts then.

Dale: What about the carotids?

Thompson: We got interested in the carotids because it was brought to our attention by a neurosurgeon who had had some dealings with Francis Murphy in Memphis in about 1956. We got our neurologist and neurosurgeons interested in this and did our first carotid on April 15, 1957. The neurosurgeons said that they really weren't interested in doing the procedures, but that they would be very happy to do the arteriograms for us, to help us study them and to care for them in any way possible.

Dale: You can't beat that!

Thompson: You can't beat that, and that's the way it has been ever since. So we had a very nice, cooperative arrangement with the radiologists, neurologists, and neurosurgeons, and we were the technicians.

Dale: Did you protect the brain in any way in the early ones?

Thompson: In the early ones, the only way we protected the brain was by doing carotid compression every day for two weeks prior to the time of the operation to see if they could tolerate carotid occlusion.

Dale: Did you have any who couldn't?

Thompson: We didn't operate on any who couldn't. But now and again . . .

Dale: You did run into some?

Thompson: Yes, you would run into some.

Dale: So you actually didn't use any shunts?

Thompson: Not at the beginning. It became obvious that this wasn't a very realistic or practical way to handle this business, so we began to use shunts because shunts were being used by some of the cardiac surgeons in some of the great vessel bypasses. We figured we could shunt the carotid, but the problem was how to do that. So our first shunts were external shunts with twelve or thirteen needles connected by a little piece of plastic intravenous tubing that we would stick in the common carotid at one end and the internal carotid at the other. But the only problem with that was that there was such a big gash in the artery that you had to close up the hole where the needle was. In those days we would go to the vascular meetings and everybody would sit around and discuss our mutual problems, so I talked this over with Frank Wheelock in Boston and he said, "Well, shoot, I think maybe you could stick a shunt inside the vessel instead of using that external shunt." He said he thought Stanley Crawford was doing this at that time, so I talked to Stanley. Although nowadays he doesn't like to admit to the fact that he was using shunts in those days, he and Mike were using shunts pretty routinely. Then I went down to Houston to see how they were doing them, and they had these shunts all cut to different sizes in sterile solution and sterile bottles. If they were going to do a carotid they just took the appropriate shunt out and stuck it in. So that is really how we started using internal shunts, after going down to Houston to see their experience with them and finding that the external shunt was really not all that satisfactory.

Dale: What's your present opinion about the shunting and non-shunting situation?

Thompson: Over the years it gradually came to be that we used the shunt routinely. Then we taught it to all our fellows and we tried various techniques—EEG monitoring and stump pressures, the adequacy of back flow, and so on. Finally, we decided that it was simple to go ahead and use shunts routinely. That is what I have always done in recent years, and it is what we have taught our fellows. That is what my whole staff does now. We do it realizing that you don't always have to, but we felt that it was satisfactory and our results have been good.

Dale: What reaction do you have to the idea that perhaps too many carotids are being done in the United States?

Thompson: I would agree that there are probably too many carotids being done in the United States. When I look at the various series that are reported and find that maybe 50 percent of somebody's series is done for asymptomatic stenosis, I think this is too much. We have been very careful in our selection over the years, and have never gone over 15 percent for asymptomatic lesions; the rest are for symptomatic lesions. Also, from time to time, when I have had to consult on cases and have had the x-rays sent to me on the carotid when someone was proposing to do it, I felt that in an asymptomatic patient there wasn't enough there to justify the operation. I think there is some justification to the claim that too many carotids are being done in some centers. This impression is hard to prove, but I honestly think it is probably true.

Dale: What about the coronary business? After all, you are not directly involved in that, so maybe your opinion is worth more there?

Thompson: Well, as I said, I don't really know about that. I would hate to comment on it because I really don't know, but you know the same thing could spill over in the coronary as you see in the carotid area. I think, too, that I have seen personal instances where patients have had femoral popliteal bypasses for claudication where I didn't think it was indicated. So I think that in some instances there have been too many femoral popliteals done for inadequate indications. That would only be from inference; as far as the coronaries go, I'd just as soon not comment on that.

Dale: I sort of have the opinion that the best surgeons of, say, the 1940s could not technically keep up with the chief residents of today. Is that true?

Thompson: Well, I think that is probably true. The chief residents today have all kinds of techniques that the surgeons in those days simply didn't have.

Dale: I look back at the fellows that I thought were the great technicians, and they would be passable by today's standards.

Thompson: We have many more efficient techniques now than we had then. Dr. Smithwick was a very careful technician, and so was Dr. Churchill, but our modern-day residents are really very good.

Dale: I recall Herm Pearse, who would do a gallbladder in about an hour, and we thought he was such a great technician. Now an assistant resident, with me helping him, takes about forty-five minutes for a gallbladder.

Thompson: Yes, we have progressed a long way technically.

Dale: How many carotids do you suppose you've done by now? Do you have any idea?

Thompson: Well over two thousand. We don't have the numbers quite up to date, but a whole lot over the period of the twenty-eight years now that we've been doing this.

Frank Veith

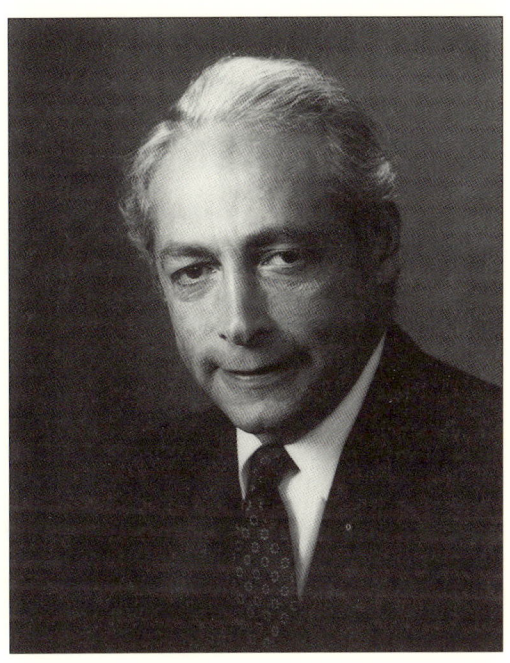

DESCENDED FROM a German immigrant who did well in business, Veith has worked in New York and Boston. He currently is chief of vascular surgery at Montefiore Hospital in New York. Respected for his early attempts at lung transplantation, he is known especially for studies on revascularization of the lower extremity. His postgraduate course attracts over a thousand participants each year, and he is noted for crisp, concise reports of current research in vascular surgery from all over the world. He was interviewed June 5, 1992.

Johnson: Frank, tell me about your early life.

Veith: I was born on August 29, 1931, in New York City and had a very undistinguished childhood. I didn't have any brothers or sisters. I went to a public school in Manhattan and I liked sports but was not particularly outstanding at any of them. I went to high school in Riverdale, where I live now. I had to ride back and forth an hour a day on the subway.

My grandfather came over from Germany as a very poor teenager and made millions of dollars in the sequin business. He brought over a half-brother from Germany, who managed to take the business away from him. We still ended up with a certain amount of family money, having started with nothing. One of my father's interests was to manage the money so that we didn't lose the rest of it, and in that he has been modestly successful. My father was a New York lawyer and was still practicing at age ninety-four. My mother had been a nurse and didn't work during my childhood. About the time I was twelve years old, they had a house in Westchester and moved up there. Manhattan and Scarsdale were the two homes I knew growing up, but it was definitely a New York City background.

I didn't consider myself a very good student. I was always joking and fooling around with the guys in the back of the room, but I must have done reasonably well because I managed to get into Cornell, even though all my high school advisors told me I had no possible chance of getting into such a good school. I did very well there, probably because my high school teachers had convinced me that I wasn't very smart and I would have to work hard in college.

I ended up going to medical school after three years, although I really don't know why. My mother, since she had been a nurse, had some influence on me and convinced me that it was a good profession to pursue. I certainly didn't want to go to law school, which was the other possibility, because I saw my father coming home every night with all his paperwork. I felt that as a doctor I probably would not have to do any paperwork; how wrong can you be! I was interested in manipulative skills. I liked to remove splinters from myself or other people and I'd had some exposure to dentistry through my uncle, who was a dentist. Medicine, like dentistry, was a way of using manual and cognitive skills to get people better. When I went to college I did take premedical courses and did pretty well. For me, one of the major forks in the road—one at which I probably made a mistake—occured when I was accepted to a number of medical schools, Harvard being one of them. I chose to go to Cornell Medical College in New York City for a number of what I consider now to be bad reasons. One was that I had a medical school scholarship there, which our family really didn't need; the other was that if I went to Harvard after three years of college I wouldn't get a Cornell degree, whereas if I went to Cornell Medical College I also got the B.A. degree, which obviously doesn't mean very much today. So I entered medical school at Cornell in 1951.

At Cornell we had a small class; it was a very personable group. I can remember living in a barracks left over from one of the Navy V-12 programs from the Second World War. It was on the East River and was a very dilapidated, run-down cardboard barracks; we used to call it "Wildwood by the Sea." I lived there for two and a half years. We had a very good group of medical students who got along very well; we used to wrestle, fight, play touch football, and do a lot of work. Medical school was a lot of work, and I was convinced in my own mind at that time that I wasn't a very good student, so I worked hard and did pretty well.

Then it came time to decide what field to go into. My uncle, the dentist, was a frustrated physician and had always been after me to go into surgery. He used to talk about one of his friends who was a general surgeon. He made general surgery sound like the be-all and end-all of careers. I guess my mother thought that that would be a reasonable thing for me to do. My father did not try to influence me, although he was very supportive. My parents never bothered me much when it came to school. That was my thing; they never helped with homework or anything like that. It was my own responsibility and it worked out pretty well. I never failed any courses or was in any trouble in school. Although I didn't graduate with honors from high school, I did quite well in college and medical school. When the time came to figure out what field I was going into, I regarded myself as somewhat of an intellectual and it appeared that most of the intellectuals in the class were going into internal medicine, worrying about lupus, collagen diseases, and so forth. That was quite interesting in medical school and I thought I would probably take my training in internal medicine.

Then we had a dog surgery course, which was very much a turning point in my thinking. I really enjoyed the manipulative aspects of operating and found that I could do it, not very well but at least to the point where I didn't consider myself a klutz. I liked the idea of doing something to get patients well, not just the idea of making a diagnosis and watching them die, or giving them some ineffective pills.

On that basis I applied for surgical internship; I was very anxious to go to Mass General, Peter Bent Brigham, or Columbia Presbyterian. As a good student, I felt I had a chance to get into the best surgical internships. I liked Boston and was oriented to New England. They had exams in those days for the internship, and I did very well at the Brigham internship exam, reasonably well at the Mass General internship exam—except for the final exam, on which I missed one rather key question that I should have known, something to do with gynecology. I listed Mass General first. Again I was in this dilemma of whether to stay in New York City or to go to Boston, and I can remember having a great deal of indecisiveness as to whether or not to go to the Brigham or Columbia as my second choice, feeling that my best chance would be to get my second choice in the match. After a lot of indecision, for personal and family reasons I chose Columbia second and have always felt I probably would have been better off going to Peter Bent Brigham and Harvard. As a medical student I had heard Dr. Francis Moore speak, and he really was quite stimulating and charismatic. He certainly turned me on to the Brigham. By the same token, in those days the Brigham was regarded as a small, intellectual, non-cutting kind of internship and residency, and that influenced me a little bit to decide against it as the leading choice. So I went to Columbia Presbyterian as an intern, along with Joe Buda. I never was really comfortable with my choice. Columbia Presbyterian was a very big, unfriendly institution, very much like Cornell had been, and had a long surgical history, but had many idols who turned out to have feet of clay. The surgical attendings there were not what I had hoped or expected them to be in many cases, although some were quite outstanding. I had feelings all along that the Brigham would have been a better choice. In those days, 1955–1956, it was arranged that surgeons either did their military duty early in their career or at the end of their residency. I applied for and was given a Berry Plan deferment to stay out of the service until I completed my residency. I thought that was a pretty good idea, but the powers that be at Columbia didn't like the idea of having their trainees stay out of the armed forces; they wanted them to go in and get their military service over. So I applied for and got a residency at the Brigham, which had always been in the back of my mind as having been a better choice than Columbia.

I had applied very early in the year. I don't remember whether I went up to see Dr. Moore, but I had done very well in the internship exam and interviews at the Brigham and I was rather quickly accepted as a first-year resident in surgery. I had spent a lot of time evaluating the place before I went and I knew many of the residents and liked them. It was with happiness that I went to the Brigham. It was an easy decision since the Columbia people weren't going to honor my Berry Plan deferment. It was the heyday of Francis Moore, and the Brigham was a smaller, friendlier place with a lot of interaction between the attending surgeons and the housestaff. I can remember very vividly when I first got there going to a party at Joe Murray's house at which the resident staff played the attending staff in softball. I remember for one reason or another I was pitching. I wasn't a star athlete, but I was a moderately good athlete, and Franny was playing for the other team. I struck him out once or twice. Franny did everything well—he was a championship yachtsman, he was a singer, he played the accordion—but I don't think he was a particularly good athlete. He was pitching and I hit a home run, so I wasn't so sure that boded well for my career.

Johnson: Was he a good surgeon?

Veith: He was an outstanding surgeon. Away from the Brigham, he had a so-so reputation as a surgeon. I can remember an argument I got into with John Najarian when we were both being awarded a Markle scholarship and were roommates. John was saying how Franny was a brilliant guy, a good speaker, and a good writer, but not such a good surgeon. We got into a big argument because John had never seen Dr. Moore operate. Dr. Moore was probably the best operating surgeon I had ever worked with. The procedures in which he was interested he performed with great gusto, balance, and tremendous skill—thyroids, abdominalperineals, gastrectomies, radical mastectomies—he was outstanding. He did those operations better than anybody else that I am aware of. Parathyroid explorations—he was terrific at those. I think somehow many of the other surgeons around the country had to reduce Franny to the size of a mere mortal, so he had the reputation of being a writing, speaking surgeon and not an operating surgeon, but he was really very, very good in the operating room. Clearly, he had a very major impact on my thinking and subsequent career.

I did moderately well at the Brigham; they had a pyramid system and I made all the various cuts. In going through the Brigham residency, one had to spend some time in the lab, and there were some very unpleasant rotations as well. We used to call these "Building and Grounds," "Basketweaving," and so forth. We had a "Laundry" rotation, and whenever the uniforms would come back with holes in them we would say it was due to the teaching laundry. However, the Brigham program was a lot of hard work; it was fun, it was good, and I really felt that I was among my peers. The men that I was with in the residency were really very compatible and I count some of them as my dear friends today.

Johnson: Who was with you then?

Veith: Not many of them are well known. Les Rudolf was a strong and good friend; so too were Alan Birtch, now at Southern Illinois, and Marty Litwin, now at Tulane, who was a provocative, interesting character but always a good friend and a very fine person. Peter Crowe became a pediatric surgeon. He had a brother named John Crowe, who was a year behind us; and Mike Eisenberg was an intern when I was a resident. We all remain good friends today. There was another really outstanding man named Danny Pugh, who ultimately committed suicide for reasons that were obscure. He was a very personable, affable, outstanding young surgeon, who must have had serious problems that at the time we didn't recognize. Jim

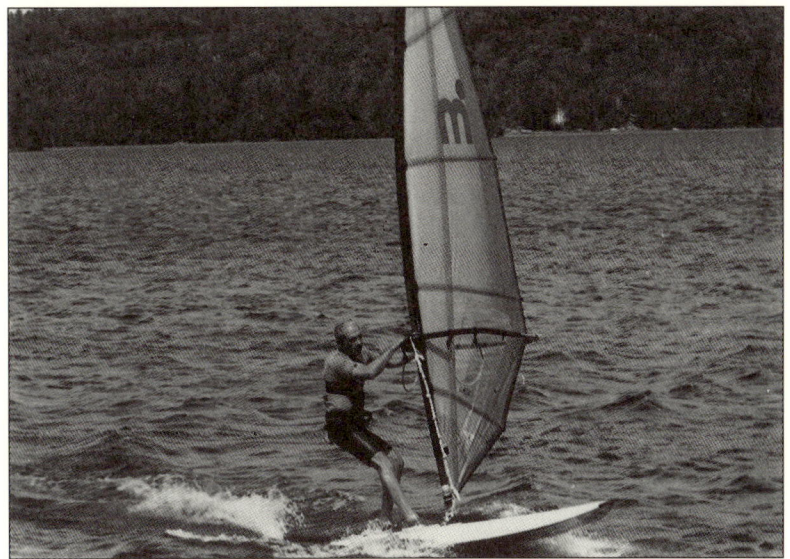

Frank is a windsurfing enthusiast.

Pierce went into transplantation with Dave Hume. I don't know what happened to Harry Demissianos. I think he went into industry sometime during the middle of his career, although he did finish his surgical internship. That was my peer group. I was also very fond of and had very good relationships with a number of the senior residents. Richard Wilson, Ed Gray, and John Kenney were some of the very influential and charismatic senior residents, and Bill Blaisdell was a junior resident rotating through the Brigham surgical program, as was Bob Rutherford. A number of young men who were destined to become important surgeons spent time at the Brigham while I was there. Of course, there were visiting professors of great preeminence: Churchill, Bob Zollinger—I got to know Bob Zollinger, Sr., very well, because the year I was the chief resident, he was the visiting professor, and we lived together for a week. I really developed quite an affection for him.

Shelton Horsley was a resident two or three years ahead of me. My wife and I had two children during the course of my time at the Brigham and our garden apartment was right next to the Horsleys, so we were very friendly with them and much influenced by Shelton and his wife, Mary. That was a very positive relationship that also added to my fondness for the Brigham and the whole residency program there. Although the work was extraordinarily hard, I felt that we were getting a superb education and background in surgery. I always compare my current trainees and resident staffs to those men. Today they just don't seem to be as supportive of each other or to be as outstanding in all ways.

The program was such that most residents spent time in the laboratory between their various rotations, during the delays when one had to wait to be promoted to the next rank. I never spent any time in the lab, probably because of the needs of the program. It was not a tightly structured program; it was loose in that there were always a number of people floating around. People would come for a year and work in the laboratory, and they might go into the residency program if there was an extra slot. The residency was really run by Dr. Moore himself, together with the chief resident. One of Dr. Moore's interesting characteristics was that he didn't appear to be very close to anyone in his attending staff and ran the program truly as a one-man show. He would use the chief resident as a colleague, ally, and sounding board rather than have someone directly under him who was his chief lieutenant. This elevated the chief resident to a very important stature. In retrospect, I think he probably did that intentionally. It was an interesting way of running things.

Johnson: Who were some of the attendings at that time?

Veith: Dick Wilson became an attending while I was there, and Chilton Crane was a very excellent attending who was really not "the" vascular surgeon but did a lot of the major vascular surgery and influenced my career greatly. He was an unflappable, solid, excellent surgeon who did a lot of aneurysm and portal hypertension work. Probably the biggest influence on my career was Dwight Harken, who had the biggest practice. In many ways the thoracic rotation made the Brigham residency, because we used to get an enormous amount of clinical operating room experience with "Uncle Dwight." He was probably the most charismatic and influential attending of all, including Franny, with regard to my career development. I watched his practice patterns and I watched his method of doing things in the operating room. There were a number of other thoracic surgeons who didn't have his style of operating, and we could compare the efficiency, speed, and effectiveness of the two different styles. Harrison Black was another thoracic attending. Both were excellent and both got great results, but they had totally different styles and one had the opportunity, because of the wealth of clinical material, to develop one's own style.

The amount of responsibility given to the surgical resident was enormous; there were no thoracic residents in those days, and I began the thoracic rotation with a great deal of fear and trepidation because I had never had a junior resident rotation and here I was thrust into a position of enormous responsibility. Dr. Harken was known as a very tough taskmaster and all the residents were in great fear of him. He usually ended up bawling them out or screaming at them for something that had gone awry. I can remember in all the two or three months I was with him on the thoracic service, he never had anything he could find fault with. The service ran extraordinarily well; I would not leave the hospital for two or three weeks at a time, sleeping only every other night, but the fact was that I managed somehow to please him. I felt that I got an enormous amount from that experience. That rotation made me feel that I really could do surgery and do it effectively. Of course, I would either in jest or in seriousness emulate Harken's mannerisms. We would jokingly say we were going to all dye our hair red, or we would lean back from the OR table and pontificate to the gallery, whether there was someone there or not. It was a lot of fun. There was a group of nurses who were real OR nurses and the working relationship was really terrific. I wish I could remember all their names. That was a real high point of the training program, although I must admit that it was physically exhausting. There were no ICUs—we used to stay up all night taking care of the patients. There were no respirators—they were just starting to come on the scene— so if we had a patient with some kind of pulmonary problem, we used to stay up all night, in shifts, squeezing a bag and ventilating the patient, because we didn't have appropriate ventilators for patients with bad lungs. There are innumerable stories. Another resident I liked, and who influenced me greatly, Alan Birtch, was actually junior to me. Alan and I were on the thoracic service together; I can remember a funny story when we had a cardiac arrest. With no

ICU, the patients were just put on the floor. Something that we would call a code today was announced, and we ran to take care of the patient. On one occasion I can remember running around a corner and Alan slipped and fell on some wet flooring. I looked back and he was on the ground, in some pain, and he couldn't get up. I said, "Don't worry, Alan, if you're hurt, you can stay there." The poor guy couldn't even stand up, so I ran away from him and went to the patient who was coding.

On another occasion they called me to donate a unit of blood for one of our patients. The patient arrested while I was giving the blood, or just at the end of the transfusion, so I had to get up and start to run to the code. I guess I was sufficiently hypovolemic that I fainted as I stood up.

Johnson: Where did you go from Boston?

Veith: After I finished my senior residency I had to go into the army. With the help of Mike Eisenberg, I volunteered to go anywhere provided they gave me a good surgical job. Nobody wanted to go to Korea and I said I'd be happy to go there. They called me up about a month before I was supposed to go in and said they had a job in Colorado Springs as chief of surgery at an army hospital if I came in the next day. I called Mike Eisenberg and through his connections he found out what the operating load per month was and that it was a good job. So I called them right back and took the job. I was not yet a trained surgeon by any manner or means because the amount of surgery at the Brigham was very limited. At the Brigham you didn't get your big surgical experience till you were chief resident, and I hadn't been chief resident. Anyhow, I went in the service and managed to convince the people in the hospital that I knew what I was doing.

There was one rather critical case involving a general's mother who was bleeding from her large intestine. Should we helicopter up to Fitzsimmons, which was ninety miles away, or should we operate where we were? I elected for one reason or another to operate on her. She was bleeding pretty vigorously; she was overweight and difficult. I didn't find any lesions, but I divided the bowel in the midportion of the transverse colon to see where the blood was coming from and ended up doing a sigmoid resection and a transverse colostomy. She stopped bleeding for a while and ultimately got better, which made me a big hero.

I used to make up for my incompetence by working very hard, taking very good care of the patients and spending a lot of time with them, so I was making rounds at six o'clock one morning and here was this poor lady with most of her small bowel out on her abdominal wall. She had dehisced through her colostomy wound. I didn't want to operate on her again, and I can remember packing the bowel back inside her abdomen and putting on a binder. She also bled postoperatively from the right colon, but it ended happily. She went on to get well.

After this I couldn't do much wrong. The colonel who ran the hospital allowed me to do whatever I wanted to do. We did a lot of cases and had a lot of fun. Colorado Springs was not an unpleasant outpost; it was a very nice place to work. I was there two years, I volunteered for everything, and I even worked for the CIA. I was very interested in the military and was thinking of staying in the army and the CIA in some way.

The army experience was a very good one and I matured a lot as a surgeon there. We had some consultants, but we didn't have any money to call them. I was friendly with a number of the surgeons in the town and one of them wanted me to go into practice with him when I got out. I was thinking of staying in, but when it came time to get out, they replaced me with a regular army lieutenant colonel, who was a terrible fellow. He tortured me enough from the military point of view that I realized this was not for me. The Brigham chief residency had opened up and Franny had written me that I could come back and be chief resident at the Brigham, which was a big deal in those days. They finished two surgical residents a year; one went to the West Roxbury VA and the other had presumably the best job, which was as chief resident at the Brigham.

I went back to the Brigham and had a very interesting time. Unlike my predecessors, I had passed my boards in the service and thought I was a pretty hotshot surgeon. The idea of calling the attendings to worry about every little thing when I had done a couple of hundred cases like that myself seemed ridiculous. Dr. Moore was a little bit turned off by that independent attitude. Whereas he thought I was appropriately conscientious and respectful before that, I believe he was a little miffed at my level of self-confidence. Anyhow, the chief resident year at the Brigham was a very good one; the chief resident was really the king of the castle and I think Franny Moore wanted it that way. Because I had done so much in the service I could afford to be very generous to my juniors and I think everybody had a pretty good time the year I was chief resident.

Johnson: Where did you go from there?

Veith: I didn't know whether I wanted an academic job or a practice job. I told Franny that I wanted to have a job just like his at some point and to do things very much the way he did. I interviewed at Lexington, Kentucky, with Ben Eiseman, but I didn't like the idea of going to Kentucky. I interviewed with Dick Karl, who had been at Cornell and had always impressed me as being a good cutting surgeon and an affable guy when I was a medical student. He had operated on my mother and had taken over an academic job at the Cornell division at Bellevue. He recruited me as his sidekick. Although he was not very well known in academic circles, this was the kind of situation that I wanted, and I took the job. I don't believe I could have stayed at the Brigham, which wasn't a terrible disappointment. I didn't like the idea of getting on the bottom of a long ladder, so I was quite willing to go to Bellevue. Little did I realize that it was going to be as much of a horror show as it was: no resources, no money, no secretaries. Everything was difficult. I didn't get to do any operating to speak of; the only cases I could hope to do were vascular cases because the chief residents did all the other cases without even an attending seeing the patient.

Johnson: You were still a general surgeon then?

Veith: I was absolutely a general surgeon, and, to back up a little bit, I should say that I've been influenced greatly by Harken, Robert Gross, and Joe Murray. I had enough transplant experience and had done a year's research in transplantation after my residency, so I felt I could qualify as a transplant surgeon, a thoracic surgeon, or a vascular surgeon. By this time I had four children and we lived in New York, in Pelham. After I got to the Cornell division at Bellevue, it became apparent that Dick Karl was the odd man out at Cornell.

Although he had an enormous practice, the Bellevue group was not very well thought of by the then-esteemed Cornell surgical faculty. I insisted on getting privileges at New York Hospital, which I received with some resistance from Frank Glenn.

Johnson: What year was this?

Veith: This was in 1964. I managed to get an NIH grant at Bellevue and got the dean to propose me for the Markle scholarship, which I was lucky enough to win. I managed to mount some kind of investigative effort on assisted oxygenation, which was based on work that I had done with Alan Birch and others at the Brigham. The Bellevue job was a very good experience in how to deal with adversity. It couldn't have been a worse place. The old Bellevue building and the office facilities were awful; we were regarded as being definitely second-class citizens by the Cornell faculty with the exception of Charlie McSherry, of whom I was very fond and with whom I worked well. The Cornell climate was not particularly favorable, although since I was at Bellevue I wasn't regarded as being a real competitor or viewed very negatively.

In any event, after about two and a half years at Bellevue, there was an administrative problem between the city of New York and Cornell and we found out, by reading the *New York Times,* that the Cornell-Bellevue affiliation had been severed, so all of us were out of a job. At that point, Marv Gliedman, who had gone to Montefiore and had previously tried unsuccessfully to recruit me there, called me up, as did a number of other people, and offered me a job. Wanting to keep my research effort alive and clearly being forced to move, we elected to move the whole operation to Montefiore, in the Bronx. It meant that we didn't have to move our family, the kids didn't have to change schools, and things like that. Montefiore Hospital and Albert Einstein had not been in my plans for the next academic move up; in fact, it seemed to me to be somewhat of a move down. I regarded it as a stepping-stone, merely a place to keep working for a year or two before going on to something bigger and better.

However, I have had a number of opportunities to leave Montefiore and the Bronx, and I haven't. We became interested in lung transplantation as a spin-off of our work on assisted oxygenation and I was able to start a clinical lung transplant program and obtain major NIH funding. Sometimes I look back and think that perhaps I should have taken a different path.

Johnson: How did you evolve into a vascular surgeon?

Veith: I went to Montefiore as a general surgeon with the charge of starting a kidney transplant program, which I did. However, there was some misunderstanding between Gliedman and me at the beginning. I had thought we had an agreement that I would run the transplant program, but as it became more and more successful, he felt that it was his program. I was never enamored with doing kidney transplants; it was, to me, very unchallenging surgery. I did get the program going and ran it, but I never was satisfied in restricting myself to that surgery; I was interested in the lung transplants. I was doing thoracic but not cardiac surgery; since one couldn't make a living doing lung transplantation, I felt I needed a clinical outlet and began to do more and more vascular surgery. When Haimovici retired in 1971, I persuaded Gliedman to make me chief of the vascular surgery service.

Johnson: Was there a service before that?

Veith: Haimovici was head of a service that had twelve general surgeons doing vascular surgery. Marvin wanted to fold vascular back into general. I persuaded him that that wasn't a good thing to do. Then over the years the vascular service evolved into something that was rather potent, forceful, and productive. In the 1970s I stopped doing general surgery and just did vascular and transplant surgery. My clinical outlet was all vascular from 1971 on.

My vascular training had largely been under Richard Warren, someone else I forgot to mention as a very positive force at the Brigham. Between Chilton Crane and him and some of the other attendings who worked at West Roxbury, we had a fairly rich vascular experience during our training period, and that served me in good stead. I never had specific vascular training or specific thoracic training, although I was able to get my thoracic boards because of my experiences with Harken and Gross.

Johnson: What is going to happen to vascular surgery as a specialty?

Veith: I believe that vascular surgery should be a stand-alone specialty linked to general surgery the way other specialties are linked to general surgery.

Johnson: What are endovascular techniques done by vascular radiologists and internists going to do to vascular surgery?

Veith: I really don't know. The diseases aren't going to go away. My own view is that although the vascular surgeons will be in competition with and threatened by the cardiologists and the invasive radiologists, those techniques will not take away all our business. If we are suitably aggressive and in the forefront, we will survive and will treat most of the patients who have vascular disease and need treatment. If they develop enough fancy hardware that works and can be put in over a wire to manage patients effectively, I think we are going to lose some of our business; but from what I have been able to see, at least in my practice, 80 percent of the cases that require invasive intervention will need an operation, even though such patients may be ministered to by radiologists at some point in their care.

Johnson: What do you foresee as happening to the government's intervention into vascular surgery, both in fees and changing practice? Will there be fewer vascular surgeons than we see applying now to the vascular programs?

Veith: We are facing a period of inhospitable conditions because there is no question that the government, reflecting society, has the impression that medicine—most prominently, surgery—has over the years been a fat cat. The mood of government, because it perceives abuses by medicine and because it has become an expensive process, will create a period of cost containment or cutbacks. This cannot occur without imposing hardships on all of us and ultimately negatively affecting the quality of the care we deliver. It is going to happen. However, vascular surgery will survive. I am optimistic about our survival and our ultimate prosperity. All of us are going to make a little less money, which may not be all bad. We will become "leaner and meaner" in the sense that industry has—by limiting abuses and by limiting the incomes of people who run poor quality, money-making vascular labs or of people who make well over $1 or 2 million in practice, sometimes doing procedures that aren't indicated. Some of the financial incentives to go into vascular surgery are going to decrease, and we will have fewer applicants for some of our programs. The people we get will be better motivated, perhaps for more altruistic reasons, to go into our specialty. Things are going to be okay.

Johnson: Do you think that all vascular surgery should be done by vascular surgeons?

Veith: I do; all vascular surgery should be done across our country in ideal circumstances by people who are comparably trained. Poor people and rich people and people in every section of the country should receive comparable care. That is an ideal system that may not be possible to put into place right away, but in the ideal circumstance I think vascular surgery should be done by people who have had comparable training. I am in accord with training our general surgeons in vascular surgery because I think they become better general surgeons, but if I were receiving care in vascular surgery I would certainly get it from someone who had optimal training. In most instances, that someone should have had a year of specialty training in vascular surgery.

Johnson: During your ten years of involvement in the vascular societies, do you think the attitude of the American Board of Surgery and the Residency Review Committee have changed so that they are beginning to understand the relationship of vascular surgeons to general surgeons?

Veith: In the beginning it was very reactionary, in that general surgery wanted to control vascular surgery and minimize its impact as a specialty. This attitude has changed somewhat, but some of those elements still exist; for example, some of the graduates of nonapproved vascular training programs can't sit for the exam, which is not right. Some of those programs provide just as adequate training as some of the approved programs. On the other hand, before the RRC became involved we may have had too many approved programs. Some of the programs were largely for the interest of the person having the fellowship and not for the interest of the trainee. I would change the system to make some of the better nonapproved program graduates eligible to take the exam. I wouldn't be quite as harsh on the requirement for general surgical residents to do as many cases as they are required to do, although I think if the cases are there, it's very nice for them to do them.

Johnson: How would you summarize the great accomplishments over your thirty years of involvement in vascular surgery?

Veith: From a personal point of view, my contribution to the field was to promote and popularize the aggressive approach to limb salvage, which really didn't exist when I started. That's been an important area to which I have actively contributed in a major way. This kind of surgery is now done universally. There has been a whole host of things that have occurred to make vascular surgery easier and better, and the limb salvage area has just been one. Advances in aneurysm surgery and in carotid surgery have really been landmarks over the last two decades. The tendency is to make what we do easier, safer, and better, and I think we are just starting on the development and evolution of procedures that are going to do that. Operations that were impossible twenty years ago are now becoming fairly safe and fairly commonplace.

Vascular surgery has been at the forefront of integrating applied science to what we do. Some of the best and brightest people are in our specialty. We have also been at the forefront of policing ourselves and organizing as a specialty to right some of the wrongs that can occur. As well as the standardization of vascular procedures for reporting, the whole thrust toward developing and credentialing vascular labs, which the vascular surgeons led, is something that they should be very proud of. I think these are major achievements that our group has accomplished. I am very proud to be a part of this specialty. Having recently become involved in the government relations business, I can see how our group compares favorably in being less self-interested, more global in our view, and more understanding of issues that may not be just in our own parochial interest. That's why we have credibility and are listened to.

Johnson: You have made a great impact in postgraduate education for the United States, not only for the people who come to the Montefiore course, but also the people who teach at the course. You have a unique concept of postgraduate education. Why did you start this?

Veith: I am proud of it. I think the bottom line is that I like to keep abreast of what is going on in developments, both scientific and clinical in the field, and I have a very difficult time doing that by reading. Frequently, things presented or written about will rise to the surface very briefly and not be noticed, so what I have done is to try to structure a meeting as an educational experience for me, and put on things that are both entertaining, practical, and important for practicing vascular surgeons to know about. I think protracted hour-long presentations that are boring and contain all sorts of irrelevant information are not particularly valuable. I like the bottom line. We have structured our meeting on the basis of what is new and important and what I want to hear about. I listen to all the talks because I want to know myself, and I think that is why other people attend our meetings.

Arthur Voorhees

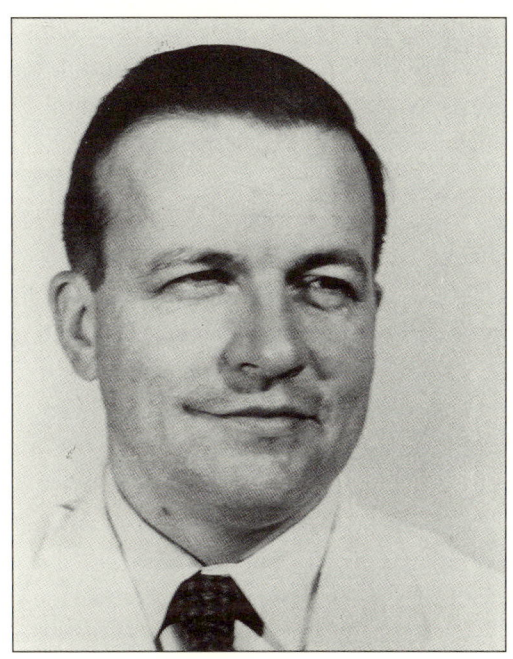

By any standard, Arthur Voorhees ranks high among the pioneers of modern vascular surgery. He calls his development of synthetic tube replacements for human arteries a serendipitous discovery. But he was already a dedicated surgical investigator and possessed the vision, determination, and courage to pursue the idea to successful use in patients.

A lung problem prematurely ended Voorhees's work in any place with air pollution, and he moved to New Mexico. He passed away on May 12, 1992. His inborn good taste and humility led him later in his life to downgrade his seminal discovery in favor of his later investigations of the cirrhotic liver, but history had already reserved a pedestal for Arthur Voorhees. He was interviewed October 30, 1987.

Dale: Arthur, tell me about your parents and your early life.

Voorhees: My early life was actually split among a number of different areas, although my parents were quite stable in one geographical area. I grew up in a small town about ten miles from Philadelphia. Moorestown was dominated by Quakers, and I may add parenthetically that I ultimately married into a Quaker family. However, my family were not Quakers.

I was born in 1921. My mother was Margaret Crow from Jacksonville, Alabama. My father's name was also Arthur Voorhees, so I'm a junior. He had grown up in Moorestown, but his family were from the New York area, where they were the ongoing descendants of a long line of Dutch settlers who first came over in 1648.

My father and mother met during World War I, at a military camp near Anniston, Alabama. After the war they married and he brought her to the North. She was a un-Reconstructed Rebel and never really accepted the ways of the North for the rest of her life. Incidentally, she is still living. She didn't accept the Yankee way of life and still feels that she was deprived of her just background.

I went to a Quaker school, the Moorestown Friends School, which has been in existence for years under the auspices of the Society of Friends. The higher schools of education that you may know of in this same system are Swarthmore College and Haverford College.

Dale: Did you attend one of those colleges?

Voorhees: No. When I went through Moorestown Friends School I began as a casual student, not zeroed in on the academic aspects but interested chiefly in athletics—soccer and baseball. I was an acceptable pitcher and was believed to be a good soccer player. But in about the ninth grade, I began to become more and more interested in academic studies and ended up at a quite high academic level. The teachers and the headmaster thought that I was destined to go to Haverford. I decided that I wanted to go to the University of Virginia, in Charlottesville, even with its reputation as a playboy country club and drinking society place. My mother thought I might go down there and learn how to be a southern gentleman. I can't think of anything in my life that was better than attending the University of Virginia. I fell under the historic spell of Thomas Jefferson and what he had bequeathed to that academic institution— the political and social thought that he held—particularly what was the first bridge that I had in my religious training. I don't know whether you have read it or not. I am speaking of "The Gospel According to Thomas Jefferson." College was a profound experience, and I enjoyed it tremendously.

Dale: Did you continue to play ball?

Voorhees: Yes, especially soccer.

Dale: What year did you enter Virginia?

Voorhees: In 1940. The war broke out in 1942, by which time I was enrolled in the premedical school program. College ended in 1943 and I went on to Columbia Medical School in New York.

Dale: What was the story of your wife and her "Flexible Flyer" connection?

Voorhees: My wife, Margaret Roberts, and I attended the same elementary and high schools, so we knew each other as children. She descended from a Quaker family who were farmers. Later they developed a business that supplied farming tools such as plows, harrows, feeders, and the like. It was a seasonal business and they needed something else to keep their work force employed during the fall and winter. One day before my wife was born, two of her cousins were watching some children sledding and saw one of the children, using a sled that was steered by the tips of the toes, bang into a tree. One cousin exclaimed, "I think I can design sleds that can be steered." From that idea came the flexible steel runner and the "Flexible Flyer" sleds. That was about 1890.

Dale: At what stage of life were you married?

Voorhees: After a prolonged courtship we became serious, so she transferred to Barnard College. I was a senior at Columbia College of Physicians and Surgeons, and we were married while I was still in medical school.

Dale: I recall that you have several children?

Voorhees: Mags and I have three children.

Dale: What influenced you to become a physician?

Voorhees: My mother's grandfather in Alabama had been a country doctor who was locally famous for his treatment of typhoid fever. He would feed his typhoid patients what was called "pot-liquor," which was the fluid in which greens or beans had been cooked. A significant number above the average survived. I think that he was probably giving them a fairly high-salt liquid diet which counteracted the problems of extensive, prolonged diarrhea. I heard a lot about him.

In 1935, when I was fourteen years old, I obtained a job as a chore boy with a physician in New York City who had a camp in Rangeley, Maine. I worked for him for about a year. He was a cardiologist, so I became interested in electrocardiograms, which were new. That intrigued me so that when it came time to make a declaration of where I was headed educationally, I put on the dotted line that I would like to go into medicine. Meanwhile, World War II started for us in 1941, and the military formed the J-12 and Army Specialized Training Program (ASTP) to keep young men in medical school as future doctors. I did not graduate from UVa but in 1943 went on to Columbia College of Physicians and Surgeons in New York. I was a small-town boy from the fields of west Jersey, and when I got up to Columbia it was all different from that or the University of Virginia with its Jefferson tradition. Frankly, I was frightened out of my pants. I suddenly found myself down at the bottom of the pile in a big city institution. I worked hard to end up in an acceptable academic position in school, and graduated in 1946.

Dale: Who was the chief of surgery?

Voorhees: Alan O. Whipple. He appointed me, but after a few weeks he retired. He told George Humphreys, "Here he is, you take him from here." George never let me forget that. I had a general surgical internship, enjoyed the hell out of it, and became absolutely enamored with one of the professors at Presbyterian Medical Center, Dr. Hugh Auchincloss. Hugh Auchincloss was a master teacher

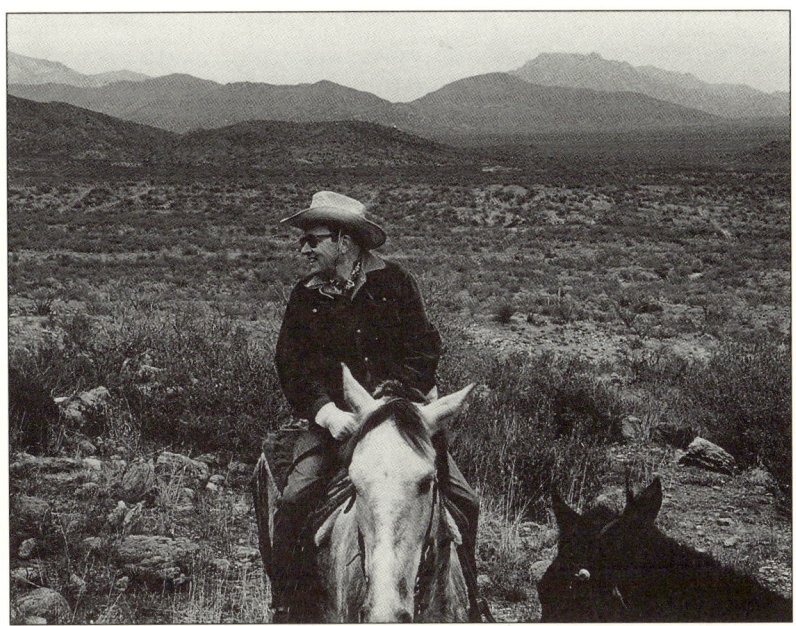

who inspired his pupils. He also was an inventor, the one surgeon I have known who had a machine shop immediately adjacent to his treatment room. In that shop he devised surgical instruments, actually making them himself. That concept appealed to me. He was one of the most influential men in my career.

Dale: Was your intern year a good one?

Voorhees: We were beginning to use a brand new drug—heparin. Arthur Blakemore was using it in cases where he was concerned about the integrity of an anastomosis. It fell upon the intern to do the Lee-White clotting time determinations on patients who were receiving heparin. One night, I got a bee in my bonnet that perhaps there might be a better way of determining how rapidly the blood could coagulate during heparin therapy, because the Lee-White test was an iffy kind of laboratory determination with great room for error. I happened to sit down with Blakemore in the dining room in the hospital that night. He was chatting about a case that we had shared and about which he was very concerned. I voiced my opinion that I thought the clotting test was wretched, particularly when I had to do it at three o'clock in the morning. I wasn't always sure of the amount of heparin that I advised on the basis of the clotting time and sometimes wondered if I was doing more harm than good. Blakemore looked at me and said, "Well, why don't you do something different? Why don't you come up with something better?" This was a typical Blakemore remark. I don't know why I said it, but I said, "Damn it, I will." He told us to come to him with ideas. This led to a wonderfully exciting period for me, because here was a man that I, frankly, idolized.

Dale: How long did you work with Dr. Blakemore?

Voorhees: The ASTP program gave me a responsibility to the military. I anticipated that the minute I finished my internship I would be inducted into military service for at least two years. But I learned that it was inconvenient at the time for the army. They told me to find some other meaningful employment or occupation during the next nine months to a year while awaiting active military service.

About that time, some of the work on blood clotting that I had started on started to pay off. It was exciting enough to make Blakemore feel that I really should continue that work. He said, "Art, why don't you come and work with me in the world of blood vessel surgery? I'll provide a fellowship for you for a year." It meant staying another year in New York, and we were not terribly enamored with the city, but it seemed to be a great opportunity, so I did it. During that time I found an elegant way of determining clotting times, but it was too sensitive and too critical to be practical, because the machinery required was three times what we thought it would be. It fizzled because of its intricacies.

Dale: What was the outcome of that work?

Voorhees: In the laboratory immediately next to where I was working, they were experimenting with arterial grafts. Robert Gross had just come out with his work in Boston, and in New York Ralph Deterling had just come to Presbyterian, where he was trying the same sort of thing with preserved human arteries. So the ferment was there.

Blakemore called me in one day and said, "Art, I know you have worked hard with this blood clotting business, and I don't want you to give it up entirely during your fellowship, but I would like you to start thinking about prosthetic mitral valves. Charles Bailey has developed the idea of going in and cracking the valve with his finger, but I don't think that's the way to go." He wanted to try to make a new valve out of the vena cava to replace sclerotic mitral valves; in other words, maybe we could replace the valve using the patient's own vena cava. It sounded like a great idea to me.

In those days there was no extracorporeal heart pump, so it had to be done in the living, beating heart. I devised a way to do this, although it was awkward and difficult. I spent an awful lot of time working on animal hearts, and subsequently spent a long time in the pathology lab with diseased mitral valves. On one occasion I made a technical error and got two silk sutures criss-crossed and left them in place inside the heart. After a couple of months, I autopsied the animal to see what had happened, and it was then that I saw that the sutures had been covered with what I thought was endocardium, although I didn't really know what it was. I went to Blakemore and told him what I saw. He listened for a while and asked, "What are you going to do with it?" I said, "What would happen if I made a prosthetic artery out of something like cloth?" He looked up at the ceiling for a minute and replied, "You just go for it." So I did.

Dale: What happened about your required time in military service?

Voorhees: I was due to serve two years. I was assigned to the Surgery Research Unit at Fort Sam Houston in San Antonio with Ed Pulaski and John Lockwood. John was sort of a godfather to the unit as head of the surgical research activities.

I was assigned to be the resident physiologist, which gave me access to research laboratory animals, an operating room, and parachute material, which was war surplus parachute nylon. My main thrust there was in the burn program, but I could pirate some of my activities away and work on the prosthetic graft. However, I was limited by a number of things. I couldn't get good histological sections. The pathology technicians were just not up to dealing with those unusual specimens. They tore everything apart and I ended up not knowing what was going on other than the fact that the people worked. During that time, John Lockwood and George Humphreys and a few others back at Presbyterian gave me a lot of encouragement. Otherwise I might have given up, because you can lose track of what your true objectives are.

Dale: Did you return to New York later?

Voorhees: Yes, to the surgical residency program at Presbyterian. George Humphreys and Blakemore suggested that I start in the surgical pathology section, so that I would have an opportunity to continue work on the arterial prostheses. One of the first steps was to explore what other things might work; after all, the parachute nylon was coarse by biologic standards.

Another chap at Presbyterian, in the Department of Orthopedics, Jim Blunt, was working on artificial tendons. He had tested all the known plastics and had implanted them as ribbons. A few of them behaved handsomely, as far as artificial tendons were concerned. He said, "I don't know how this may help you, but Vinyon is nonirritating, so why don't you go and see whether the Union Carbide people have any sort of a fabric that might help." I replied, "Great," and went sailing off downtown to a fine engineer with Union Carbide who heard my story and was sympathetic and helpful.

Dale: What was his name?

Voorhees: I don't know. He said, "Vinyon is a strange material. It is so inert that it will not take an aniline dye and therefore is of no value commercially to Union Carbide, but if you can use it . . ." and reached over his desk and pulled out a standard bolt thirty or forty inches wide and God knows how many yards long, and said, "Here, take this if you wish." Well, I took the stuff and it was beautiful, with an exquisite silk finish of a neutral brownish color. I remember taking that bolt uptown on the Eighth Avenue subway. Over the next year we used this as prostheses. Vinyon was the one and only cloth used for the first twenty human implantations. We didn't know how it was made, or how many strands to the inch, or anything else. It all came from that first bolt. After we had done this for about two years in dogs the results were exciting, but there had been no human use.

One night while I was a senior resident, but not chief, a man came in with a ruptured aneurysm. He was about seventy-five years old. I called "Blake" [Blakemore] and said, "We have this particular problem; would you come in?" We took the fellow to the operating room and opened his belly. He had a circumscribed retroperitoneal hematoma due to a perforated arteriosclerotic aneurysm of the aorta, which promptly ruptured so widely that we had to clamp his aorta to control the severe bleeding. We called the New York Blood Vessel Bank, which was located in the New York Hospital, only to be told that there were no homologous human arteries available that night.

Meanwhile, Blake had arrived and joined the surgical team. He turned to me and said in his marvelously soft Virginian accent, "Art, why don't you get some of that cloth and put it in?" That, of course, was a command, for in 1952 no one worried about hospital committees, permits, lawsuits, but only what was best for a patient. I scurried upstairs to the lab and sewed up a couple of tubes of Vinyon, which I hoped would be the right size. They were sterilized by steam in the autoclave and used to replace the aorta. The graft functioned perfectly, just as it had in dogs. But the man had already lost so much blood that he died on the operating table despite our efforts to save him.

Later that year, several other patients were similarly grafted, and lived. They were the first successful placements of synthetic grafts. Our report to the American Surgical Association in 1952 aroused great interest.

Dale: To say the least! Why was Vinyon-N not used later?

Voorhees: We viewed it as one material which worked but recognized that others might be better. Soon many other synthetics were tested.

The Union Carbide people were great. They took the position that although Vinyon-N had no value to them, they would make it if it would help people. That was generous, because a bolt would cost them $20,000 or $30,000 in 1953.

Dale: That is interesting, especially since DuPont refused to cooperate in any way when we requested their help. Soon the other synthetics were being investigated, to the extent that any young vascular surgeon worth his salt had his own particular prosthesis.

Voorhees: Yes, nylon, then Teflon, then Dacron became favorites during a decade of investigation of the various available materials. At every meeting there were new and exciting reports. You were part of it.

Dale: What an exciting time. We all aspired to the stars! Now let me ask about some other matters. Arthur, what thoughts do you have about efforts to control health care costs?

Voorhees: One thing that I saw so much of in New York is the need to stop providing high-technology care for inappropriate clinical situations. There is no reason to admit an individual first to a renal dialysis program and subsequently to renal transplant. The costs are enormous and are borne by the public. I have no sympathy for individuals who got that way because of drug addiction.

Dale: How can we control that?

Voorhees: I think that we are primarily dealing with a social problem and not a medical problem, so to reduce medical costs, I think we actually need to correct social behavior. In our hospital, which was an average general hospital in a large urban center, the costs for the excesses of humanity—speed in auto accidents, violence due to drug abuse, alcoholism, as well as obesity—the costs are astounding.

Dale: Do you favor legalization of drugs?

Voorhees: I do. It is probably the only solution for our society. China's harsh and deadly solution has been extremely effective, but it could never be applied in the U.S. social structure.

Dale: What about euthanasia? Recently there have been reports of its legalization under certain circumstances in Europe.

Voorhees: I have always been a bit confused about euthanasia. I've never had a sense of what my own response should be. It is difficult to conceive of a situation where I personally would deliberately do something to shorten a person's life, such as giving him an excessive dose of morphine. On the other hand, I see no moral justification for prolonging life where the outcome is known and where one is merely prolonging the agony of that individual's life.

Dale: I imagine you have had occasion personally to "pull the plug" or stop a respirator?

Voorhees: Yes, but that is not euthanasia. It is simply stopping our meddling.

During part of my I life was involved in working with problems associated with liver disease. Actually, I hope that my main contribution was there. I spent the first ten years of my post-residency career working with vascular disease and I spent the remaining twenty years in liver disease.

Dale: Working with cirrhotics?

Voorhees: Yes. That had a profound effect on me because of the knowledge that in so many instances I was dealing with people who were biologically disadvantaged.

Dale: How do we know that the majority of these are alcoholic cirrhotics? Why aren't most of them post-hepatitis patients who happen to drink a lot of alcohol?

Voorhees: That is quite probable. I think that some day we will be able to pick up markers that will give us far more information, but I agree with you. I am not at all sure that it is a pure alcohol problem. Alcohol may be an accelerator.

James Yao

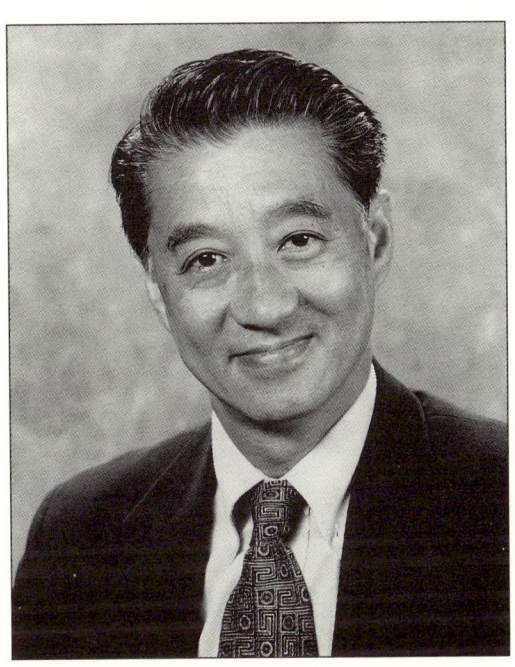

J IMMY YAO (Yao See-Tao) is an example of what can be accomplished by working hard and taking advantage of opportunity. His election as president of the Society for Vascular Surgery reflects the respect and prestige he has from his peers. Yao's high standards of excellence for himself, his fellow surgeons, and his patients' care have served him well. He was interviewed June 3, 1990.

501

Johnson: Jimmy, tell me about the boy from South China who made good.

Yao: I was born on October 14, 1935, in Canton, China, which is in the southern part of China, very close to Hong Kong. When I was four, the Japanese invaded China, and my family moved to Macao, which is a Portuguese colony. I grew up and went to high school in Macao.

When I graduated from high school, the communists took over China. As a result, I was looking for a place to finish my higher education, so I went to Taiwan and attended the National Taiwan University Medical School as an overseas student. I didn't go back to China until I returned in 1984 at the invitation of the Chinese government. That's the first time I visited Beijing.

I came to the United States in 1961 looking for a rotating internship. Cook County, where I ended up, was a pretty well-known place. I became interested in surgery and was lucky that Bob Freeark offered me a position as a surgical resident. I enjoyed my residency very, very much—not just learning surgery, but associating with the residents. We were much closer than the residents are today and got to do our own things. The hospital was busy, with a lot of patients and a lot of independent operating. I did strictly general surgery with a lot of trauma cases.

I also met my wife Louise while I was at Cook County. She was a nurse when I met her, and we were married in Chicago in 1967.

Johnson: What did you do at the end of the five years at Cook County?

Yao: I decided I'd like to pursue some specialty training. I was looking for a place to go, and I talked to a visiting orthopedic surgeon from England. He said there was a very well-known professor in England, W. T. Irvine, who was his personal friend, and told me, "You should go over there. I'm going to write you a letter of introduction. Maybe you can take a fellowship and learn something about surgical physiology and vascular surgery." Irvine was a general surgeon with an interest in investigation. That was the start of my career: The orthopedic surgeon wrote a letter, and I was lucky to be accepted in a research assistant job at St. Mary's Hospital in London to work in the blood flow laboratory.

At that time there was no specialty training in vascular surgery, but I was quite interested in it and took this job as a research position. I knew St. Mary's had an excellent reputation in vascular surgery, with Charles Rob and Felix Eastcott. I had an opportunity to do some basic work that was really attractive to me.

I had a wonderful time in London. I made a lot of friends there, was treated well, and learned a lot. The professor told me, "If you go back to the United States, you will need an additional degree to make you more special. If you ever want to go into academic surgery, get a postgraduate Ph.D., which will give you much stronger support in your academic area." He encouraged me to register at the University of London to work on a Ph.D. thesis and at the same time observe what they were doing in clinical surgery. I assisted on vascular operations now and then, but I didn't do a lot of surgery. I had a wonderful experience, a good combination of clinical and basic research.

We started with measurements of blood flow by strain gauge plethysmography. Doppler ultrasound was introduced in 1961. I still remember when Mr. Parks demonstrated the equipment to us in London. It sounded very useful. Strandness and David Sumner were the first to introduce this instrument for use in vascular disease. I was aware of the measurement of ankle pressure by Travis Windsor and Eugene Strandness, so we started working on ankle pressure measurement with Doppler ultrasound. We bought the equipment and compared the ankle pressure measurement with the plethysmographic technique. We correlated muscle flow as measured by plethysmography to that measured by xenon, including the effects of exercise. I finished the ankle pressure project, wrote an article, and sent it to the *British Journal of Surgery*. Mr. Felix Eastcott, who was editor of the *Journal* at that time, read the article. He didn't know that we were doing ankle pressure measurement by ultrasound and only learned this through the *Journal*. One morning he talked to me about ankle pressure measurement. I wondered how he knew about it, because we had been quietly working on this project. He said, "I'm the editor, and I knew about this through the article you submitted." That was how I got to know Felix. Gradually we developed a very good working relationship. I learned about vascular surgery by watching Felix perform vascular operations. He has been very supportive of my work.

My thesis was on the comparison of plethysmography with ultrasound-derived ankle pressure, measuring blood flow with and without exercise, drug treatments, or surgical treatment.

Johnson: Was anybody doing primarily vascular surgery?

Yao: Mr. Eastcott was; he also performed general surgical procedures. John Hobbs, another person I met, helped me a lot in my investigations. It was a good exposure to vascular surgery, to medicine, and to physiology. Also, it was good to see a different medical system. I was appointed lecturer in surgery in the medical school and did a little bit of teaching.

Johnson: Did you operate?

Yao: Not independently—I assisted most of the time. Performing operations was not the primary reason for my being there, but I became involved in many surgery procedures. Mr. Eastcott didn't do a lot of carotid operations or distal bypasses, but did do a lot of aortic aneurysm operations. I still remember the femoral bypass procedures—we would never go below the knee.

I watched Mr. Eastcott do carotid endarterectomies under hypothermia, cooling the patient down in a tank with ice. It would take about an hour and a half to cool to the temperature at which we would operate. Mr. Eastcott measured stump pressure with a manometer. This was in 1962 or 1963. When you look back, you realize that there have been significant changes in the practice of vascular surgery.

I was assigned to Professor Irvine of the surgical unit. Mr. Eastcott was the consultant and was independent of the surgical unit. I knew he was a famous and well-known vascular surgeon, so I would talk to him frequently and observe his operations even though I was not in his group.

Johnson: In 1971 you finished your Ph.D. What university was associated with St. Mary's?

Yao: The University of London. You had to present a thesis and be examined by the examiner. I was lucky to pass the examination. I never went to the ceremony.

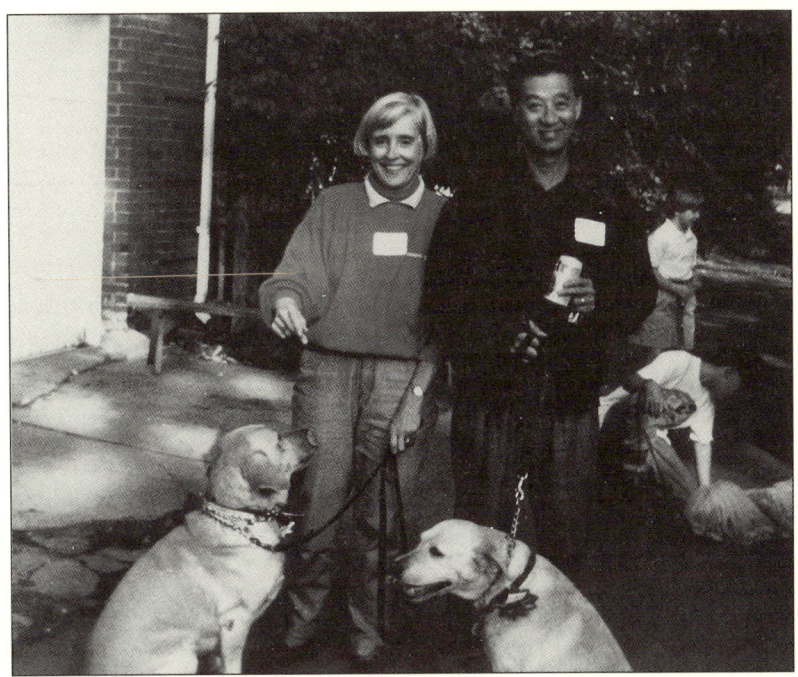

Louise and Jimmy with "Bonnie" and "Max."

Johnson: Was there anyone else in London doing vascular surgery at that time besides Felix Eastcott?

Yao: Yes. Felix was one of the major forces then, but Mr. Peter Martin at Hammersmith Hospital and Professor Gerald Taylor at St. Bartholomew's Hospital were also performing vascular surgery. I went to see Peter Martin operate on the profunda femoral artery and went to see Professor Taylor regarding electromagnetic flow measurement. John Kinmonth at St. Thomas was working on lymphatics. I had an opportunity to meet all of those pioneers at work.

Johnson: What did you do after the three years in London?

Yao: I was looking for a job in the United States. Through Professor Irvine I made arrangements to go to Detroit to work with Alexander Walt at Wayne State University. This was about ten months before I moved back to Chicago. Alexander Walt was at Detroit Receiving Hospital and Emerick Szilagyi was at Henry Ford Hospital.

Johnson: Did you see Dr. Szilagyi then?

Yao: I asked for an appointment to see him to learn about vascular surgery at Henry Ford Hospital, and I was told to show up at the vascular conference. So I showed up at the vascular conference, shook Emerick's hand, sat in the back row, heard him discuss cases, and that was it. Later, Dr. Joseph Elliott showed me around the hospital. I paid my homage to Henry Ford Hospital in 1971.

Also in 1971, I went to Philadelphia for the June vascular meeting at the Warwick Hotel, where I met John Bergan. I had been on the Northwestern University Service and had been appointed as an instructor in surgery at Northwestern University when I was at Cook County, so I knew a few people at Northwestern. When John Bergan asked me if I would like to come back to Northwestern, join him in practice, and develop the laboratory, I grabbed the opportunity and replied, "Yes, I would be very interested." He was doing transplantation and vascular surgery. He had someone working with him on transplantation, but I don't think he had anybody working with him on vascular surgery.

John Beal was chairman of the Department of Surgery. Bergan doubled up on transplant and vascular surgery. Dr. Otto Trippel was at the VA Hospital. There wasn't a special division for vascular surgery at that time. Julie Conn was doing general and vascular surgery at Provident Hospital. That is how I was exposed to these three individuals. I more or less joined John Bergan at Wesley and practiced vascular surgery exclusively.

In 1973 or 1974, after I had been at Northwestern for two years, John Bergan proposed to John Beal that we establish a division of vascular surgery. John Beal approved, and that's how the whole thing started.

Johnson: Tell me about the early days of vascular surgery at Northwestern.

Yao: We were using woven grafts and were doing a lot with above-the-knee bypass. We really hadn't started doing any below-the-knee work; I was very busy working on the vascular laboratory at that time.

The laboratory was at Wesley. We continued what I had done at St. Mary's Hospital. I concentrated on the development of Doppler ultrasound and was also involved with training general surgeons in vascular surgery, which we began doing in 1976, after we had established the division. John Beal was pleased. Bergan realized we had a service and could offer some specialty training. He thought that vascular surgery was really being handled poorly by many surgeons. General surgeons were too busy, and nobody really paid much attention to the vascular cases. Cardiac surgeons were more interested in the heart, and vascular surgery was always performed last on the list. I agreed with Jack Wylie. We needed to give better care to the vascular patients because they were not being handled well. I think that was the bottom line—to provide better care to this group of patients. We followed the vascular fellowship model that Jack Wylie established in San Francisco. We had Dick Dean as the first fellow, which was lucky; Dr. William Scott of Vanderbilt University recommended him to John Bergan. We worked together very nicely and had fun together. Dick is an outstanding person, and he helped out a lot with the program.

We had two fellows. Dick was on the university side and Paul Stanton was at the VA. The program was one year. The following year, the program called for six months at the VA and six months at Wesley. The fellows participated in a large number of cases at the VA. They worked with us in the laboratory and helped with cases at Wesley. Recently we changed the fellowship to a two-year program. We primarily followed the guidelines of the Residency Review Committee.

There didn't seem to be any conflicts between the general surgeon and the vascular fellow at this early stage. We had a lot of cases, and John had a good reputation, which attracted referrals. We were doing clinical investigations and were also working hard at writing, publishing, and presenting. We established our identity as vascular surgeons, which I think was very important to our success. We became known as vascular surgeons who cared for vascular patients only. Many patients came to John as private patients. He is the one who really started the practice.

Johnson: Tell me the history of the December postgraduate program.

Yao: We started in 1978. At that time, Geza de Takats was an outstanding surgeon, and we wanted to do something to honor him.

Geza was on the faculty at Northwestern a long time ago, and he ran the vascular clinic. John and I got together with Geza for lunch at the Tavern Club, Geza's private club. We said, "Geza, we need to do something for you." So we talked, and we settled on venous problems. Venous disease was always Geza's baby. We invited all outstanding experts in the field in this country and abroad to pay tribute to Geza. That's how the December symposium was started at Northwestern. Once it was started, we thought it was a good idea, so we kept on doing it.

Geza seldom came to our conferences after his retirement, but we had a nice working relationship. He was an outstanding person and was very supportive of my career. When I first returned to Chicago, he came to visit me and wanted to know about my work. We continued to exchange ideas and discuss articles. He was really nice to younger people. I was a nobody, but Geza was very nice to me. He knew the literature and I learned a lot from him.

The next year the conference was on carotid artery disease. We didn't have a book at that time. We put the presentations on videotape, but they never really materialized. Then, a year later, we did lower extremity revascularization and decided to have a book at the time of the meeting. In the beginning we had some grants from the Scholl Foundation. The next year we may have made a little money. Generally speaking, those events do not make a lot of money; they just meet expenses. The first meeting had about two or three hundred people attending. Now we limit it to five hundred. We started at the Drake Hotel, but it's too small now.

Johnson: How do you decide what the topic is going to be?

Yao: John and I talk about it. He and I both come up with some ideas. We compare notes and then develop a program. We think it's better to pick a topic instead of trying to cover everything. We decide the format very early. We cover venous and carotid artery problems, and lower extremity and aortic problems, and then repeat the order. The success is due to the speakers. We owe a lot to people like you, Andy Dale, Jim DeWeese, Stanley Crawford, Michael DeBakey, and all the leaders in vascular surgery who come. It would be naive to say the attendance is due to John or me. I think that most of those attending come because of the faculty. Instead of having three or four speakers, we like to get the best for a particular topic. I think that's another key to the success.

Johnson: You've been involved in the national arena of vascular surgery and its endeavors over the period of time when it has evolved from just another operation to one that requires a lot of expertise. What are some of your observations?

Yao: I have seen measurement in vascular surgery. We have spent a lot of time critically analyzing our results by measurement. We have been objective. This information guides our treatment. We know how good the operations we perform are, and we can recommend them to patients very honestly, not just because we think so but because we can measure the success of the operation. That is one of the major things that vascular surgery has accomplished. We talk about patency, but we have the ability to measure the function of the bypass objectively.

Vascular surgery has made great strides not only in measurement but also in basic science research. The investigation of problems at the molecular level in the last five or six years is another exciting area. Mind you, you can measure so much, you can do so many tests, but now in the last five or six years, we have started looking into what the cell does, and why and how it does it I think it's exciting. Take aneurysms, for instance. Why do patients form aneurysms? We are getting into the molecular level to find the abnormalities in elastin and collagen. Vascular surgery will move nicely into this type of research. We have developed all sorts of surgical procedures, and we have mastered many surgical skills. I am very happy to see much more effort directed to the basic sciences. As I see it, in the next decade molecular biology will dominate research in our area. I am not degrading, but we have done enough with measurements. Even though you now can add color to the scanner, it will not change the basic problems. Work on the molecular level will move our specialty another step ahead. I think measurements and molecular biology are the two greatest things that I have seen during the last two decades.

Johnson: What do you think your major contributions have been to the evolution to the vascular surgery in the last two decades?

Yao: I don't know if I contributed anything, but I think we are able to measure blood flow in a more objective fashion. Also, I think we have dedicated a lot to the educational effort, training people to do the right thing. I think we have a fellowship program that is able to produce that type of physician. These are the things to which I feel I have contributed. Right now I am trying to develop basic science research in our program. We are working with other basic scientists in molecular biology in our center. We are also developing an endovascular study group to work with radiologists, cardiologists, and cardiac surgeons in evaluating new endovascular techniques. I think we have to move ahead to adjust our practice to newer techniques.

Johnson: Do you think that the vascular societies are supporting your endeavors in molecular biology?

Yao: I think we should do more. I think the vascular societies, especially the Lifeline Foundation of the SVS, should do more to stimulate these efforts. The challenge is working with other groups of physicians to learn and become involved in new technology. We can stand on the sidelines and complain about lasers and all the new devices that may replace vascular operations, or we can adjust and develop physicians and surgeons interested in research.

We have to be involved. At Northwestern we have formed an endovascular study group composed of radiologists, cardiologists, cardiac surgeons, and me, so everybody can talk to each other and do things together. I think we vascular surgeons have to adjust to new techniques and position ourselves into the field so that we can influence those techniques, and not just withdraw and say, "Those mercenary physicians are doing this and that." I think we have to get in there and use all the influence we have. We have been teaching vascular disease, and we need to continue to be involved in the process. If we don't, we are going to be left behind. I think we need to change our attitude and not just talk to each other. We need to talk to other specialists. We need to start educating the public.

Johnson: You and John Bergan were associated for many years.

Yao: I am indebted to him for opportunity. He never dominated me or my work but was supportive and helped me develop. He wanted one to do things for vascular surgery, and he wanted me to be a partner in the big picture. The best quality he had was to develop other people. He wanted one to be equal as a partner, not just to say, "I'm your boss."

Johnson: You have had a fascinating life, from Canton to the pinnacle of Chicago.

Yao: You won't believe it: I have just been elected president of the Chicago Surgical Society. That's a great honor. On special occasions like this, I can't help but think back. When I came here, I didn't know anything.

Johnson: Who do you think influenced your life the most?

Yao: My mother. She was more or less a leader in the family.

Johnson: Is that typical of the Chinese?

Yao: I don't know if it's typical of the Chinese, but the father tends to be doing things outside, and is never really around the home. I was more attached to my mother. She encouraged us to be better, to do good things, to move upward. That had a strong influence. It was my upbringing to be better all the time. So I think that she was the major influence on my life. She taught us how to be generous to people. That's one thing I always remember. Not just people above you, but people who work under you. You have to be nice, even to the people who clean the room. You have to be nice to everybody, not just somebody higher than you. That's the basic thing.

ABOUT THE BOOK

Band of Brothers was designed and typeset in Quark XPress on a Mac-Intosh by Kachergis Book Design, Pittsboro, North Carolina. The typeface, Adobe Minion, was designed by Robert Slimbach and reflects the classical typography of the late Renaissance.

This book was printed on sixty-pound Booktext Natural and bound by BookCrafters, Chelsea, Michigan.